Neurological illness in pregnancy

Principles and practice

This book is dedicated to Autumn Klein's daughter, Cianna.

Neurological illness in pregnancy

Principles and practice

EDITED BY

Autumn Klein

University of Pittsburgh Medical Center, Pittsburgh, PA, USA

M. Angela O'Neal

Brigham and Women's Hospital, Harvard Medical School, Boston, MA, USA

Christina Scifres

University of Oklahoma College of Medicine, Oklahoma City, OK, USA

Janet F. R. Waters

Magee Women's Hospital, University of Pittsburgh Medical Center, Pittsburgh, PA, USA

Jonathan H. Waters

Magee Women's Hospital, University of Pittsburgh Medical Center, Pittsburgh, PA, USA

WILEY Blackwell

Registered office: John Wiley & Sons, Ltd, The Atrium, Southern Gate, Chichester,
West Sussex, PO19 8SQ, UK

Editorial offices: 9600 Garsington Road, Oxford, OX4 2DQ, UK
The Atrium, Southern Gate, Chichester, West Sussex, PO19 8SQ, UK
111 River Street, Hoboken, NJ 07030-5774, USA

For details of our global editorial offices, for customer services and for information about how to apply for
permission to reuse the copyright material in this book please see our website at
www.wiley.com/wiley-blackwell

Library of Congress Cataloging-in-Publication Data

Neurological illness in pregnancy : principles and practice / edited by Autumn Klein, M. Angela O'Neal,
Christina Scifres, Janet F. R. Waters, Jonathan H. Waters.
   p. ; cm.
Includes bibliographical references and index.
ISBN 978-0-470-67043-9 (cloth)
  I. Klein, Autumn, editor.   II. O'Neal, M. Angela, editor.   III. Scifres, Christina, editor.
IV. Waters, Janet F. R. (Physician), editor.   V. Waters, Jonathan H., editor.
  [DNLM: 1. Nervous System Diseases.   2. Pregnancy Complications.   WQ 240]
  RG580.N47
  618.3–dc23

                                                                                              2015015026

A catalogue record for this book is available from the British Library.

Set in 8.5/12pt Meridien by Aptara Inc., New Delhi, India
Printed and bound in Malaysia by Vivar Printing Sdn Bhd

1   2016

Contents

Notes on contributors

Valérie Biousse
Professor of Ophthalmology and Neurology
Emory University School of Medicine
Atlanta, GA, USA

Yvette M. Bordelon
Associate Clinical Professor of Neurology
David Geffen School of Medicine at the
University of California, Los Angeles
Los Angeles, CA, USA

Benjamin M. Brucker
Assistant Professor of Urology
New York University School of Medicine
New York, NY, USA

Anil Can
Doctoral Research Fellow
Department of Neurosurgery
Brigham and Women's Hospital
Harvard Medical School
Boston, MA, USA

Louis R. Caplan
Professor of Neurology
Beth Israel Deaconess Medical Center
Harvard Medical School
Boston, MA, USA

Kathy Chuang
Clinical Fellow in Neuromuscular Medicine
Brigham and Women's Hospital
Harvard Medical School
Boston, MA, USA

Anne Davis
Associate Professor of Obstetrics and Gynecology
Columbia University Medical Center
New York, NY, USA

William T. Delfyett
Assistant Professor of Neuroradiology
University of Pittsburgh School of Medicine
Pittsburgh, PA, USA

Rose Du
Associate Professor of Neurosurgery
Brigham and Women's Hospital
Harvard Medical School
Boston, MA, USA

Kimberly L. Ferrante
Assistant Professor of Obstetrics and Gynecology
New York University School of Medicine
New York, NY, USA

David T. Fetzer
Assistant Professor of Radiology
University of Texas Southwestern Medical Center
Dallas, TX, USA

Nancy Foldvary-Schaefer
Professor of Neurology
Cleveland Clinic Lerner College of Medicine
Cleveland, OH, USA

Elizabeth R. Gerstner
Assistant Professor of Neurology
Massachusetts General Hospital
Harvard Medical School
Boston, MA, USA

Diogo C. Haussen
Assistant Professor of Neurology
Emory University School of Medicine
Atlanta, GA, USA

Aiden Haghikia
Scientific Assistant
Department of Neuroanatomy and
Molecular Brain Research
Ruhr University
Bochum, Germany

Kerstin Hellwig
Senior Consultant
Department of Neurology
St. Josef Hospital
Ruhr University
Bochum, Germany

Sally Ibrahim
Assistant Professor of Medicine
Cleveland Clinic Sleep Disorder Center
Cleveland Clinic Lerner College of Medicine
Cleveland, OH, USA

Linda P. Kelley
Fellow, Neuro-ophthalmology
Emory University School of Medicine
Atlanta, GA, USA

Jennifer L. Lyons
Assistant Professor of Neurology
Brigham and Women's Hospital
Harvard Medical School
Boston, MA, USA

Olajide Kowe
Consultant Anesthesiologist
Yorktown Regional Hospital
Saskatchewan, Canada

Mark E. Molitch
Martha Leland Sherwin Professor of Medicine
Division of Endocrinology, Metabolism and Molecular
Medicine
Northwestern University Feinberg School of Medicine
Chicago, IL, USA

Shibani S. Mukerji
Clinical Fellow in Neurology
Massachusetts General Hospital
Harvard Medical School
Boston, MA, USA

Page B. Pennell
Associate Professor of Neurology
Brigham and Women's Hospital
Harvard Medical School
Boston, MA, USA

Sathiji Nageshwaran
Division of Brain Sciences
University College London School of Medicine
London, UK

Nancy J. Newman
Professor of Ophthalmology, Neurology and
Neurological Surgery
Emory University School of Medicine
Atlanta, GA, USA

Victor W. Nitti
Professor of Urology and Obstetrics and Gynecology
New York University School of Medicine
New York, NY, USA

M. Angela O'Neal
Instructor in Neurology
Brigham and Women's Hospital
Harvard Medical School
Boston, MA, USA

Mohammad Kian Salajegheh
Assistant Professor of Neurology
Brigham and Women's Hospital
Harvard Medical School
Boston, MA, USA

Soma Sengupta
Instructor, Division of Neuro-Oncology
Beth Israel Deaconess Medical Center
Harvard Medical School
Boston, MA, USA

Huma Sheikh
Instructor in Neurology
Faulkner Headache Division
Brigham and Women's Hospital
Harvard Medical School
Boston, MA, USA

Marsha Smith
Department of Neurology
Southern Ohio Medical Center
Portsmouth, OH, USA

Janet F. R. Waters
Clinical Assistant Professor in Neurology
Magee Women's Hospital
University of Pittsburgh Medical Center
Pittsburgh, PA, USA

Jonathan H. Waters
Professor, Department of Anesthesiology and
Bioengineering
Magee Women's Hospital
University of Pittsburgh Medical Center
Pittsburgh, PA, USA

Judith M. Wong
Pediatric Fellow
Department of Neurosurgery
University of California Los Angeles
Los Angeles, CA, USA

Mark S. Yerby
Associate Clinical Professor of Public Health
North Pacific Epilepsy Research
Oregon Health Sciences University
Portland, OR, USA

Preface

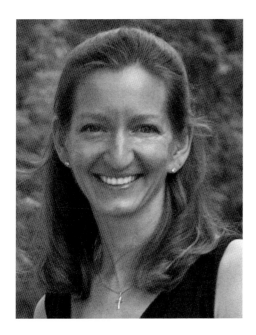

Dr. Autumn Klein

The creation of this textbook was initiated by Dr. Autumn Klein, a pioneer of women's neurology. She developed the format and carefully chose the authors from an elite group of specialists from across the United States and abroad. She unexpectedly passed away on April 17, 2013, before the completion of the book. In her memory, the authors of the book chose to complete the textbook as a legacy to her passion for the field of women's neurology.

Dr. Klein began her education by studying gender and neuroscience at Amherst College where she earned her BA magna cum laude. She went on to obtain a PhD in neuroscience and an MD from Boston University School of Medicine. After an internship in internal medicine at Brown University, she completed her residency in the Harvard Neurology Residency Program at Brigham and Women's Hospital and Massachusetts General Hospital, where she served as chief resident in her final year.

She completed a fellowship in clinical neurophysiology and epilepsy and then went on to establish the Division of Women's Neurology at Brigham and Women's Hospital. She subsequently moved to Pittsburgh where she founded the Division of Women's Neurology within the Departments of Neurology and Obstetrics at the University of Pittsburgh. From its inception, Dr. Klein served as the chief of this unique subspecialty of neurology. The division served and continues to serve as an interdisciplinary program bridging neurology with obstetrics, gynecology, and women's medicine. It focuses on gender differences in medical evaluation, diagnosis, and implementation of treatment and care. In addition to the creation of this division, she created an epilepsy monitoring unit for the treatment of pregnant women with epilepsy.

Autumn is fondly remembered for her selfless devotion to the patients for whom she cared. She made herself available for consultation on obstetrical patients 24/7. It was always reassuring to have her respond to an unexpected neurologic event. She educated her patients about their neurologic disease and about what to expect during pregnancy and motherhood. She collaborated extensively with obstetricians, anesthesiologists, and epilepsy staff to provide comprehensive patient care. With this first edition of *Neurological Illness in Pregnancy*, we hope that Autumn's vision will be fulfilled and that it will create a legacy that carries on for generations to come.

M. Angela O'Neal

Christina Scifres

Janet F. R. Waters

Jonathan H. Waters

CHAPTER 1

The history and examination

Mary A. O'Neal

Brigham and Women's Hospital, Harvard Medical School, Boston, MA, USA

Introduction

The focus of this chapter will be on the information most helpful to understand, counsel, and treat female neurology patients in their reproductive years. The key elements of the neurologic history and examination will be systematically reviewed with emphasis on gender differences. It will conclude with a few clinical cases. The goal is to enable neurologists to develop the knowledge and skills to maximize care for their female patients with regard to family planning and pregnancy. The objective of this chapter is to help physicians to perform a history and examination that focuses on and identifies the specific family planning concerns of the female patient and how these concerns relate to their neurologic disease.

Many common neurological diseases preferentially affect young women. How we, as neurologists, approach treatment depends on our patients' needs at that point in her life cycle. This is different for each disease process.

Migraine is a very common disorder with lifetime prevalence in women of up to 25%. Because of hormonal influences, the ratio of affected women over men is 3:1 [1]. The history should include usual triggers, of which menses and ovulation are common. Birth control pills (BCPs) have a variable influence on migraine frequency and in some women may aggravate the disorder [2]. However, many women with menstrual headaches report that cycle suppression (which can be obtained using the subdermal implant, injectable contraception, a pill, patch, or ring) improves their symptoms. The type of migraine is important when discussing contraception. Women with classic migraines should be counseled to avoid estrogen-containing contraceptives (e.g., the pill, patch, or ring), given the increased risk of ischemic stroke. However, common migraine does not preclude use of estrogen-containing contraceptives unless associated with other cerebrovascular risk factors such as an underlying hypercoaguable state. [3] Furthermore, when choosing medications (abortive or prophylactic), you should take into account, whether the woman are trying to get pregnant, or, if not trying to conceive, what birth control they are utilizing. For instance, topiramate in doses above 200 mg/day may reduce the effectiveness of oral contraceptives [4]. Does the patient have regular menses? Could she have polycystic ovarian syndrome? If so, Valproate would not be a good choice as a prophylactic medication [5]. Another concern with patients already predisposed to obesity is that many prophylactic medications can contribute to weight gain.

Multiple sclerosis is another example of a neurologic disease that affects women in their childbearing years [6]. Many of these patients are on an immunomodulatory medication. Interferons are pregnancy class C, copaxone pregnancy class B, and methotrexate a pregnancy class D medication. Because Immunomodulatory

Neurological Illness in Pregnancy: Principles and Practice, First Edition.
Edited by Autumn Klein, M. Angela O'Neal, Christina Scifres, Janet F. R. Waters and Jonathan H. Waters.
© 2016 John Wiley & Sons, Ltd. Published 2016 by John Wiley & Sons, Ltd.

medications are not recommended during pregnancy, birth control should be discussed if the woman is not planning pregnancy. What should we recommend to our patients who would like to become pregnant? [7] They should discontinue their immunomodulatory medication when they discontinue their hormonal or intrauterine contraceptive, as the only contraceptive that typically delays return to fertility is depot medroxyprogesterone acetate. They should be counseled that pregnancy does not worsen overall MS disability [8] Treatment needs to be appropriately adjusted to best address our patient's needs at each particular point in her life cycle.

Past medical history

Patients' medical background allows us to frame a more accurate diagnosis for their current complaints. The disorders from which women suffer are different from those that affect men. A woman's reproductive desire adds an additional layer of complexity. The medical illnesses more common in women influence which is the most probable neurologic disorder. The following is a brief snap shot of some of the disorders that are more prevalent or occur exclusively in women and how that shapes their care.

The psychiatric problems of depression, anxiety, and borderline personality disorder are more frequent in women [9, 10]. Thus, their neurological problems may be a consequence of somatization, conversion, or have an overlay due to these conditions. These women are at risk for over testing and noncompliance, as well as poor maternal weight gain, poor infant bonding, substance abuse, and postpartum depression [11, 12]. The medications we choose need to take these factors into account.

Autoimmune disorders also affect women more frequently. They may have neurologic complications directly due to their rheumatologic problem, like lupus flares [13, 14]. In addition, their neurologic problem may be due to a

result of an underlying hypercoaguable state or as a consequence of their immunosuppressant medications. The recommendations and concerns for these women during pregnancy are highly specialized.

Cardiovascular concerns are important though they are uncommon in premenopausal women. Although estrogen before the menopausal transition is likely protective against cardiovascular disease, we cannot ignore women with a strong family history of vascular disease especially if associated with other risk factors such as tobacco use and migraines [15]. These women do suffer from cardiovascular complications and need advice about risk factor modification. Women with congenital or acquired cardiac disease will need specialized care to appropriately manage the physiologic changes that occur during pregnancy and labor.

An obstetrical and lactation history is extraordinarily important. The number of pregnancies, the gestational stage of the current pregnancy, and the history of either planned or spontaneous abortions predict which obstetrical and neurological diseases are most likely. These factors also determine how, if necessary, to image and what medications are appropriate. For instance, the association with antiphospholipid antibody syndrome and spontaneous miscarriages is well established [16]. A history of eclampsia should be sought. There is good evidence that prior eclampsia predicts eclampsia in future pregnancies as well as increases risk of future maternal hypertension [17, 18]. Other obstetrical issues such as preterm premature rupture of membranes and placenta previa should be asked about directly as these patients are predisposed for recurrence in future pregnancies [19]. A woman with a history of recurrent fetal loss needs an obstetrical referral to help planning/monitoring in future pregnancies.

Bone health is often neglected. The medications we choose should reflect this concern [20]. In addition, many neurologic patients' disability may limit weight bearing [21]. It is

Table 1.1 Drugs that may have adverse effects on bone metabolism

Anticoagulants
  Warfarin
Cyclosporine
Steroids
Medroxyprogesterone acetate
Vitamin A and synthetic retinoids
Loop diuretics
Antiepileptic drugs
  Phenytoin
  Carbamazepine
  Phenobarbital
Chemotherapeutic drugs
  Aromatase inhibitors
  Methotrexate
  Ifosfamide
  Imatinib
Proton pump inhibitors
Antidepressants
  Selective serotonin reuptake inhibitors (SSRIs)
  Tricyclics
Thiazolidinediones
Antiretroviral therapy

important to be aware of the effects of medication on bone health; as the long-term use of many medications increase the risk of osteoporosis [22] (see Table 1.1). Examples of commonly used medications that promote bone loss include the anticonvulsants, phenytoin, and carbamazepine. Counseling about the benefits of exercise as well as recommending daily calcium and vitamin D intake is helpful to avoid these complications.

A history of an underlying hypercoaguable disorder is an extremely important historical data in pregnancy planning. During pregnancy there is an increase in factors I, II, VII, VIII, IX, and X as well as a decrease in protein S. The net result is that normal pregnancy is a hypercoaguable state. If a woman has a preexisting hypercoaguable disorder, her chance of having a clotting complication is high and anticoagulation during her pregnancy should be recommended [23].

Surgeries such as those involving the lower spine may make epidural anesthesia more challenging or complicated. For example, a lumbar peritoneal shunt depending on the location may preclude an epidural. Other patients with severe scoliosis, obesity, or lumbar fusion may make neuroaxial anesthesia challenging. A personal or family history of anesthetic complications is an additional historical piece to be obtained. A prior history of postdural headache should be inquired about as this increases a patient risk for recurrence [24]. Anything that would make the patient at risk for anesthesia should warrant an early consult to an obstetrical anesthesiologist.

Medication considerations

Contraception is a topic that neurologists tend to neglect. It is important to provide patients with recommendations on which contraception options are most appropriate. The most effective contraceptives are the subdermal implant and intrauterine contraceptives, which have been estimated to be 20 times as effective as oral contraceptives and surgical sterilization. There is a myriad of contraceptive choices and they are generally chosen due to personal preference, efficacy, and safety. In our patients, efficacy may be affected by medication interactions (e.g., topiramate) or at times disability. For instance, young women whose disability involves the spinal cord may not be good candidates for certain barrier methods of contraception due to difficulty in positioning or with peroneal sensory loss. In other women, certain types of contraception are contraindicated by safety concerns. For women who have had a stroke, significant cardiovascular risk factors, an underlying hypercoaguable state, and migraine with aura, combined estrogen containing pills, patch, or ring are not recommended [3]. However, progestin-only methods including the subdermal implant, intrauterine contraceptive, the injectable contraceptive, or progestin-only pills (e.g., Micronor) are safe.

When choosing to prescribe medications to women of childbearing age, it is important counsel the patient on risks and benefits of treatment. We are prescribing medications to young women who may or may not be planning on pregnancy at the time of consultation. Knowledge of the pregnancy class of the medication prescribed and what that means to your patient is essential in order to counsel them on the risks of taking that medication during pregnancy and what to do with the medication if they get pregnant. The Mother to Baby website (www.mothertobaby.org) and hotline is a useful source for information on medication use during pregnancy; free information on medication use during lactation is available from Lactmed (http://toxnet.nlm.nih.gov/cgi-bin/sis/htmlgen?LACT). Is there any influence of the medication on their method of birth control? Should they be taking higher doses of folate (e.g., 5 mg/day)? The potential effect of *in vitro* fertilization on the underlying neurological disease may need to be discussed especially for women with migraines [25]. The effects of medication on the long-term gender-specific health issues such as weight and bone health should also be considered.

The issues around fertility are complex. What are the potential risks of fertility treatment? Are there alternatives? The available options for these women require discussion, planning, and individualization for best care. A number of medications may affect fertility. The mechanisms are diverse, but weight gain is the most common. Additional weight contributes to the metabolic syndrome and polycystic ovarian syndrome. In addition, to weight gain, valproate may also influence androgen levels making contraception more problematic [26]. It has also been associated with neural tube defects. Therefore, if there is a reasonable alternative medication that controls the neurological disorder in women of childbearing age that would be preferred.

Family history and genetics

Family history is a critical component to the history. It tells us which disease processes are likely, so we can appropriately screen and counsel patients to minimize risk. Women with a strong family history of coronary artery disease, hypertension, or diabetes need to be made aware of increased risk of vascular disease associated with obesity, sedentary life style, smoking, and estrogen. Pregnancy may add to risk factors.

Do they have a genetic disorder? What is the mode of inheritance? Is there a reliable genetic test? These are important factors to help women make informed decisions about pregnancy. The more information the patients have the better equipped they are to make appropriate choices. It is a mistake to assume a patient understands the disease, simply because it runs in their family. For example, a young woman presented to clinic with a family history of maternal Huntington's disease. Her mother had tested negative. She did not understand that she was not at risk for inheriting the disorder. Knowledge is a powerful tool.

Habits

The habits (good and bad) that women employ before and during pregnancy affect their cardiovascular risk. During pregnancy, these risks are magnified. Moreover, it is hard to over emphasize the benefits of exercise on managing stress, weight, depression, and sleep. The effects on heart and brain health are well documented. Barriers for routine monitoring including health screening like mammograms and Pap smears need to be recognized. These may be cultural, socioeconomic, or driven by the patient's disability. For example, consider a patient with multiple sclerosis who attempted to obtain a gynecologic examination. If she is paraplegic, she may be unable to transfer onto her internist's examination table.

Review of systems

A review of systems there should include special attention to a number of issues for female patients. Are they at their ideal weight? Has there been weight loss or gain? Their weight influences their risks, as well as what medications should be chosen or avoided. Obesity increases the risk for gestational diabetes, hypertension, and eclampsia [27–29]. Irregular menses may indicate an underlying hormonal imbalance, influence fertility, and determine which medications are most appropriately employed. Menorrhagia and iron deficiency are common problems in young women that can be effectively treated with use of the levonorgestrel-containing intrauterine system. Iron deficiency is often compounded during pregnancy exacerbating conditions such as restless leg syndrome. Breast masses or discharge are key elements/components that deserve to direct query of our female patients.

Examination

Gender does not affect the neurologic examination. The areas on which to focus are determined by the patient's history. The history of the present illness, medical background, and physiologic state of the woman allows the physician to generate a list of the most likely possibilities. The findings on examination help to narrow and/or confirm this differential. The most important elements of the medical examination include blood pressure and weight. The other necessary pieces of the medical examination are patient-specific and dependent on the history.

Cases studies

Below are vignettes that demonstrate the importance of a gender-based history and how this will guide a therapeutic approach. These cases are based on actual patients.

Case 1

A 24-year-old woman comes in for evaluation of her headaches. She has two kinds of headaches. The first is a daily constant aching headache worst at the end of the day. It is aggravated by stress and is associated with bilateral neck pain. This headache has been present for past 1 year, but worse over the last several months. She takes acetaminophen or ibuprofen about six tablets of either everyday for this headache.

The second headache is hemicranial throbbing and much more severe. She has nausea, rare vomiting, and light sensitivity with this headache. She denies any other symptoms. During this headache she has to lie down. The frequency varies from one to three times a month. It occurs always 1–2 days prior to her menses. She has noted that red wine can trigger it. The headache lasts usually 1 day. These headaches began in her teens. Her mother and sister have similar headaches. She has never been treated for her headaches.

Her past medical and surgical history is unremarkable.

Medications include: acetaminophen prn, ibuprofen prn

She drinks four to six caffeinated beverages a day.

She recently stopped her oral contraceptives as she wants to become pregnant.

Pertinent social history is that she is engaged to be married in 2 months. They are planning on starting a family as soon as possible. She has no history of tobacco use, alcohol use, or illicit drugs, but she does not exercise on a regular basis.

Her family history is positive for migraine in mother and sister. In addition, her mother and an aunt had breast cancer.

On review of systems she endorses the following: She has lost ten pounds over the last 2 months. She has regular menses and normal breasts; she has not had an obstetrics and gynecology (OB/GYN) examination for 2 years. Her sleep is poor with difficulty falling asleep. She says she has been quite anxious about her upcoming wedding.

The history is consistent with a diagnosis of chronic daily headaches of the tension type and common migraine. Her triggers, factors that are provoking her headaches, and her desire to conceive all frame the therapeutic approach. In this case, education about analgesic rebound, overuse of caffeine, and poor sleep will need to be addressed. Stress management including a regular exercise program and its importance and relation to headache and sleep. She needs education on which medications are considered safe in pregnancy and the importance for women with a family history of breast cancer to have regular examinations. Prophylactic medication is less appropriate as she is actively trying to conceive. Abortive therapy may be an option, providing the medication is not contraindicated during pregnancy, it is also important to avoid the potential pitfall of analgesic rebound.

Case 2

A 28-year-old woman gravida 7 para 3, 24 weeks pregnant with chronic hypertension comes in for evaluation of headaches. The headache began 3 weeks ago. They were initially intermittent, but over the last 10 days they have become constant. They are worse in the morning or if she coughs. She has no clear relieving factors. Her blood pressure has not been well controlled with systolic pressures recorded as high as 220. Her labetalol was increased and her blood pressures have improved. They have been running around 140–150/90. Over the last week, she has been having blurred vision and worsening headache. Over the last 2 days, she has noted some double vision with the images side by side. The diplopia is worse when she looks far away and while watching television. She denies any other neurologic problems. She does not usually suffer from headaches. She underwent a 24-hour urine protein which was normal, suggesting that preeclampsia was not the source of her headache. CBC including platelet count was normal. Liver enzymes were also normal. She had a brain MRI and MR venogram 10 days ago which were normal.

Her past medical history is remarkable for hypertension, renal stone, history of requiring a nephrostomy tube during her last pregnancy, and a history of herpes simplex virus.

She is taking multivitamins and labetalol only.

Her review of systems is notable for weight gain of 30 pounds since the start of the pregnancy. She has no diabetes and no sleep problems.

The history is concerning for elevated intracranial pressure causing a sixth nerve palsy in the second trimester of pregnancy with a 30 lb. weight gain. Of note is that she had recent normal imaging. She had gained a significant amount of weight which makes idiopathic intracranial hypertension (IIH) a concern. The hypercoaguability associated with pregnancy causing cerebral venous thrombosis is also in this differential, but less likely given her normal venogram. Neurologic consequences of hypertension such as stroke (ischemic or hemorrhagic) are unlikely given her history and normal imaging studies. Posterior reversible encephalopathy syndrome would also be less likely given her history of worsening headache with improved blood pressure control. On examination, her blood pressure was 120/90. Her weight was 205 lbs. and height 61 inches. The neurological examination confirmed a left sixth nerve palsy and papilledema. A repeat brain MRI and MR venogram was done. The MR venogram was normal. The repeat brain MRI showed dilatation of the subarachnoid space around the optic nerve sheath a finding seen in IIH (Figure 1.1) Her CSF opening pressure was 550 mm. The testing confirms a diagnosis of IIH.

These cases illustrate how to individualize the history in order to consider gender differences and allow us to better treat our female patients. It is important to anticipate our patient's risks for disease based on their genetic makeup, lifestyle choices, and preexisting medical conditions. In this setting, clinicians must also be aware of the patient's desires for conception present and future. This will allow our patients to achieve their life goals with minimal health risk.

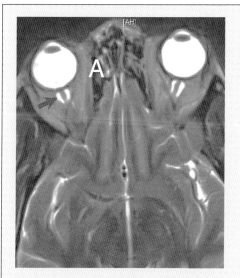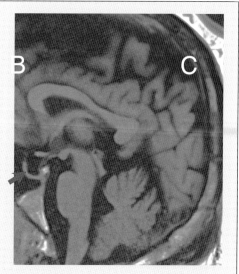

Figure 1.1 The axial T_2 image on the left shows dilatation of the subarachnoid space around the optic nerves. On the right is a sagittal T_1 image depicting an empty sella.

References

1 Lipton RB, Bigal ME, Diamond M, et al. Migraine prevalence, disease burden and the need for preventive therapy. *Neurology.* 2007;68:343.

2 Aegidius K, Zwart JA, Hagen K, Schei B, Stovner LJ. Oral contraceptives and increased headache prevalence: The Head-HUNT Study. *Neurology.* 2006;66(3):349.

3 Chang CL, Donaghy M, Poulter N. Migraine and stroke in young women: case-control study. The World Health Organization Collaborative Study of Cardiovascular Disease and Steroid Hormone Contraception. *BMJ.* 1999;318(7175):13.

4 Gaffield M, Culwell K, Lee R. The use of hormonal contraception among women taking anticonvulsant therapy. *Contraception.* 2011;83(1):16.

5 Nelson-DeGrave VL, Wickenheisser JK, Cockrell JE, et al. Valproate potentiates androgen biosynthesis in human ovarian theca cells. *Endocrinology.* 2004;145(2):799.

6 Cook SD, Troiano R, Bansil S, Dowling PC. Multiple sclerosis and pregnancy. *Adv Neurol* 1994;64:83.

7 Boskovic R, Wide R, Wolpin J, et al. The reproductive effects of beta interferon therapy in pregnancy: a longitudinal cohort. *Neurology.* 2005;65:807.

8 Confavreux C, Hutchinson M, Marie Hours M, Cortinovis-Tourniaire P, Moreau T, and the Pregnancy in Multiple Sclerosis Group. Rate of pregnancy-related relapse in multiple sclerosis. *N Eng J Med.* 1998;339:285–291.

9 American Psychiatric Association. *Diagnostic and Statistical Manual of Mental Disorders (DSM-IV-TR),* Fourth edition, Text revision, American Psychiatric Association, Washington, DC, 2000, no abstract available.

10 Grant BF, Cho SP, Goldstein RB, et al. Prevalence, correlates, disability, and comorbidity of DSM-IV borderline personality disorder: results from the Wave 2 National Epidemiologic Survey on Alcohol and Related Conditions. *J Clin Psychiatry.* 2008;69(4):533.

11 Larsson C, Sydsjö G, Josefsson A. Health, sociodemographic data, and pregnancy outcome in women with antepartum depressive symptoms. *Obstet Gynecol.* 2004 104(3):459–466.

12 Bonari L, Pinto N, Ahn E, et al. Perinatal risks of untreated depression during pregnancy. *Can J Psychiatry.* 2004;49:726.

13 Dugowson CE, Koepsell TD, Voigt LF, et al. Rheumatoid arthritis in women. Incidence rates in group health cooperative, Seattle, Washington, 1987–1989. *Arthritis Rheum.* 1991;34:1502.

14 Costenbader KH, Feskanich D, Stampfer MJ, Karlson EW. Reproductive and menopausal factors and risk of systemic lupus erythematosus in women. *Arthritis Rheum.* 2007;56:1251.

15 MacClellan LR, Giles W, Cole J. Probable migraine with visual aura and risk of ischemic stroke: the stroke prevention in young women study. *Stroke.* 2007;38:2438–2445.

16 Cervera R, Balasch J. Autoimmunity and recurrent pregnancy losses. *Clin Rev Allergy Immunol.* 2010;39:148.

17 Chesley SC, Annitto JE, Cosgrove RA. The remote prognosis of eclamptic women. Sixth periodic report. *Am J Obstet Gynecol.* 1976;124:446.

18 Sibai BM, el-Nazer A, Gonzalez-Ruiz A. Severe preeclampsia-eclampsia in young primigravid women: subsequent pregnancy outcome and remote prognosis. *Am J Obstet Gynecol.* 1986;155:1011.S.

19 Lee T, Carpenter MW, Heber WW, Silver HM. Preterm premature rupture of membranes: risks of recurrent complications in the next pregnancy among a population-based sample of gravid women. *Am J Obstet Gynecol.* 2003;188:209.

20 Pack AM, Morrell MJ. Epilepsy and bone health in adults. *Epilepsy Behav.* 2004;5(Suppl 2):S24.

21 Cummings SR, Nevitt MC, Browner WS, et al. Risk factors for hip fracture in white women. Study of Osteoporotic Fractures Research Group. *NEJM.* 1995;332:767.

22 Crawford P, Chadwick DJ, Martin C, Tjia J, Back DJ, Orme M. The interaction of phenytoin and carbamazepine with combined oral contraceptive steroids. *Br J Clin Pharmacol.* 1990;30(6):892.

23 Bates SM, Greer IA, Middeldorp S, et al. VTE, thrombophilia, antithrombotic therapy, and pregnancy: Antithrombotic Therapy and Prevention of Thrombosis, 9th ed: American College of Chest Physicians Evidence-Based Clinical Practice Guidelines. *Chest.* 2012;141:e691S.

24 Kuntz KM, Kokmen E, Stevens JC, et al. Post-lumbar puncture headaches: experience in 501 consecutive procedures. *Neurology.* 1992;42:1884.

25 Martin VT, Behbehani M. Ovarian hormones and migraine headache: understanding mechanisms and pathogenesis–part I. *Headache.* 2006;46:3.

26 Herzog AG. Menstrual disorders in women with epilepsy. *Neurology.* 2006;66(6 Suppl 3):S23.

27 Garbaciak JA Jr, Richter M, Miller S, Barton JJ. Maternal weight and pregnancy complications. *Am J Obstet Gynecol.* 1985;152:238.

28 Gaugler-Senden IP, Berends AL, de Groot CJ, Steegers EA. Severe, very early onset preeclampsia: subsequent pregnancies and future parental cardiovascular health. *Eur J Obstet Gynecol Reprod Biol.* 2008;140 (2):171–177.

29 Gross T, Sokol RJ, King KC. Obesity in pregnancy: risks and outcome. *Obstet Gynecol.* 1980;56:446.

CHAPTER 2

Hormonal and physiologic changes in pregnancy

Janet F. R. Waters
Magee Women's Hospital, University of Pittsburgh Medical Center, Pittsburgh, PA, USA

Physiologic and endocrine changes are necessary to support the growth and health of the fetus during pregnancy and to assure the health of the mother up to and beyond delivery. Copious production of polypeptide and steroid hormones by the fetal/placental unit produces physiologic adaptations of virtually every maternal organ system [1]. This chapter will review what is currently understood about the flood of hormonal changes that occur in the various phases of pregnancy.

Embryology

At 3–4 weeks gestation, in the absence of a Y chromosome, the gonad begins to form an ovary. Primordial germ cells proliferate and migrate through the dorsal mesentery reaching the gonadal ridge at 6 weeks gestation. These premiotic cells continue to proliferate and are referred to as oogonia. At 10–12 weeks, some oogonia begin meiosis and arrest in prophase I and become primary oocytes. By 16 weeks, primordial follicles develop and by 20 weeks a peak of 6–7 million germ cells are formed. During the second half of gestation, atresia leads to reduction in the number of oocytes to 1–2 million at birth. No further oocytes develop after birth and follicular atresia continues throughout childhood. Most girls will enter puberty with 300,000 to 400,000 oocytes in their ovaries [1].

Menstrual cycle

The menstrual cycle is produced through complex hormonal feedback loops involving the ovary and the hypothalamic–pituitary axis. There are two phases that occur in the ovary during the menstrual cycle: the follicular phase and the luteal phase. The endometrium undergoes three phases that are triggered by hormones produced in the ovary. These phases include the proliferative phase, secretive phase, and degenerative phase. During the ovarian follicular phase, the ovary secretes estradiol that stimulates proliferation of the endometrium, which lines the uterus. At the beginning of the menstrual cycle, the endometrium is thin but as ovulation nears, estrogen stimulates growth and enhanced blood supply. After ovulation, the ovary secretes progesterone which inhibits further endometrial proliferation. During the luteal phase, progesterone stimulates endometrial changes that cause it to be more edematous as a result of increased capillary permeability. Endometrial cells enlarge and produce prostaglandins that play an important role in implantation, pregnancy, and menstruation. This endometrial stage is known as the secretory phase. If implantation does not occur, the endometrium enters the degenerative phase. Estrogen and progesterone withdrawal leads to prostaglandin production leading to endometrial ischemia and reperfusion

Neurological Illness in Pregnancy: Principles and Practice, First Edition.
Edited by Autumn Klein, M. Angela O'Neal, Christina Scifres, Janet F. R. Waters and Jonathan H. Waters.
© 2016 John Wiley & Sons, Ltd. Published 2016 by John Wiley & Sons, Ltd.

injury. The endometrium becomes necrotic and sloughs away. Blood loss can vary from 25 to 60 mL [1].

If conception occurs, implantation takes place in the mid-portion of the secretary phase of the endometrium, and the luteal phase of the ovary. The embryo invades the uterus 8 to 10 days after ovulation and fertilization. The syncytiotrophoblast secretes human chorionic gonadotropin (hCG) which preserves the corpus luteum and maintains production of progesterone and other hormones to allow the development of the decidua, the endometrium of pregnancy.

Hormonal changes in pregnancy

Ovarian hormones of the corpus luteum

The corpus luteum produces several hormones that are crucial to maintaining pregnancy in the first 6 weeks of gestation. Hormones produced include estradiol, progesterone, 17-hydroxy progesterone, and relaxin. Removal of the corpus luteum in the first trimester of pregnancy leads to a drop in progesterone and estradiol which could induce abortion. Primate studies have shown that relaxin plays several roles in maintaining pregnancy. It increases vascularization of the endometrium and stimulates differentiation of endometrial stromal cells into predecidual cells. Its presence also stimulates insulin-like growth factor-binding protein and prolactin which in turn promotes the development of the decidua [2]. It also softens the pubic symphysis and acts in synergy with progesterone to inhibit contractions.

Polypeptide hormones

A role of the placenta is to facilitate communication between the mother and the developing fetus while maintaining the immune and genetic integrity of both. Initially, the placenta alone provides endocrine function. As the fetus matures, it begins to contribute and by the end of the first trimester, it will provide hormonal precursors to the placenta [3].

Human chorionic gonadotropin

In the first 6 weeks of gestation, hCG levels double every 1.7 to 2 days. Its plasma half-life is 24 hours and can be detected in the maternal peripheral circulation within 24 hours of implantation. Maternal plasma hCG concentration peaks in the 10th week of pregnancy and then declines gradually in the third trimester. hCG is a glycoprotein consisting of 237 amino acids and has two chains, an alpha chain and a beta chain. The alpha chain is identical to the alpha chain of TSH, FSH, and LH. The beta chain is similar to the beta chain found in luteal hormone (LH) but has an additional 30 proteins. It plays a role in the establishment of maternal blood flow in the intervillous space.

Human placental lactogen

Human placental lactogen (HPL) is produced by early trophoblasts and is detectable in maternal circulation at 4–5 weeks gestation. It is a protein of 190 amino acids and is structured similarly to growth hormone and prolactin. HPL alters maternal glucose metabolism and mobilizes free fatty acids. It contributes to the peripheral insulin resistance of pregnancy. It has not been shown to promote lactation.

Other placental peptide hormones

A number of peptides have been isolated from placental tissues. Placental growth factor and vascular endothelial growth factor play a role in placental angiogenesis and fetal growth and may be involved in the cascade of events that lead to preeclampsia and eclampsia. Activin, inhibin, corticotropin-releasing hormone, fibroblast growth factor, epidermal growth factor, platelet-derived growth factor, all have been identified in placental tissue but the mechanism of their function has yet to be elucidated.

Steroid hormones

Steroid hormones are crucial to the establishment and maintenance of pregnancy. Included in this group are estrogens, progestins, glucocorticoids, mineral corticoids, and androgens. The precursor for all steroids is the 27 carbon-containing cholesterol molecule, a lipid composed of four fused rings with associated side chains [4]. Modification of the side chains, and at locations along the steroid back bone alters bioactivity. The placenta is unable to synthesize steroid hormones *de novo*, but it is able to convert steroids derived from fetal and maternal precursors [3].

Progesterone

Progesterone is necessary for the maintenance of pregnancy. It is produced by the corpus luteum during the first 6–8 weeks of pregnancy in response to the stimulus LH, and later in response to the stimulus of placental hCG. Following involution of the corpus luteum, the placenta is the major site of synthesis of progesterone from cholesterol precursors. The principle source of precursors is maternally derived circulating low-density lipoprotein (LDL). The LDL can also be synthesized *de novo* in the fetal liver and adrenal glands [5]. Enzymes in the placenta cleave the cholesterol side chain to produce pregnenolone which is subsequently isomerized to create progesterone. In total, 250–350 mg of progesterone are produced daily by the placenta in the third trimester [3]. Progesterone has a number of important roles including preparation of the endometrium for implantation and preparation of the breasts for lactation. Progesterone in conjunction with relaxin and nitrous oxide prevents uterine contraction during pregnancy. Progesterone causes hyperpolarization of myometrial cells decreasing the amplitude of action potentials. Progesterone also inhibits T-cell-mediated allograft reduction and may play a role in immunologic tolerance in the uterus. Insufficient progesterone production can lead to preterm labor and spontaneous abortion [6].

Estrogen

Estrogens oppose many of the actions of progesterone. It has a role in softening the cervix in advance of delivery. Estrogen also promotes uterine contractility. It increases the number of uterine oxytocin receptors and myometrial gap junctions to produce effective contractions during labor. Estrogen also stimulates an increase in lactotrophs in the pituitary and raises the prolactin level to its peak just prior to delivery. Estrogen is produced by the placenta primarily by converting fetal dehydroepiandrosterone (DHEA) sulfate to estriol. 16a-hydroxy-DHEA sulfate is produced in the fetal adrenal and liver. In the placenta, this substrate undergoes desulfation and aromatization to produce the weak estrogen, estriol. During pregnancy, levels of estriol increase 1000-fold. Fetal DHEA sulfate is also a precursor to estrone and estradiol. In the placenta, fetal DHEA sulfatase is converted by placental sulfatase to free DHEA and then is enzymatically converted to the androgens, androstenedione, and testosterone. They are aromatized in the placenta to estrone and estradiol, respectively [3]. Estrone is 10 times more potent than estriol and estradiol is 100 times more potent. Levels of estrone and estriol increase during pregnancy by 50-fold.

Endocrine changes during pregnancy

Pituitary gland

The pituitary gland increases in size during pregnancy by approximately one-third. This increase is due primarily to the increase in lactotrophs for the production of prolactin. Prolactin rises progressively during pregnancy and increases following meals and at night. Increased pituitary size and elevation in prolactin persists in breast-feeding mothers. In non-lactating women, pituitary size and prolactin levels return to baseline 3 months after delivery. Serum FSH and LSH drop to near undetectable levels during pregnancy. Growth hormone, ACTH, and TSH secretion remain unchanged.

Pancreas

The role of insulin and glucagon is to expedite intracellular transport of glucose, amino acids, and fatty acids. In early pregnancy, insulin levels remain unchanged or drop into the low range of normal. As the pregnancy progresses, secreting beta cells undergo hyperplasia and pancreatic islets increase in size. In the second trimester, insulin levels rise due to increased secretion. Insulin secretion in response to meals is accelerated. Pregnancy becomes a hyperinsulinemic state, with resistance to its peripheral metabolic state. Fasting glucose levels are maintained at low-normal levels and excess carbohydrates are converted to fat [3].

Adrenal cortex

Cortisol levels increase throughout pregnancy reaching a threefold increase by the third trimester. Elevated cortisol levels likely contribute to insulin resistance during pregnancy and may also contribute to the development of striae. Despite the rise of cortisol levels to that seen in Cushing's syndrome, no other manifestations of Cushing's syndrome are seen. High levels of progesterone may be exercising antagonist actions to minimize the glucocorticoid effects.

Estrogen stimulates increased hepatic synthesis of renin. Renin is then converted to aldosterone resulting in an eightfold increase in aldosterone production in the zona glomerulosa. Renin, aldosterone, and angiotensin all become elevated during pregnancy. Nevertheless, no blood pressure elevation, hypokalemia, or hypernatremia occurs. Progesterone is a competitive inhibitor of mineral corticoids and likely mitigates the response to higher levels.

Thyroid gland

The thyroid gland enlarges during the first trimester of pregnancy. Estrogen stimulates an increase in thyroid-binding globulin that results in an elevation in total serum thyroxin. Free thyroxin and triiodothyronine remain in the normal range. The polypeptide hormone hCG has weak TSH-like activity and can produce transient biochemical hyperthyroidism in early gestation.

Parathyroid gland

Fetal skeletal development requires on average 30 g of calcium prior to delivery at term. To facilitate this, the maternal parathyroid becomes hyperplastic and serum PTH levels become elevated. Maternal serum calcium levels decline between 28 and 32 weeks gestation due to fetal bone formation as well as hypoalbuminemia of pregnancy. Ionized calcium is maintained at normal serum levels throughout pregnancy.

Physiologic changes in pregnancy

The prodigious output of polypeptide and steroid hormones by the fetal–placental unit results in physiologic alteration of virtually every maternal organ system [3]. Some of these striking changes are summarized below.

Weight

There is wide variation in total weight gain in women during pregnancy. On average, a gain of 25 pounds occurs, but in some individuals, weight gain is considerably greater. Obesity during pregnancy has increased dramatically in the past 20 years in the United States and is associated with increased risk of a number of adverse outcomes including gestational diabetes, venous thromboembolism, congenital defects, fetal demise, and surgical morbidity [3]. In the neurologic setting, obesity in pregnancy is associated with increased risk of preeclampsia and eclampsia and idiopathic increased intracranial pressure (pseudotumor cerebri). These complications will be discussed in detail in subsequent chapters.

Blood

Blood volume increases dramatically during pregnancy. During the second trimester, blood volume reaches a level of 150% of prepregnancy volume. Because the plasma volume expands faster than does the red cell mass, a relative anemia of pregnancy is seen. A 20% drop in hematocrit is not uncommon. Similarly, a drop in platelet count occurs but the overall mass of platelets increases. Fibrinogen increases by up to 40%. All coagulation factors increase during pregnancy except for Factors 11 and 13 and there is a decrease in Protein C and S. With all of these changes, in the last trimester, a relatively hypercoaguable state exists. As such, there is an increased risk of thrombotic events in the last trimester and peripartum period, particularly in women with a preexisting propensity for thrombosis.

Cardiovascular

In the pregnant woman, blood pressure gradually declines until 34 weeks gestation where it drops by 10% of prepregnancy levels. It gradually increases in the last month of pregnancy to its baseline level. Heart rate increases during pregnancy by 20%. Cardiac output rises rapidly in the first trimester by 20% and continues to increase by an additional 10% by the 28th week of pregnancy. Peripheral vascular resistance declines throughout pregnancy and peripheral venous distention increases until delivery.

Pulmonary

While respiratory rate remains stable, tidal volume and respiratory minute volume increase by 40%. Expiratory reserve gradually declines by 40%. Vital capacity remains unchanged.

Renal

Due to blood volume expansion, renal flow increases 25–50%. Glomerular filtration rate increases early in pregnancy then plateaus at 40% above prepregnancy levels.

Gastrointestinal

Gastric emptying time slows progressively throughout pregnancy, reaching a low of 50%

below baseline by 36 weeks. Heartburn in the third trimester is not uncommon. Esophageal sphincter tone decreases during pregnancy.

Endocrine control of parturition

The precise factors that trigger parturition in humans remain elusive. In animal models, there is a drop in progesterone levels at the onset of labor. This interrupts the quiescence of the uterus and onset of labor takes place. A drop in progesterone levels at the onset of parturition has not been demonstrated in human studies [7]. It has been postulated that progesterone function may be diminished through decreases in functional progesterone receptors, sequestration by a circulating progesterone-binding protein, inactivation of local progesterone activity by myometrial cells, or production of an endogenous progesterone antagonist. In humans, circulating estrogen increases at mid-gestation and continues to rise until birth [8–10]. Decrease in progesterone function releases myometrial inhibition allowing it to become more responsive to the effects of circulating estrogen. Sporadic, painless uterine contractions begin to occur and the lower uterine segment and cervix become softer and thinner, known as effacement [3]. An increase in the estrogen/progesterone ratio increases the number of oxytocin receptors and myometrial gap junctions. This leads to coordinated, effective contractions resulting in labor and delivery.

Endocrinology and physiology of the postpartum patient

Endocrine changes

Twenty-four hours after delivery, progesterone levels drop to luteal phase levels and after several days, return to follicular phase levels. Twenty-four to seventy-two hours after delivery, estradiol declines to follicular phase levels. Both FSH and LH remain low during the first few weeks of the puerperum. In the non-lactating female, FSH and LH return to follicular phase levels 3–4 weeks after delivery.

Physiologic changes

Blood volume declines to 80% of the pre-delivery levels by the third postpartum day. Cardiovascular changes influence liver and renal function including clearance of hormones. Hypertrophic myometrial cells decrease in size and the uterus gradually returns to a prepregnant size over a 6-week period after delivery. The endometrium which was sloughed at delivery regenerates by the seventh postpartum day.

Lactation

Prolactin is released by the pituitary gland and increases throughout pregnancy. Prolactin in conjunction with estrogen, progesterone, growth hormone, and glucocorticoids each play a role in the development of breast alveolar lobules. Delivery is associated with a surge in prolactin levels. Although prolactin reaches high levels in the third trimester, lactopoesis does not occur until unconjugated estrogens drop to prepregnancy levels 36–48 hours after delivery [3]. During breastfeeding, suckling leads to the release of oxytocin which results in contraction of the smooth muscle fibers surrounding the alveolar gland ductules. Suckling also leads to increased release of prolactin from the pituitary which supports lactogenesis. Surges of prolactin are believed to inhibit the release of gonadotropin-releasing hormone by the hypothalamus preventing ovulation. If breastfeeding does not occur, prolactin levels drop, lactogenesis ceases, and breasts development returns to a nonpregnant state. Gonadatropin-releasing hormone levels rise and the normal menstrual cycle is initiated.

References

1 Rosen MP, Cedars MI. Female reproductive endocrinology and infertility. In: Gardner DG, Shobeck D, eds. *Greenspan's Basic & Clinical Endocrinology*, 9th ed. New York: McGraw Hill, 2011; pp. 423–477.

2 Goldsmith LT, Weiss G. Relaxin in human pregnancy. *Ann N Y Acad Sci.* 2009;1160:130–135.

3 Taylor RN, Badell ML. Endocrinology of pregnancy. In: Gardner DG, Shobeck D, eds. *Greenspan's Basic & Clinical Endocrinology*, 9th ed. New York: McGraw Hill, 2011; pp. 553–571.

4 Kallen CB. Steroid hormone synthesis in pregnancy. *Obstet Gynecol Clin North AM.* 2004;31:795–816.

5 Miller WL. Steroidogenic enzymes. *Endocr Dev.* 2008;13:1–17.

6 Meis PJ, Aleman A. Progesterone treatment to prevent preterm birth. *Drugs.* 2004;64:784–795.

7 Mesiano S, Welsh TN. Steroid hormone control of myometrial contractility and parturition. *Semin Cell Dev Biol.* 2007;18:321–331.

8 Boroditsky RS, Reyes FI, Winter JS, Faiman C. Maternal serum estrogen and progesterone concentration preceding normal labor. *Obstet Gynecol.* 1978;51:686–691.

9 Tulchinsky D, Hobel CJ, Yaeger D, Marshall JR. Plasma estrone, estradiol, estriol, progesterone, and 17-hydroxyprogesterone in human pregnancy. *Am J Obstet Gynecol.* 1972;112:1095–1100.

10 Walsh SW, Stanczyk FZ, Novy MJ. Daily hormonal changes in the maternal, fetal and amniotic fluid compartments before parturition in primate species. *J Clin Endocrinol Metab.* 1984;58:629–639.

CHAPTER 3

Neuroimaging

William T. Delfyett[1] & David T. Fetzer[2]

[1] University of Pittsburgh School of Medicine, Pittsburgh, PA, USA
[2] University of Texas Southwestern Medical Center, Dallas, TX, USA

Introduction

Throughout pregnancy and the puerperium, hormonal, physiologic, and potentially pathologic changes may result in a variety of neurologic symptoms and clinical findings. Pregnancy-related changes may also influence preexisting medical conditions or bring previously unknown neurologic conditions to clinical attention. When a pregnant patient presents with a neurologic complaint or clinical sign, a physician must consider broad diagnostic categories in order to expedite diagnosis and management of treatable causes as neurologic pathology contributes to up to 20% of maternal deaths [1]. Neuroradiologic imaging is frequently utilized as part of this diagnostic evaluation. This chapter will review the physiologic changes most germane to the imaging of neurologic conditions, safety issues related to diagnostic imaging during pregnancy, and the imaging findings of a spectrum of neurologic conditions with common clinical presentations.

KEY POINTS

1 The health of the mother is the single most important factor in safeguarding the health of the fetus.

2 Radiation and intravenous contrast concerns, though important, should not delay the execution of critical imaging examinations.

3 Careful selection of an imaging workup when evaluating the pregnant patient can minimize potential adverse effects to the fetus without sacrificing diagnostic power.

4 The potential radiation dose associated with diagnostic imaging should be minimized whenever possible, following As Low As Reasonably Achievable (ALARA) principles.

5 Fetal radiation doses of less than 5 rad (50 mGy) have not been shown to increase rates of fetal abnormality or pregnancy loss.

6 Both iodinated and gadolinium-based contrast agents may be administered during pregnancy or the puerperium in appropriate clinical circumstances.

7 Recognition of the imaging features of pregnancy-associated conditions may allow for rapid initiation of therapy, minimizing potential adverse effects for both mother and fetus.

Anatomic and physiologic changes of pregnancy

The following is a review of the specific physiologic, hormonal, immunologic, and hemodynamic physiologic changes in pregnancy to which many anatomic and pathologic processes are generally attributed, and thus most pertinent to neuroimaging (Table 3.1). Many of these changes may influence the imaging appearance

Neurological Illness in Pregnancy: Principles and Practice, First Edition.
Edited by Autumn Klein, M. Angela O'Neal, Christina Scifres, Janet F. R. Waters and Jonathan H. Waters.
© 2016 John Wiley & Sons, Ltd. Published 2016 by John Wiley & Sons, Ltd.

Table 3.1 Physiologic changes in pregnancy

Hormonal	Metabolic	Immunologic	Hemodynamic	Hematologic
↑ hCG, prolactin; ↑ Estrogen and progesterone precursors and products; ↑ ACTH	↑ Cholesterol turnover; ↑ circulating triglycerides (Weeks 20–40): ↑ insulin resistance; ↑ glycogen synthesis and storage	↑ Cortisol; ↑ progesterone-induced T-cell inhibitors	↑ Heart rate and stroke volume with ↑ cardiac output 40–60%; ↑ blood volume (50% plasma and 10–30% red cell mass resulting in pseudo-anemia of pregnancy)	↑ Levels of coagulations factors (VII, IV, V, fibrinogen; ↑ platelet aggregability; ↑ heparin neutralization; ↑ protein C inhibitors
↓ LH and FSH	(Weeks 1–20): ↓ insulin resistance; ↓ glycogen synthesis and storage		↓ Systemic vascular resistance and ↓ blood pressure	↓ Fibrinolytic activity, antithrombin III levels; ↓ protein S inhibitor

Reproduced from Reference [2] with permission of Elsevier.
hCG, human chorionic gonadotropin; ACTH, adrenocorticotropic hormone; LH, luteinizing hormone; FSH, follicle-stimulating hormone.

of normal structures outside the pelvis. For instance, hemodynamic and cellular changes related to hormonal influences may affect organ size including an increasing size of the heart, kidneys, and thyroid [3]. In addition, a decrease in brain size has been observed *in vivo*, both with the administration of high dose exogenous steroids as well as in both healthy and preeclamptic patients over the course of pregnancy, with return to baseline by 6-month postpartum [4, 5].

Fluctuations in pituitary gland function throughout the course of pregnancy may influence its anatomic appearance. Adenohypophyseal enlargement is attributed to lactotroph hypertrophy and may account for up to 30% increase in gland weight and mean volume increase of 120%, as seen in Figure 3.1 [6]. The degree of craniocaudal enlargement may reach 9 mm in the third trimester, and up to 12 mm in the immediate postpartum period. Pituitary enlargement often resolves by 6 months postpartum [7].

Changes in circulating adrenocorticotropic hormone (ACTH), prolactin, and estrogen products have been associated with a trophic effect on neoplasms such as pituitary adenomas, hemangioblastomas, schwannomas, and meningiomas, as well as malignancies such as choriocarcinoma, melanoma, and breast carcinoma, all of which may present with intracranial metastases [8, 9]. Meningiomas, one of the most frequently encountered intracranial

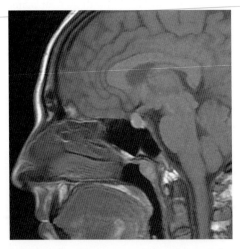

Figure 3.1 34 y/o female, 1-week postpartum, with severe headache. Physiologic hypertrophy with a sagittal T_1-weighted image demonstrating a homogenous, enlarged pituitary gland with convex superior margin, measuring 1.0 cm in height. Reproduced from Reference 2 with permission of Elsevier.

masses, have been shown to express numerous growth factor receptors including those for sex hormones, as have schwannomas [10–14]. In meningiomas, the presence of estrogen receptors has been associated with a more aggressive clinical course, recurrence, and clinical progression [12] Changes in meningioma size have been reported following modulation of hormonal replacement therapy, further validating the potential hormonal trophic effect [15]. However, regarding schwannomas, recent work examining immunohistochemical stains for growth factor receptors has raised questions regarding the veracity of the widely reported potential hormonal trophic effect on these lesions [16–19].

Selective immunosuppression during pregnancy, primarily from increased levels of circulating cortisol, as well as progesterone-induced T-cell inhibition, may have an inhibitory effect on autoimmune disorders such as multiple sclerosis, discussed in detail elsewhere in this volume.

The hypercoagulable state during pregnancy, due in part to increased circulating fibrinogen and other clotting factor levels, as well as increased platelet aggregability, is compounded by the reduction in fibrinolytic activity due to decreased endogenous anticoagulants such as protein S and antithrombin III [8, 9, 20]. Surprisingly, randomized studies have shown that there is not an increased risk of stroke during pregnancy, however, a significantly increased risk is evident in the peri- and postpartum periods (Figure 3.2) [9, 21], especially in the setting of hypertension, diabetes, hyperlipidemia, and premature atherosclerosis formation. The risk of arterial dissection or deep venous thrombosis during a prolonged or difficult labor also increases the risk of embolic infarction.

Hormonal and hemodynamic changes may also be involved in the growth or development of intracranial aneurysms. Increased levels of relaxin, upregulation of collagenase, and collagen remodeling may affect vessel wall integrity. The risk of subarachnoid hemorrhage (SAH),

a leading cause of maternal mortality, has been reported up to five times greater during pregnancy than in a nonpregnant woman [8, 22]. Despite a potential underlying physiologic mechanism, this reported increased risk may be the subject of some controversy as other authors have not shown such a difference in risk [23,24]. Aneurysm rupture has been widely reported as a leading cause of SAH, but some studies suggest that hypertensive disorders may be just as likely an underlying cause [22, 24].

Imaging the pregnant patient

There are up to six million pregnancies in the United States annually, with up to two million ending in pregnancy loss [25]. Physicians across many disciplines encounter pregnant patients in both acute and more chronic care settings, including those presenting with neurologic signs or symptoms. While many conditions may be benign and self-limited, the exclusion of potentially serious conditions often involves diagnostic neuroimaging. In choosing the most appropriate imaging study, diagnostic utility must be weighed against any potential adverse effects to the mother or fetus. With modern imaging techniques and the utilization of available guidelines, both diagnostic efficacy and patient safety can be maximized.

The American College of Radiology (ACR), the European Society of Urogenital Radiology (ESUR), and the American Congress of Obstetricians and Gynecologists (ACOG) have published guidelines regarding imaging of the pregnant patient [26–28]. For both the optimization of patient care and management of potential medico-legal issues, hospitals and radiology departments should formalize their own policies regarding the imaging of pregnant patients, incorporating the available practice guidelines generated by consensus expert panels. In many cases, a well-documented risk–benefit analysis should be performed and informed consent

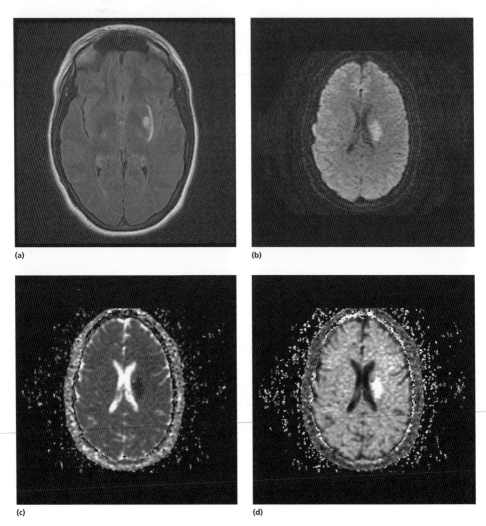

Figure 3.2 33 y/o peripartum female with acute onset right-sided weakness and difficult speaking. Axial FLAIR through the basal ganglia (a) demonstrates abnormal T_2 signal within the left basal ganglia and internal capsule; diffuse weighted image (b) also demonstrates increased signal while the corresponding ADC (c) and exponential-ADC (d) maps confirm restriction of water diffusion, signifying acute infarction. Reproduced from Reference 2 with permission of Elsevier.

obtained. In emergent situations, the health of the mother and fetus may obviate this process.

Radiation exposure

All medical imaging devices involve the production and detection of energy. Ultrasonography, for instance, relies on the transmission of mechanical waves (sound) into the body with images produced by recording the reflected waves (echoes). Most other modalities rely on electromagnetic waves or radiation. Magnetic resonance imaging (MRI) is performed in a large superconducting magnet; however, images are produced using relatively low-energy radiofrequency pulses, a form of nonionizing radiation. Ionizing radiation, on the other hand, as used in radiography, fluoroscopy, and computed tomography (CT), involves high-energy photons (quanta of electromagnetic radiation; i.e., x-rays). When absorbed by the body, these photons may interact with atoms in tissue and fluid, liberate a particle (electron), and potentially result in alterations of chemical bonds and production of reactive ions (radicals) that are chemically reactive and biologically harmful.

Radiation exposure is expressed in coulombs per kilogram, while absorbed dose is expressed in rads or gray (Gy) [29]. Equivalent and effective dose, expressed in sieverts (Sv), take into account the radiation type and radiosensitivity of the exposed tissue, respectively. Natural background radiation for an adult is 3 mSv per year. For a fetus, however, the estimated dose is 0.5–1.0 mSv during the 9-month gestation. The National Council on Radiation Protection and Measurements (NCRP) has instituted a maximum permissible fetal dose in pregnant radiation workers of 5 mSv.

Two types of biologic effects, deterministic and stochastic, must be considered when discussing ionizing radiation exposure to any patient. Deterministic effects from direct tissue damage are associated with specific threshold values of exposure. Such effects have been reported in clinical practice, including skin burns during prolonged fluoroscopic procedures, hair loss in adults undergoing multiple CT perfusion examinations or cataract formation following excessive lens exposure (Table 3.2) [30, 31]. For deterministic effects specific to the fetus, exposures prior to 2 weeks of gestation are characterized by an "all or none" phenomenon, with either failure of implantation/spontaneous loss or a complete absence of detectable effect. The most radiation-sensitive period for the fetus, however, is between weeks 2 and 15, the primary period for organogenesis, during which time reported deterministic effects may included miscarriage, organ malformation, and mental retardation [26, 32]. Intrauterine growth retardation and neurologic effects such as low IQ may be seen in exposures later in pregnancy

Table 3.2 Threshold doses for deterministic radiation effects

Effect	Dose (acute exposure)
Temporary epilation and erythema	2–5 Gy
Prolonged erythema, permanent partial epilation	5–10 Gy
Skin desquamation and necrosis	>10 Gy
Cataracts	2 Gy (5 Gy chronically)

[Administration, 2012]
http://www.fda.gov/Radiation-EmittingProducts/
RadiationSafety/RadiationDoseReduction

(Table 3.3). While individual diagnostic examination doses may be well within an acceptable range, fetal cumulative dose from multiple sequential examinations may reach threshold doses for various deterministic effects.

Stochastic effects, however, occur by chance, occur without any defined threshold, and are believed to occur at any level of radiation exposure; these effects primarily include genetic effects and cancer risk. Childhood malignancy following radiation exposure and leukemia is the most commonly discussed stochastic effects [33, 34]. Numerous reports on high-level radiation exposure have discussed the potential risk of ionizing radiation in animal models as well as following *in utero* exposures [35–42]. For example, longitudinal registries of the survivors of atomic bomb explosions have included children younger than the age of 6 and those *in utero* at the time of the exposure; both groups demonstrated dose-related increases in solid cancer rates [40]. According to the International Commission on Radiation Protection, the best quantitative estimate of stochastic risk is about 1 cancer per 500 fetuses exposed to 30 mGy, or 0.2%; the ACR practice guidelines state that a dose of 20 mGy represents an increased risk of 40 additional cancers per 5000 births, or 0.8% [43]. An excess relative risk of leukemia has also been reported following multiple types of radiation exposures [44], while the estimation of relative

Table 3.3 Suspected in utero deterministic radiation effects

Gestational age	<5 rad (50 mGy)	5–10 rad (50–100 mGy)	>10 rad (100 mGy)
0–2 weeks	None	None	None
3–4 weeks	None	Probably none; theoretical failure of implantation	Possible spontaneous abortion
5–10 weeks	None	Possible effects are scientifically uncertain and may be too subtle to be detected clinically	Possible malformations, increasing likelihood with increasing dose
11–17 weeks	None	Possible effects are scientifically uncertain and may be too subtle to be detected clinically	IUGR; increased risk of microcephaly and IQ deficits, increasing frequency and severity with increasing dose
18–27 weeks	None	None	IQ deficits not detectable at diagnostic doses
>27 weeks	None	None	None applicable to diagnostic medicine

Reproduced from Reference 26 with permission of the American College of Radiology.
IUGR, intrauterine growth retardation; IQ, intelligence quotient.

risk of leukemia varies, the dose-dependent risk has been estimated at approximately 6% per 100 rad exposure (1 Gy) *in utero* [37]. First trimester exposure appears to convey greater risk than second or third trimester exposure.

In practice, fetal doses of less than 5 rad (50 mGy) have not been shown to measurably increased rates of fetal anomalies or spontaneous loss. Practice guidelines published by the ACR regarding the use of ionizing radiation in adolescent and potentially pregnant patients address risk in reference to this exposure limit of 5 rad (50 mGy). At absorbed doses between 5 and 15 rad (150 mGy), possible fetal effects may exist; however, effects specifically due to radiation exposure in this range may be too subtle to detect considering congenital defects exist in 5–10% of births without a history of radiation exposure [26, 45].

The levels of ionizing radiation encountered in modern diagnostic imaging are typically orders of magnitude less than the exposures discussed above. In any case, these studies and guidelines do not obviate the need to consider radiation exposures in every case. Remember: with the potential for stochastic effects, no level of ionizing radiation exposure can be deemed completely "safe." Since there is no theoretical exposure level below which stochastic effects would not occur, the protection paradigm summarized in the acronym "ALARA" (As Low As Reasonably Achievable) was developed [26]. It is important to consider, however, the balance of exposure reduction with diagnostic quality in order to maintain examination efficacy and certainty.

Computed tomography

Medical imaging has surpassed natural background radiation as the largest contributor to an individual's yearly radiation exposure, with computed tomography (CT) representing the largest fraction. The fetal ionizing radiation dose associated with CT varies with maternal size, exam parameters, and whether the fetus is directly irradiated. With cervical spine or cranial imaging, for instance, the fetus is only exposed via internal scatter radiation and radiation dose is considered to be less than 0.01 rad (0.1 mGy) [34, 46, 47]. Direct irradiation could occur with a lumbar spine or abdominal CT that may be obtained for pain or in the setting of trauma. Though *in vivo* fetal absorbed doses cannot be measured directly, a lumbar spine CT dose to the fetus has been estimated to be 0.28–2.4 rad (2.8–24 mGy) and the dose associated with a CT of the abdomen and pelvis may be up to 3 rad (30 mGy) [48–51]. An effective dose, a measure that takes into account the fetus' increased sensitivity to radiation damage, can also be estimated; in a number of simulations for abdominopelvic CT, the estimated effective fetal doses range from 0.73 to 1.4 rad/100 mAs (7.3–14.3 mGy/100 mAs) [52].

Advances in dose reduction technology include dynamic modulation of the radiation exposure depending on body part size and composition [53]. Additionally, varying image processing techniques, such as iterative reconstruction, offer consistent diagnostic image quality while allowing for even further dose reduction, [54–56]. While radiation doses may be significantly lowered by a combination of techniques, utilization of CT imaging is increasing nationwide, including in pregnant patients [57]. Radiation doses can be included in the patient's medical record in order to increase physician awareness of the cumulative radiation dose; many radiology departments include CT doses (typically reported as dose-length product, or DLP) and fluoroscopic exam times in their examination reports. A record of these data also allows radiation safety officers to calculate the best estimates of fetal dosages and provide the most appropriate counseling for any given patient, if needed [58].

Magnetic resonance

Magnetic resonance imaging (MRI) utilizes a strong magnetic field, fluctuating magnetic gradients, and radiofrequency pulses (nonionizing radiation). No current evidence exists to suggest harm to the fetus exposed to magnetic fields up to 3 Tesla (T). Tissue heating, as a result of energy deposition from radiofrequency pulses, and acoustic noise exposure have been reported as potential concerns regarding MRI; however, limited data are available. The ACR practice guidelines suggest deferring elective examinations due to these potential concerns, though

advocate the use of MRI if the results could have a direct benefit to the health of the patient or fetus [59]. For example, fetal imaging for antenatal diagnoses using MRI is endorsed with guidelines established jointly by the ACR and the Society of Pediatric Radiology.

Contrast administration

Contrast-enhanced imaging is often desired for improved diagnostic utility; however, safety concerns must be considered. Intravenous contrast may include iodinated-based agents utilized in CT and gadolinium chelates in MRI. There has been no proven teratogenic effect associated with the intravenous administration of iodinated CT contrast during pregnancy. However, fetal thyroid exposure to iodinated contrast could potentially be associated with neonatal hypothyroidism. If it is not possible to defer contrast administration, written informed consent should be obtained along with subsequent attention to the fetal thyroid function markers on routine neonatal screening [60, 61].

Gadolinium chelates used in MRI have been shown to cross the placenta, enter fetal circulation, and pass into the amniotic fluid following fetal renal excretion before complete clearing. Given this exposure, the administration of MR contrast agents should also be deferred during pregnancy whenever possible. While animal studies have demonstrated developmental abnormalities following gadolinium exposure, this occurs at concentrations far higher than would be used in clinical settings. Therefore, MR contrast administration may be considered when absolutely clinically warranted. It is advisable that any decision involving the administration of gadolinium-based agents to the pregnant patient should follow a well-documented risk benefit analysis, with signed informed consent obtained [59].

Some iodinated contrast agents and extremely small amounts of gadolinium-based agents are excreted into breast milk (<1%), and even smaller quantities are absorbed by the infant gastrointestinal tract (<1%); at these small doses, no association with any adverse outcome has been identified. The ACOG and ACR guidelines do not advocate any interruption of breastfeeding following the administration of iodinated CT contrast nor gadolinium MR contrast [27]. A 24-hour period of interruption of breastfeeding ("pump and dump") may be offered as an option to allay maternal concern, a practice the European Society of Urogenital Radiology supports following the administration of any gadolinium agent [28].

Neuropathology and associated imaging findings

Headache is one of the most common neurological complaints. Widespread incidence of headaches in reproductive age women has been reported, and it follows that headaches will be encountered in the pregnant patient [62–64]. Unfortunately, varied causes, both benign and potentially life-threatening, may present with this nonspecific symptom.

Primary headache disorders, migraine headaches with or without an aura, may be up to three times more common in females following puberty; [65]. The exact underlying physiology of migraines is not completely understood, though estrogen hormonal influences play a role. Increasing estrogen levels during the menstrual cycle are associated with improving symptoms and falling levels with worsening symptoms [62, 66]. During pregnancy, consistently elevated estrogen levels are also associated with improvement in certain migraine headaches, with 11%, 53%, and 79% of women reporting improvement in headaches symptoms during first, second, and third trimesters, respectively [67, 68]. A pregnant patient with a known headache disorder may require no neurologic imaging when presenting with headache, though a variety of superimposed signs or symptoms may warrant further evaluation.

Secondary headaches, or headaches relating to an actionable underlying cause such as in pseudotumor cerebri (Figure 3.3), may represent the earliest warning sign of a treatable or even life-threatening illness. Intracranial mass lesion or hemorrhage, ruptured aneurysm, dural venous thrombosis, and central nervous system infection among others could all present with headache. Numerous studies and reviews have examined the varying headache presentations in attempt to better discern headaches that will ultimately be categorized as a primary headache disorder from those associated with a significant secondary cause, usually focusing on key "red flags." That a patient presenting with headache is pregnant often considered justification enough for further evaluation [69]. Of all reported factors, acute sudden onset, shorter duration of presenting symptoms, and association with a focal neurologic examination all seem to warrant the search for secondary causes [69]. Additionally, in determining the need for neurologic imaging, cluster-type headache, abnormal finding on neurologic examination, undefined headache, headache with aura, headache exacerbated by exertion or valsalva, and headache with vomiting were found to be predictive of an underlying intracranial abnormality, to varying degree. However, no clinical features reliably exclude secondary intracranial conditions [70]. A potential algorithm developed by DeLuca and Bartleson in Seminars in Neurology, 2010, for the utilization of neuroimaging in the patient presenting with headache is reproduced in Table 3.4.

In the pregnant patient presenting with an acute, sudden onset headache, a non-contrast CT of the head is generally the first imaging study of choice, aimed at the detection or exclusion of intracranial hemorrhage, fluid collections, intracranial masses, stroke, the sequelae of trauma, as well as assessing possible sinus or mastoid infections [69]. With the performance of a head CT, the fetus is far removed from the x-ray beam and external body shielding is not needed; internally scattered radiation

Neuroimaging   **23**

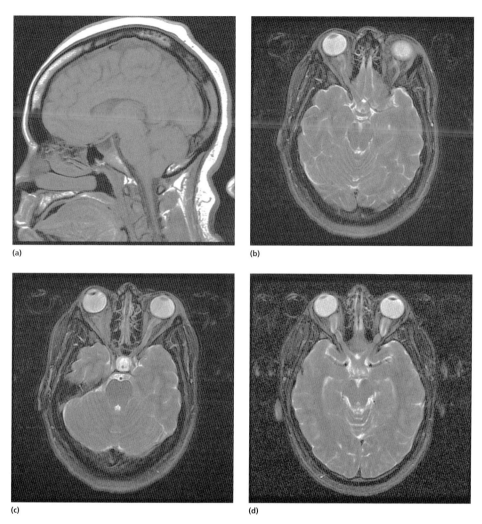

(a)

(b)

(c)

(d)

Figure 3.3 33 y/o female, 10 days postpartum, with persistent headaches. Sagittal T_1 (a) demonstrates flattening of the pituitary gland and settling of the posterior fossa contents. Axial T_2 images (b,c) demonstrate an "empty sella" as well as optic nerve tortuosity and circumferential CSF space prominence. Imaging findings of increased intracranial pressure, in combination with a lumbar puncture opening pressure of 45 mm water and papilledema on ophthalmologic examination, were consistent with pseudotumor cerebri. In a different patient, 21 y/o female with pseudotumor cerebri, MRI demonstrates tortuous optic nerves with marked dilatation of the CSF spaces with flattening of the optic disc (d). Reproduced from Reference 2 with permission of Elsevier.

contributes to an estimated fetal dose of 0.01 rad (0.1 mGy).

For many patients, the presentation may be more protracted or raise concern for vascular disease, neoplasm, or infection. Additionally, there may be persistent clinical concerns, even following a negative CT examination. In these cases, an MRI of the brain should be considered. The improved soft tissue characterization, the availability of exquisitely sensitive

Table 3.4 Preferred imaging modality in evaluating suspected underlying cause of headache

MRI preferred	Vascular disease: cerebral infarction and venous infarct Neoplasm: primary and metastatic tumors, skull base tumors, carcinomatosis, and pituitary tumors Infections: cerebritis, brain abscess, encephalitis, and meningitis Chiari malformations Intracranial hypotension/CSF leaks Pituitary apoplexy Rare encephalopathies: CADASIL, MELAS, and SMART
CT preferred	Fractures Trauma Acute hemorrhage: subarachnoid, intraparenchymal, epidural, and subdural Sinus and mastoid disease
MRI and CT equivalent	MR/CT arteriography: vasculitis, aneurysms, carotid, and vertebral dissection MR/CT venography: cerebral venous thrombosis

Reproduced from Reference 71 with permission of Mayo Foundation for Medical Education and Research. CADASIL, cerebral autosomal dominant arteriopathy with subcortical infarcts and leukoencephalopathy; MELAS, mitochondrial encephalomyopathy, lactic acidosis, and stroke like episodes; SMART, stroke-like migraine attacks after radiation therapy; MRI, magnetic resonance imaging; CT, computed tomography.

diffusion weighted imaging, and the ability to obtain both arterial and venous angiographic images without exogenous contrast are distinct advantages of MRI over CT [71]. Administration of gadolinium-based contrast agents is reserved for specific situations in which the risks and benefits have been carefully considered [59]. When considering dural venous thrombosis or other vascular causes such as vasculitis, vasospasm, or aneurysm, iodinated contrast may be used for both CT angiographic and conventional catheter-based interventions, both

of which provide improved reproducibility and spatial resolution over MRI.

Intracranial hemorrhage

The pregnant patient presenting acutely with severe headache, focal neurologic deficits, or meningismus will frequently undergo a non-contrast CT of the head, which in some cases will reveal intracranial hemorrhage.

Extra-axial hemorrhage

Epidural and subdural hematomas in pregnancy are typically the result of trauma, as in the nonpregnant population. Subdural hemorrhages are an uncommon complication of dural puncture and have been described in postpartum patients following spinal-epidural anesthesia (Figure 3.4) [72].

Subarachnoid hemorrhage has been reported up to five times more likely during pregnancy than in the nonpregnant population, though some authors have not shown this difference in certain populations [22, 24]. Subarachnoid hemorrhage and its sequelae represent the third leading cause of non-obstetric-related maternal death [21]. Primigravida, increased maternal age, and advanced gestation age convey even greater risk [73]. Aneurysm rupture and hypertensive disorders have been variably reported as the leading underlying cause [8, 9, 22, 24, 74].

Non-contrast CT is the first-line examination with sensitivity greater than 90% (Figure 3.5). However, if clinical suspicion persists, lumbar puncture may be performed; though invasive, lumbar puncture remains the gold standard. Computed tomography is the preferred modality to follow up hemorrhage and monitor for complications such as intraparenchymal extension and hydrocephalus [21].

Catheter angiography remains the gold standard to determine the cause of hemorrhage. When readily available, MR angiography (MRA) should be considered as non-contrast three-dimensional time-of-flight imaging may be performed. Recent advances in MRA, including the use of higher magnetic field strengths, continue

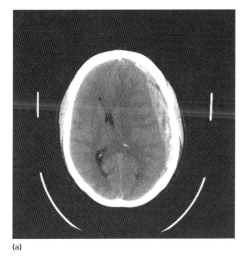 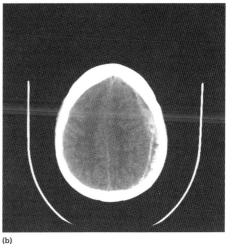

(a)   (b)

Figure 3.4 31 y/o female, 1 day following cesarean section for arrested labor and chorioamnionitis, with sudden onset headache with rapid deterioration of mental status. Examination revealed fixed and dilated pupils. Non-contrast CT images (a,b) demonstrate a hyperdense, lentiform extra-axial (subdural) collection over the left hemisphere with marked mass effect and midline shift. Reproduced from Reference 2 with permission of Elsevier.

to improve MRI performance. In the search for a suspected intracranial aneurysm, studies suggest that 90% of angiographically confirmed aneurysms greater than 3 mm in size can be identified with MRA. Magnetic resonance angiography may perform less well when considering small aneurysms, complex aneurysms, or those adjacent to bony structures of the skull base.

Advances in CT have increased CT angiography (CTA) speed and sensitivity and many radiologists favor CTA to MRA in the evaluation of intracranial aneurysms due to the increased spatial resolution and superior reproducibility [75–77]. However, ionizing radiation is involved and intravenous contrast administration is required.

Magnetic resonance angiography allows for the assessment and follow-up of non-ruptured aneurysms without radiation exposure, though both MRA and CTA may be used for treatment planning. Important findings include aneurysm size, location, and additional characteristics such as neck size (narrow vs. wide), proximity to vessel origins, and orientation of the aneurysm apex in relation to its base. Studies have shown that treatment of ruptured aneurysms is beneficial to both mother and fetus (52% reduction and 22% reduction in mortality rates, respectively). Both endovascular coiling and surgical clipping may be attempted, depending on aneurysm size, location, and other characteristics. For incidentally identified unruptured aneurysms, treatment is typically considered for symptomatic or enlarging lesions [74]. Debate exists regarding delivery options, with cesarean section typically recommended to decrease the risk of increasing intracranial pressure during labor and delivery, however, rupture incidence of untreated or incompletely treated aneurysms between vaginal and cesarean delivery are not significantly different, and similar to the background population.

Primary nonaneurysmal SAH is a diagnosis of exclusion. Rarely SAH may be identified by non-contrast CT or lumbar puncture with no aneurysm identified, even by catheter

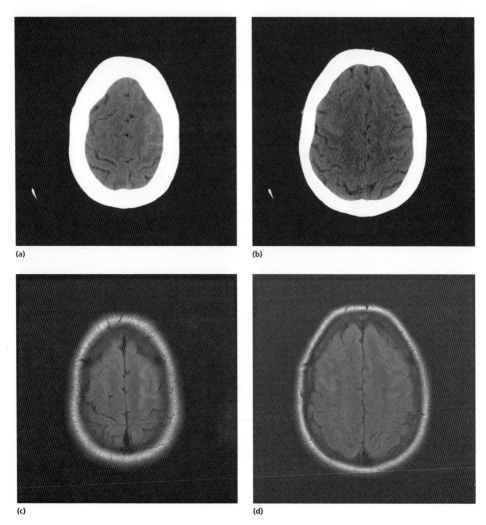

Figure 3.5 30 y/o female with preeclampsia developed acute onset severe headaches following childbirth. Non-contrast CT images (a,b) demonstrate linear sulcal hyperdensity consistent with acute subarachnoid hemorrhage; corroborating MR images demonstrate loss of normal FLAIR CSF suppression (c,d) as well as blooming artifact on susceptibility-weighted images (e,f), all findings of subarachnoid blood products. Reproduced from Reference 2 with permission of Elsevier.

angiography. Nonaneurysmal SAH is typically induced by hypertension and may relate to failure of intracranial autoregulation and rupture of the relatively thin-walled pial veins [78]. A spinal MR may be attempted and repeat cerebral catheter angiography may be considered if initial examinations fail to identify an underlying cause.

Intra-axial hemorrhage
Hemorrhagic infarction

Despite the physiologic changes associated with pregnancy, multicenter randomized trials have not shown an increased risk of ischemic or hemorrhagic infarction during pregnancy. However, in the first several weeks following delivery, the risk of infarction is markedly increased.

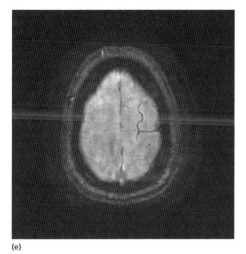

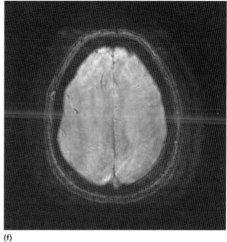

(e)   (f)

Figure 3.5 (*Continued*)

Hemorrhagic infarctions (intra-axial parenchymal hemorrhages) are less common than SAH and may result from a variety of pathologies.

Venous thrombosis

Pregnancy is a hypercoagulable state and the elevated risk of cerebral venous thrombosis (CVT) is greatest in the first 2–4 weeks following delivery. Cerebral venous thrombosis is reported to account for up to 6% of maternal deaths. Common presenting symptoms include headache, seizure, papilledema, encephalopathy, focal neurologic deficit, and symptoms of idiopathic intracranial hypertension (IIH) as 20–40% of patients with CVT may demonstrate elevated intracranial pressure. Venous infarction, an important cause of parenchymal hemorrhage, may occur following sinus thrombosis, tends to be peripheral, does not respect arterial territories, and may involve deep brain structures. Both the degree of collateral drainage and thrombus recanalization can contribute to waxing and waning clinical symptoms, parenchymal changes, and simultaneous occurrence of both vasogenic and cytotoxic edema [79–82].

In the case of suspected CVT, a non-contrast CT is an important initial examination to quickly exclude hemorrhage, however, it is often normal. The classic finding of a hyperdense venous sinus on non-contrast CT (Figure 3.6) is only seen in a minority of cases, reportedly up to 25% [83]. Dehydration, elevated hematocrit, adjacent hemorrhage, motion, or streak artifact could all mimic this finding. Cytotoxic or vasogenic edema, parenchymal hemorrhage, subdural hemorrhage, and findings suggestive of IIH are potential secondary CT findings [84].

Though catheter angiography remains the gold standard, both CT and MR angiographic imaging techniques are widely utilized in the evaluation of suspected CVT. On CT venography, a focal venous cutoff or filling defect in an otherwise normally enhancing dural sinus are common findings of venous thrombosis. One must ensure that a venous-phase of contrast enhancement is acquired as mixing of opacified and non-opacified dural venous blood, sometimes seen on an arterial acquisition, may simulate a non-occlusive thrombus (Table 3.5). While CT is essentially equivalent to MRI in the detection of thromboses of the dural sinuses, MR imaging techniques may be superior to CT for assessing cortical veins [85].

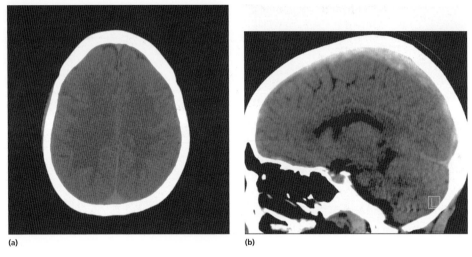

(a)   (b)

Figure 3.6 45 y/o postpartum female with 9 days of headache. Axial (a) and reconstructed sagittal (b) non-contrast CT images demonstrate a hyperattenuating, expanded sagittal dural venous sinus consistent with acute thrombosis. Reproduced from Reference 2 with permission of Elsevier.

Given the lack of ionizing radiation and requirement for exogenous contrast, MRI is often preferred in the cases of suspected CVT during pregnancy. The venous sinuses can be evaluated on both anatomic images and non-contrast venographic techniques (Figure 3.7). Venous sinuses should appear as flow voids on routine anatomic sequences, the loss of which could be consistent thrombosis. However, technical factors and normal anatomic variations contribute to potential pitfalls when relying on anatomic MR images alone (Table 3.5) [86]. Slow or turbulent flow may result in an incomplete flow void, simulating CVT, though may also be encountered with a recanalized or partially thrombosed sinus [82]. In addition, the

Table 3.5 Pitfalls in CT and MR venography

Anatomic concerns applicable to both CT and MRI	CT venography	MR venography
Numerous variations in the pattern of venous sinuses	Errors in exam timing compromising venous opacification	Slow and heterogeneous flow in venous sinuses mimicking thrombosis
Left to right asymmetries	Contrast related issues, including poor IV access compromising venous opacification	Longer imaging, and user defined velocity thresholds in phase contrast techniques
Venous sinus septations and inconstant patterns of contributing veins		
Presence of arachnoid granulations as filling defects	Streak artifact from skull	Loss of signal due to saturation effects with in-plane flow
Variation in anatomy and hemodynamic effects	Beam hardening causing the spurious appearance of hypodense parenchyma	Intrinsic T_1 signal related to thrombus simulating flow
Partially recanalized thrombosed sinuses		Contrast related issues in contrast enhanced MRV

MRI, magnetic resonance imaging; CT, computed tomography.

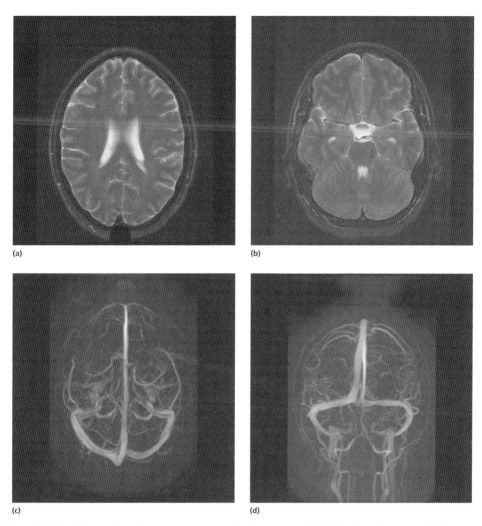

(a) (b)

(c) (d)

Figure 3.7 22 y/o female, first trimester, presenting with headache. Axial T_2 MR through the sagittal (a) and transverse (b) sinuses demonstrate a normal flow void. Three-dimensional phase-contrast (non-contrast) MR venography (c–e) confirms normal flow-related signal, signifying patent venous sinuses. Reproduced from Reference 2 with permission of Elsevier.

signal intensity of a venous thrombus can vary over time depending on the presence or absence of variable hemoglobin breakdown products [82, 87–89].

Certain GRE or T_2*, susceptibility weighted MR sequences are especially sensitive to blood products and can be helpful in acute cases of thrombosis or when T_1 and T_2 signal abnormalities are varied or subtle. The increased sensitivity of these sequences contributes to the superiority of MRI in diagnosing thromboses of the small cortical veins (Figure 3.8) [85, 88]. Diffusion weighted images, on the other hand, are not helpful as thrombosed dural sinuses may have a widely variable appearance [80, 87, 90, 91]. The addition of MR venography may be beneficial to the diagnosis of CVT.

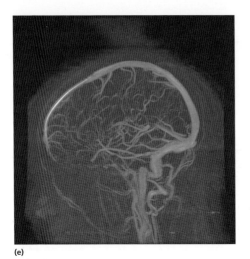

(e)

Figure 3.7 (*Continued*)

The MR venography may consist of post-contrast imaging; however, phase contrast and time-of-flight techniques, as seen in MR angiography (Figure 3.9), are often used to evaluate the major cerebral veins and dural venous sinuses in a pregnant patient as they can be performed without contrast. Venographic images from these techniques are created by maximizing signal from patent dural venous sinuses while minimizing signal from the parenchyma and other stationary structures. Flow-related signal is expected from patent vascular structures. However, a number of technical concerns may contribute to pitfalls when relying on these sequences as well (Table 3.5) (Figure 3.10). In time-of-flight imaging, the in-plane flow may result in loss of flow-related signal. For phase-contrast imaging, a velocity range must be selected for each acquisition. If venous flow is significantly slow or fast, velocities falling outside the expected range may result in a signal gap, simulating CVT. Finally, venous septations, turbulent flow, or the angle of slice selection may all result in artifacts [92], these artifactual signal gaps may be noted in up to 31% of normal MR venographic cases.

Normal anatomic variations in the pattern of superficial draining veins or the dural venous sinuses may contribute to potential pitfalls when utilizing either CT venography or MR venographic techniques (Figure 3.11) [86]. Therefore, findings from a variety of imaging techniques must be analyzed in combination. The addition of contrast-enhanced MR venography may eliminate some artifacts and increase diagnostic sensitivity and specificity, with a variety of techniques described (Figure 3.12) [93–95]. However, given potential concern regarding contrast administration in the pregnant patient, these techniques should be reserved for the postpartum period unless absolutely necessary.

Amniotic fluid embolism

Amniotic fluid embolism is a fairly rare peripartum entity with incidence of about 1 in 20,000 deliveries, however, accounts for 5–10% of maternal mortality in the United States. Mortality reaches 60% and most survivors suffer from significant neurologic morbidity. The pathophysiology is poorly understood; however, is felt to require ruptured membranes, breach of uterine or cervical veins, and a pressure gradient between the uterus and venous drainage allowing for passage of amniotic fluid, fetal cells, and other debris into the maternal circulation. There is typically a dramatic onset of cardiorespiratory collapse; clinical presentation of anaphylaxis has led some to suggest the term anaphylactoid syndrome of pregnancy. Imaging findings are nonspecific with areas of restricted diffusion and associated vasogenic edema and possible hemorrhage within multiple vascular territories, suggesting an embolic event (Figure 3.13).

Eclampsia, encephalopathy syndrome, and angiopathy

Rarely, conditions such as eclampsia and the related posterior reversible encephalopathy syndrome (PRES), also known as reversible posterior leukoencephalopathy syndrome (RPLS), as well as postpartum cerebral angiopathy (PCA) may present with intracranial hemorrhage. The

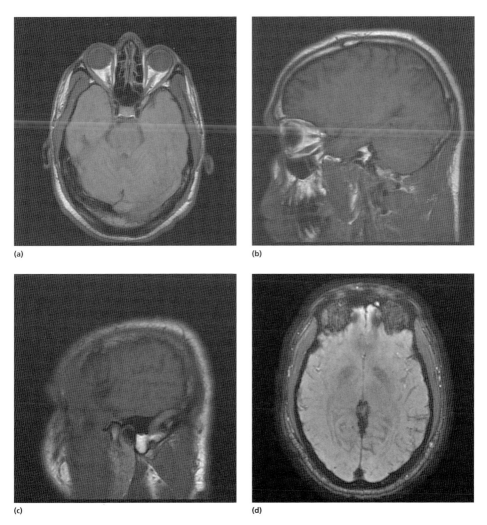

(a)

(b)

(c)

(d)

Figure 3.8 Non-contrast MR with axial proton density (a) and sagittal T_1 (b,c) MR images demonstrate loss of the expected flow void within the left transverse sinus, compared to the contralateral side; axial susceptibility-weighted images (d–f) demonstrate "blooming" artifact from acute thrombosis of the vein of Galen and transverse sinus with additional blooming within the deep cerebral and small cortical veins, likely from additional thrombosis or extremely slow flow; left occipital parenchymal hemorrhage is also present; axial (g) and sagittal (h) T_1-weighted images demonstrate a filling defect with the dural venous sinuses. Reproduced from Reference 2 with permission of Elsevier.

more common clinical presentation of these entities, however, is without hemorrhage.

An additional cause for intra-axial hemorrhage is from an underlying mass lesion, classically from choriocarcinoma; however, many primary and metastatic lesions may present with headache and intracranial hemorrhage. These are discussed in detail later in this chapter.

Encephalopathy

Though headache may be the most common presenting neurological complaint during

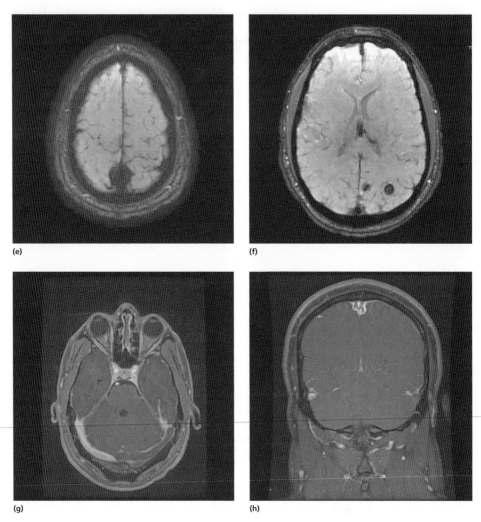

Figure 3.8 (*Continued*)

pregnancy, encephalopathy, though also non-specific, may indicate a more severe underlying neuropathology. The most common causes are eclampsia and etiologies defined by hypertensive episodes with imaging findings of PRES/RPLS.

Eclampsia/preeclampsia and hypertensive encephalopathy

Preeclampsia is a complex clinical syndrome affecting 5–10% of all pregnancies (up to 30%

of twin gestations) and is defined by the presence of hypertension, proteinuria, and peripheral edema, typically presenting around the 20th week of gestation [21, 96]. Patients may present clinically with headaches, visual disturbances, confusion, and right upper quadrant pain.

If a preeclamptic patient presents with seizures or coma, the diagnosis of eclampsia is made. This life-threatening condition is treated medically with hypertension control

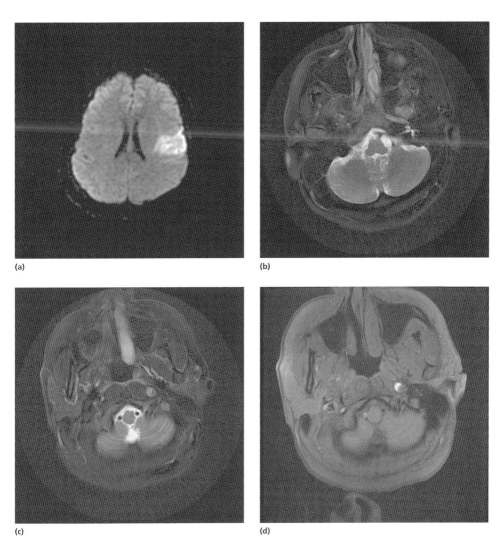

(a)

(b)

(c)

(d)

Figure 3.9 Non-contrast MR angiography in a 42 y/o female, 4 weeks pregnant, with acute-onset right arm weakness and numbness. Diffusion-weighted imaging (a), with ADC maps (not shown) confirmed acute infarction; axial T_2 through the skull base (b,c) demonstrate loss of the expected left internal carotid artery (ICA) flow void, while T_1 fat-suppressed image through the distal internal carotid (d) demonstrates crescentic hyperintense mural thrombus; maximum-intensity projection (MIP) reformatted image from 2D time-of-flight imaging through the neck (e) demonstrates loss of the expected flow-related signal from the left internal carotid with "string sign;" axial 3D time-of-flight images (f,g) confirm loss of flow-related signal from the left internal carotid; MIP reformatted image (h) demonstrates rapid flame-shaped tapering of the distal ICA. Reproduced from Reference 2 with permission of Elsevier.

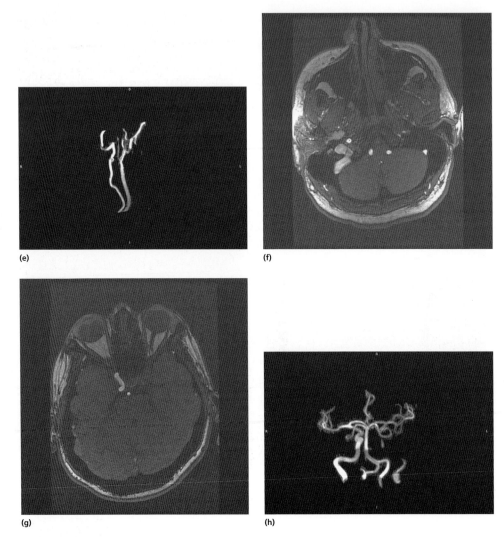

(e)

(f)

(g)

(h)

Figure 3.9 (*Continued*)

and seizure prophylaxis with magnesium sulfate. However, if seizure activity persists, emergent delivery may be required as symptoms typically resolve shortly following delivery of the placenta. Patients may also present with hemolytic anemia, elevated liver function tests, and low platelets, part of the HELLP syndrome. Patients with preeclampsia/eclampsia may present with clinical findings identical to those seen in hypertensive encephalopathy in nonpregnant patients. A specific etiology is unknown, however, some theorize that placental-derived cytotoxic factors contribute to widespread vascular derangements, disruption of autoregulation, and breakdown of the blood–brain barrier leading to vasogenic cerebral edema [21, 96]. Though typically self-limited, uncontrolled hypertension may also be accompanied by vasospasm and intracranial hemorrhage [8].

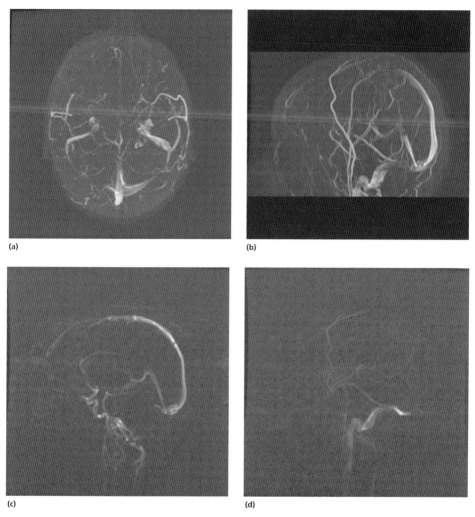

(a)

(b)

(c)

(d)

Figure 3.10 Non-contrast 2D phase-contrast MR venography with axial (a) and sagittal (b) MIP-reformatted images demonstrate signal gaps (lack of flow-related enhancement) within the sagittal and transverse venous sinuses due to in-plane flow artifact; 2D time-of-flight venography demonstrates flow-related signal within the sagittal sinus (c), however, a signal gap is seen within the right transverse sinus (d). Reproduced from Reference 2 with permission of Elsevier.

Posterior reversible encephalopathy syndrome/reversible posterior leukoencephalopathy syndrome

Imaging findings of preeclampsia/eclampsia are inseparable from those of PRES, also known as reversible posterior leukoencephalopathy syndrome (RPLS), in the nonpregnant patient [9]. The PRES/RPLS is also associated with systemic lupus erythematosus (SLE) and thrombotic thrombocytopenic purpura (TTP) and seen in patients receiving cyclosporine, tacrolimus, and chemotherapy. Regarding the pregnant patient, it is typically identified between the third trimester and 6–8 week postpartum period following an episode of significant hypertension. Patients may present with

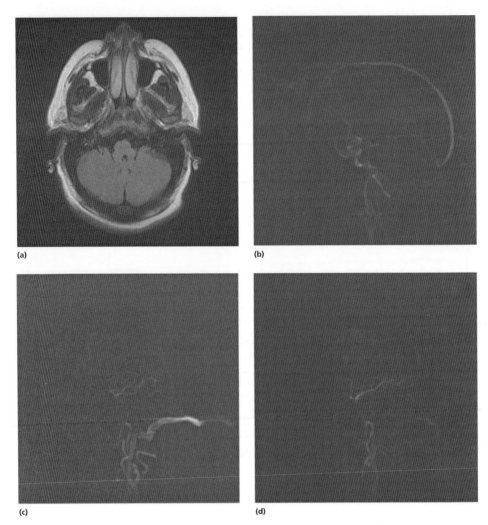

(a)   (b)

(c)   (d)

Figure 3.11 42 y/o postpartum female, diagnosed with preeclampsia, presenting with dizziness. Axial FLAIR MR image (a) demonstrates the expected dural venous sinus flow voids (open arrow); MIP reformatted images from 2D phase-contrast MR venography through the sagittal (b) and transverse venous sinuses (c,d) demonstrates absent flow-related signal from the right transverse sinus; similar findings on 3D phase-contrast venography with sagittal (e), coronal (f), and axial (g) MIP images, likely due to slow flow within normal a variant; subsequent contrast-enhanced CT venography with axial (h) and MIP reformatted images (i,j) demonstrate a patent sinus. Reproduced from Reference 2 with permission of Elsevier.

self-limited severe headache, seizures, and cortical blindness.

Computed tomography findings are nonspecific with areas of patchy white matter hypoattenuation; watershed regions are the most affected, particularly in the occipital regions,

however, the frontal and parietal lobes may also be involved [21]. On CT, areas of hyperattenuation likely signify subarachnoid or even parenchymal hemorrhage. On MRI, the patchy areas of T_1 hypointensity and T_2 hyperintensity, most conspicuous on FLAIR sequences, affect

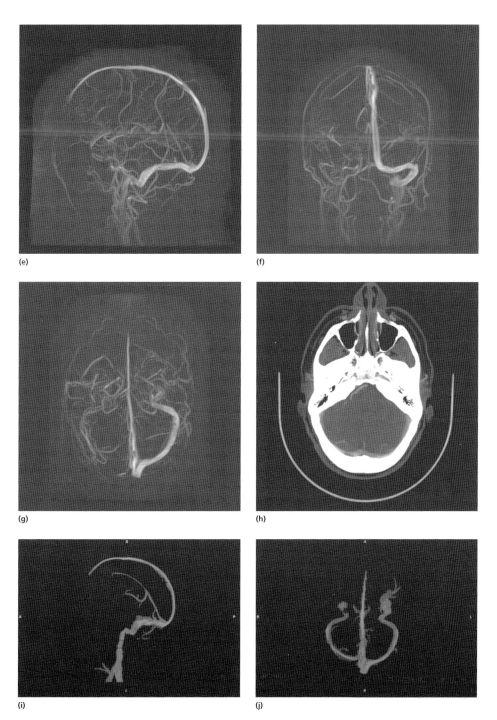

(e)

(f)

(g)

(h)

(i)

(j)

Figure 3.11 (*Continued*)

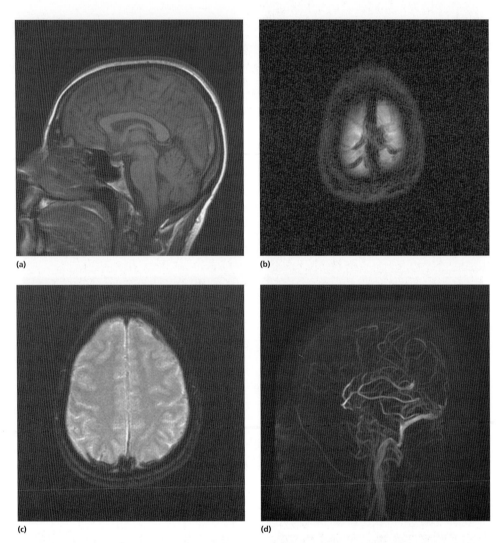

(a)

(b)

(c)

(d)

Figure 3.12 45 y/o female with 9 day history of a persistent postpartum headache. Sagittal T_1 MR (a) demonstrates loss of the expected sagittal sinus flow void; axial susceptibility-weighted images (b,c) demonstrate blooming artifact within the sagittal sinus; 3D phase-contrast venography with sagittal (d) and coronal (e) MIP reformatted images demonstrate loss of flow-related signal from the sagittal sinus; axial (f,g), coronal (h), and sagittal (i) post-contrast MR venography demonstrate filling defect within the sagittal sinus, confirming thrombosis. Reproduced from Reference 2 with permission of Elsevier.

the subcortical parietoocciptal regions, however, may also involve the frontal lobes, basal ganglia, pons, and brainstem; cortical involvement may also be seen (Figure 3.14). Facilitated diffusion may result in increased signal on diffusion weighted imaging and would correspond to areas of increased pixel values on ADC maps; true areas of parenchymal infarction may occur and would demonstrate decreased values on ADC maps (Figure 3.15). Hemorrhage may be seen as well, and variable enhancement is a known imaging finding [21]. Angiography

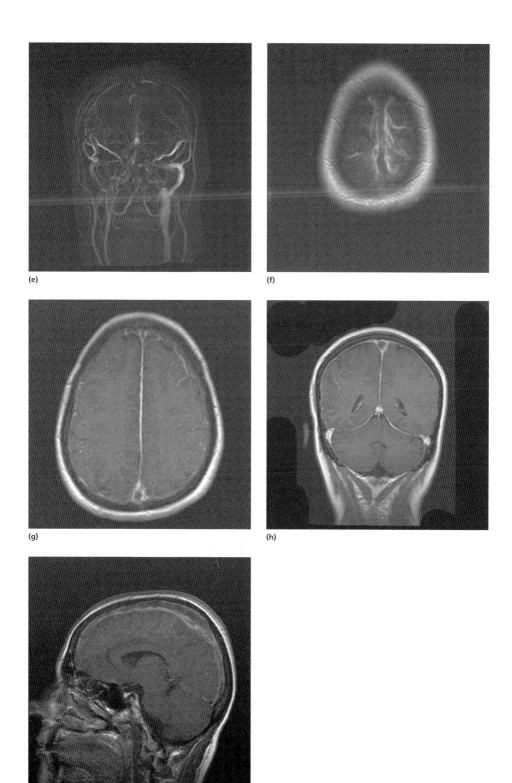

(e)

(f)

(g)

(h)

(i)

Figure 3.12 (*Continued*)

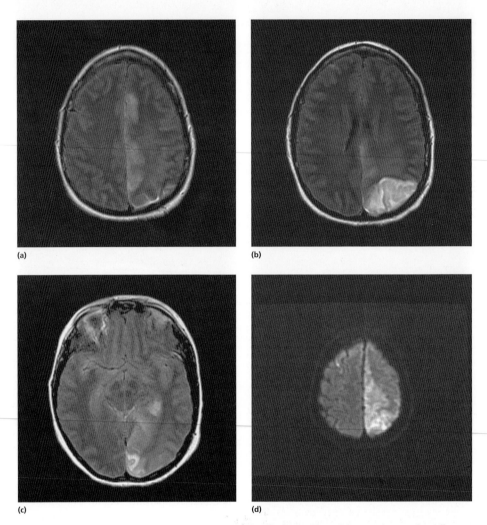

(a)   (b)

(c)   (d)

Figure 3.13 33 y/o female with acute-onset confusion and tachycardia during labor, cardiovascular collapse ensued and patient became comatose. An emergent cesarean section was performed and the patient was presented for imaging. FLAIR MR images (a–c) demonstrate multiple cortical and subcortical regions of T_2 signal abnormality across multiple vascular territories; DWI (d) demonstrate confluent restricted diffusion within the posterior left hemisphere with a contralateral punctate focus of signal abnormality—findings concerning for an embolic event; (e) ADC map demonstrates both infarction by decreased pixel values and vasogenic edema by increased pixel values. Reproduced from Reference 2 with permission of Elsevier.

may demonstrate vasospasm of the medium and large cerebral arteries, particularly involving the basilar artery.

Postpartum angiopathy

Postpartum cerebral angiopathy (PCA), also known as peripartum cerebral angiopathy or vasculopathy, is indistinguishable from eclampsia and PRES/RPLS on imaging. Postpartum cerebral angiopathy also presents with severe headaches, seizures, and focal neurological deficits clinically, however, occurs in normotensive women without proteinuria, typically in the 4-week postpartum period [8, 97, 98].

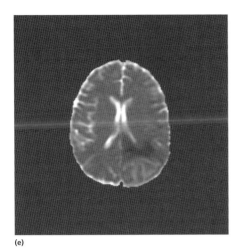

(e)

Figure 3.13 (*Continued*)

Clinical information is often required to differentiate these diagnoses; however, some authors believe that postpartum angiopathy, eclampsia, hypertensive encephalopathy, and PRES/RPLS are different manifestations of the same underlying pathophysiologic process. The idiopathic form of PCA is typically reversible and non-relapsing [9]. An iatrogenic form of PCA has been linked to the administration of bromocriptine (lactation suppression), ergot alkaloids (postpartum hemorrhage), and sympathomimetics (often found in cold medication and nasal decongestants) [9, 99].

Imaging features are similar to PRES with patchy T_2 hyperintense white matter lesions in the watershed areas. Catheter angiography may demonstrate multifocal and reversible stenoses (arterial beading) primarily within the anterior circulation. Treatment is typically supportive, steroids are often provided, and intracranial angioplasty is rarely required. Rarely infarction and intracranial hemorrhage may also be seen.

Wernicke's encephalopathy

Wernicke's encephalopathy is a potentially life-threatening condition resulting from severe deficiency in thiamine [100]. Most frequently, Wernicke's encephalopathy occurs in the setting of alcoholism and associated malnutrition (Figure 3.16), however, can occur in other conditions including hyperemesis gravidarum as seen in pregnancy. In the setting of severe thiamine deficiency, brain metabolism is impaired, lactic acidic accumulation ensues, osmotic gradients develop, and integrity of the blood–brain barrier may be impaired. This abnormality is prone to occur in regions where thiamine-dependent glucose metabolism is highest, accounting for the fairly distinct appearance on MRI.

Wernicke's encephalopathy is characterized by abnormal elevated T_2 signal at the medial thalami, mammillary bodies, periaqueductal gray matter, floor of the fourth ventricle, and superior cerebellar vermis. Restricted diffusion on DWI may also be seen, along with abnormal enhancement of the affected structures following contrast administration. Consideration of this diagnosis and the recognition of the fairly characteristic imaging findings may facilitate a prompt diagnosis and early initiation of life-saving therapy in a patient population where the diagnosis might not otherwise be as suspected.

Seizures

As discussed earlier, there are many potential etiologies of seizures in the pregnant, peripartum, and postpartum patient. Both intra- and extra-axial hemorrhage may be a cause for or represent an underlying cause of seizure activity; headache and seizure may be the initial clinical findings for venous thrombosis. Also, the dramatic clinical presentation of amniotic fluid embolism may include seizures. An initial non-contrast CT head may assist in the exclusion of intracranial hemorrhage, as discussed earlier.

A first- or second-trimester patient with hyperemesis gravidarum presenting with seizures may be suffering from Wernicke's encephalopathy from thiamine deficiency; clinical suspicion must remain high as prompt initiation of treatment is critical. Imaging findings are discussed earlier.

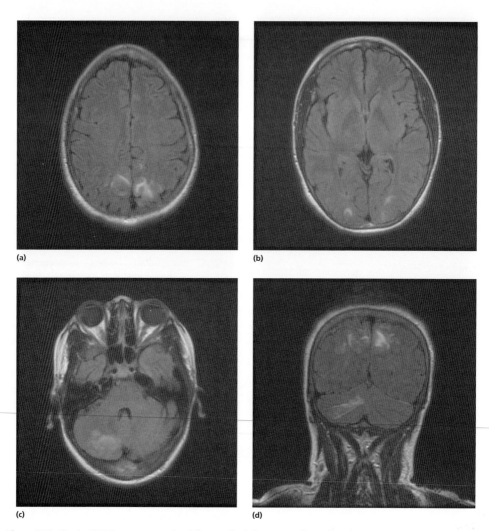

(a)   (b)   (c)   (d)

Figure 3.14 35 y/o, G3P2, postpartum day 9 from twin delivery, re-admitted with tonic–clonic seizures. History of hypertension and several days of headache. Axial (a–c) and sagittal (d) FLAIR MR images demonstrate patchy areas of juxtacortical, primarily white matter T_2 hyperintensity involving the parietal and occipital lobes and cerebellum, typical locations for hypertensive encephalopathy or PRES/PRLS. Reproduced from Reference 2 with permission of Elsevier.

A patient with preeclampsia presenting with seizures is diagnosed with eclampsia and aggressive medical management is required to prevent manifestations of hypertensive encephalopathy and PRES/PRLS, as discussed earlier. After delivery, a normotensive patient with PCA may also present with seizures.

In addition, seizure activity may rarely be the presenting sign of an intracranial mass lesion. Classically, this may be an enlarging meningioma; however, any intracranial mass, whether responding to pregnancy-related hormone changes or not, may come to clinical attention during pregnancy. Details regarding some of these lesions are discussed later.

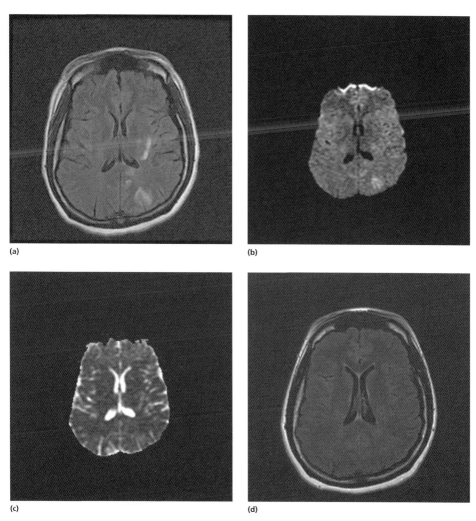

(a)

(b)

(c)

(d)

Figure 3.15 36 y/o female, one day following cesarean section at 33 weeks for severe preeclampsia, presenting with cortical blindness. Magnetic resonance imaging confirms findings of hypertensive encephalopathy with axial FLAIR through the lateral ventricles (a) demonstrates abnormal T_2 signal within the occipital periventricular and juxtacortical white matter, as well as within the left internal capsule; diffusion-weight image (b) demonstrates associated increased signal within the occipital regions, however, the corresponding ADC map (c) reveals facilitated diffusion, as opposed to infarction. A follow-up MRI (d) demonstrates complete signal alteration resolution. Reproduced from Reference 2 with permission of Elsevier.

Epilepsy and seizure disorders

In pregnant patients with primary seizure disorders who were enrolled in a large European registry (EURAP), baseline seizure control was maintained without change in symptoms in 63.6% of women, with approximately 93% being seizure-free throughout pregnancy. Approximately 17% and 16% of women had an increase and decrease in their seizure frequency, respectively. While the majority of women with epilepsy experience no change in seizures, there are conflicting reports regarding incidence of

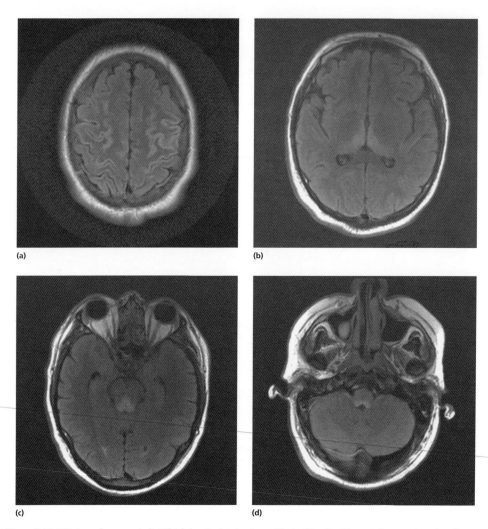

Figure 3.16 27 y/o male presented with abdominal pain at outside facility. Rapid mental status deterioration necessitated transfer. Axial FLAIR (a–d) demonstrates abnormal increased T_2 signal within the posterior frontal cortex, medial thalami, periaqueductal gray matter, and floor of the fourth ventricle. Areas of true restricted diffusion (e,f) were confirmed by ADC maps (g). Patient became comatose, was unresponsive to medical management, and died. Postmortem examination demonstrated macrophage-rich infiltration of the periaqueductal brainstem, medial thalamus, hypothalamus, and mammillary bodies consistent with Wernicke's encephalopathy. Reproduced from Reference 2 with permission of Elsevier.

complications of pregnancy [101–103]. There are known potential teratogenic effects of a variety of anti-epileptic drugs (AEDs), with variations in classes of drugs and dosages influencing teratogenic potential [104–106]. Balancing the risks of various classes of AED therapy with those associated with uncontrolled seizures should be the primary management dilemma, rather than imaging.

There is little need to alter established seizure and epilepsy MRI protocols when considering a pregnant patient. Thin-section volumetric

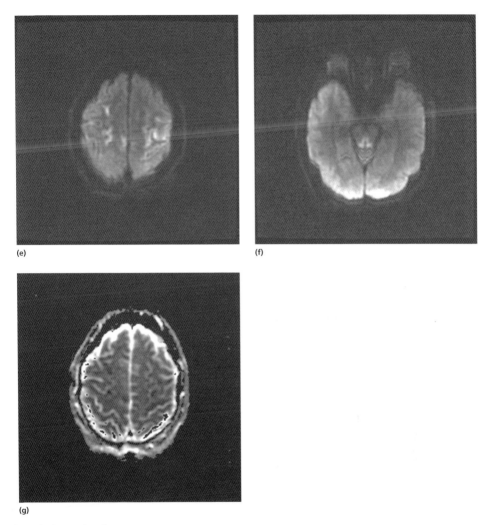

(e)

(f)

(g)

Figure 3.16 (*Continued*)

acquisition of T_1-weighted sequences allows for detailed evaluation of anatomy, cortical gyral patterns, and detection of heterotopic gray matter. T_2-weighted and FLAIR sequences may be used without modification for evaluation of hippocampal, mesial temporal, and other parenchymal signal abnormalities.

In established seizure patients, MRI evaluation, when required, is most frequently performed without contrast. While a primary seizure disorder could initially present during pregnancy, a host of other potential causes of seizure is often considered, for which contrast administration may be typically ordered. For the evaluation of meningitis, encephalitis, inflammatory parenchymal changes, metastatic disease, and underlying parenchymal lesions, for instance, contrast administration may be beneficial, though likely not essential. In addition, though diagnostic accuracy for venous thrombosis is improved with contrast-enhanced imaging, a host of non-contrast MR techniques exist

[82]. In fact, most conditions can be confidently excluded with non-contrast MR imaging. Only in a minority of cases, when making a definitive diagnosis proves troublesome, should contrast administration be considered, at which time the decision returns to a careful risk versus benefit analysis.

Focal neurological deficits
Cranial neuropathies

Many cranial neuropathies may be idiopathic and attributed to hormonal changes during pregnancy [107]. Other neuropathies may result from mass effect along their peripheral course or parenchymal abnormalities centrally. For example, meningiomas can arise along the intracranial dural reflections and are commonly seen at the orbital apex, parasellar regions, cerebellopontine angle cistern, and basilar cisterns. The trophic effect of pregnancy on meningiomas has been previously discussed (Figure 3.17). Direct impression on any of the cranial nerves due to accelerated growth could produce clinical symptoms and it would not be surprising to discover that a meningioma is the culprit for any presenting cranial neuropathy. Other common potential causes of distinct cranial neuropathies are listed further.

Contrast-enhanced MRI is generally preferred for the evaluation of cranial neuropathies, though thin-section CT may be an acceptable substitute in select cases.

Cranial nerve II—optic nerve

When considering the pregnant or puerperal patient that presents with a visual complaint, the practitioner must consider all components of the visual pathway. Ischemic or hemorrhagic stroke, venous infarctions associated with dural sinus thrombosis, PRES, or PCA could all cause visual impairment or blindness due to involvement of the visual cortex or portions of the optic tracts. Though the elevated estrogen and immunosuppressive state of pregnancy have been associated with a decrease in relapse rate in multiple sclerosis, demyelination could still be considered [108–110]. Rebound relapses of demyelination could be considered in the postpartum patient, with involvement possibly occurring along the optic tracts or the optic nerve, presenting as an acute optic neuritis [111]. Neuromyelitis optica has also been shown to be influenced by pregnancy with increased rate of relapses following delivery [112, 113]. Generally, MRI is the preferred imaging modality, though CT may be performed in especially acute presentations.

Pituitary adenomas, meningiomas, and other sellar or supra-sellar masses can cause compressive symptoms on the optic chiasm, prechiasmatic optic nerves, and proximal optic tracts, causing distinct visual field defects (Figure 3.17). Benign physiologic pituitary enlargement may also occasionally cause chiasmal compression. Acute visual changes could relate to rapid pituitary enlargement in the cases of apoplexy while embolic phenomena can occur in the setting of carotid dissection or cardiac abnormalities such as atrial fibrillation.

Cranial nerves III, IV, V, and VI

Anatomically, cranial nerve III originates anteriorly from the midbrain, IV from the dorsal midbrain and courses anteriorly, V from the anterolateral pons, and VI from the anterior pontomedullary junction, and all may be affected by lesions in these regions. For example, extraaxial masses such as nerve sheath tumors may exert increasing mass effect during pregnancy and come to clinical attention (Figure 3.18).

Cranial nerves III, IV, V2, and V3 course along the lateral aspect of the cavernous sinus, variably occurring within the sinus or between layers of dura. The abducens nerve, the most medial of these structures, is closely related to the cavernous carotid artery (Figure 3.19). Given the course of these cranial nerves, they are subject to possible compression by enlarging pituitary adenomas or in pituitary apoplexy during pregnancy. Additional sellar and suprasellar masses, such as meningiomas and even hemangiomas, may be effected by hormonal and hemodynamic changes of pregnancy and exert

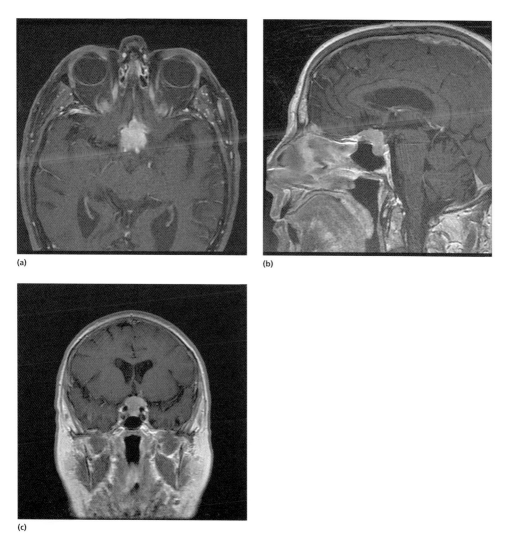

(a)

(b)

(c)

Figure 3.17 76 y/o female with 6 months of blurry vision, bilateral temporal hemianopsia. Axial (a), sagittal (b), and coronal (c) post-contrast T_1 MR images demonstrate a homogenously enhancing supra-sellar meningioma exerting upward mass effect upon the optic chiasm. Reproduced from Reference 2 with permission of Elsevier.

variable mass affect upon these cranial nerves (Figure 3.20).

Idiopathic oculomotor nerve palsies have been reported during pregnancy and have been attributed to hormonal changes, often resolving postpartum [107]. Transient palsies of the trigeminal nerves have also been reported following spinal–epidural anesthesia. Abducens nerve palsies have been reported as a presenting symptom of preeclampsia, as well as following spinal/epidural anesthesia with subsequent development of low intracranial pressure [114,115]. Magnetic resonance imaging may be performed in the evaluation of these disorders,

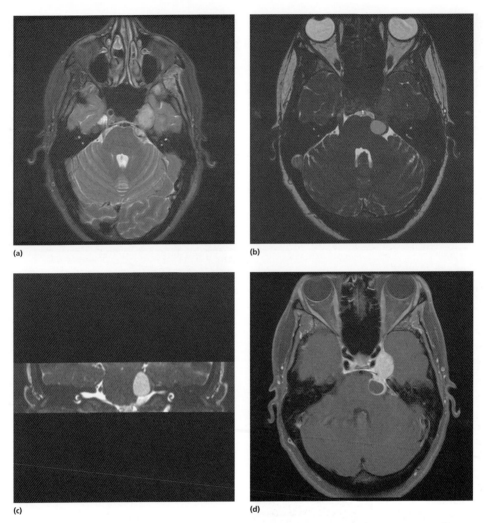

(a)

(b)

(c)

(d)

Figure 3.18 38 y/o female with left facial numbness, facial droop, and jaw pain. Axial T_2 MR (a), as well as 3D thin-slice gradient echo (b,c) demonstrates a part solid, part cystic mass along the expected course of the left trigeminal nerve, expanding Meckel's cave; post-contrast axial (d) and coronal (e) T_1 MR images demonstrate homogenous enhancement of the soft tissue component, again filling Meckel's cave, with lack of enhancement within the cystic portion. Biopsy confirmed a trigeminal schwannoma. Reproduced from Reference 2 with permission of Elsevier.

potentially detecting signs of decreased intracranial pressure (Figure 3.30) [116].

Imaging plays a crucial role in evaluating some of the more serious causes of cranial nerve palsies, including pituitary apoplexy and intracranial aneurysms. Non-contrast MRA may accompany a brain MRI as part of the clinical evaluation. Likewise, CTA sensitivity allows for rapid and reproducible evaluation of symptomatic patients [75–77]. Catheter angiography remains the gold standard in excluding a possible intracranial aneurysm, especially

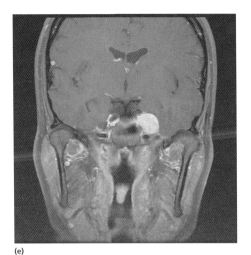

(e)

Figure 3.18 (*Continued*)

considering the high rate of mortality associated with an untreated ruptured aneurysm.

Cranial nerves VII and VIII

Bell's palsy, or paralysis of the facial nerve, is often idiopathic with sudden, rapid onset and is often self-limited [117]. Bell's palsy has

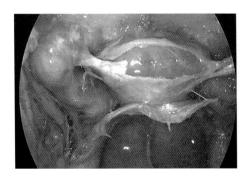

Figure 3.19 Photograph from an endonasal trans-sphenoid sellar dissection (Image courtesy Dr. Juan Fernandez-Miranda MD) demonstrating an opening in the dural reflections covering the pituitary gland, the adjacent cavernous carotid, the abducens nerve laterally, and the lateral-most aspect of the cavernous sinus containing cranial nerves III, IV, V2, and V3. Reproduced from Reference 2 with permission of Elsevier.

been reported extensively in pregnant patients, though the exact prevalence remains uncertain [118–120]. Typical Bell's palsy requires no imaging evaluation though imaging may be obtained in atypical cases. There is little indication for CT; the usual MRI findings include abnormal enhancement of the facial nerve within the internal auditory canal and at the labyrinthine segment of the facial nerve, and prominent asymmetric enhancement at the geniculate ganglion and the tympanic portions of the facial nerve (Figure 3.21). Other than the typical idiopathic palsy, important differential considerations for an abnormally enhancing facial nerve include Lyme disease, leptomeningeal disease, and retrograde perineural spread of parotid neoplasms. The imaging diagnosis essentially relies on the administration of contrast. In the pregnant patient, benefits of contrast administration may be outweighed by the potential risks for what is usually a self-limited condition.

Cranial nerves VII and VIII also may be subject to compressive effects of meningiomas and vestibular schwannomas, enlargement of which is reported during pregnancy (Figure 3.22) [8, 9].

Cranial nerves IX, X, XI, and XII

Similar to cranial nerves VII and VIII, cranial nerves IX, X, and XI may be affected by meningiomas or schwannomas as they course from the brainstem to the jugular foramen. Although more commonly associated with jugular foramen tumors, cranial neuropathies of IX and XI (Vernet's syndrome) have been reported in association with venous thrombosis at the jugular foramen [121]. Hypoglossal cranial nerve palsies may accompany meningioma enlargement though have also been reported in association with preeclampsia [122].

Pituitary tumors

When considering cranial neuropathies of II, III, IV, V, and VI, tumors of the pituitary gland, micro- (<10 mm) and macroadenomas (>10

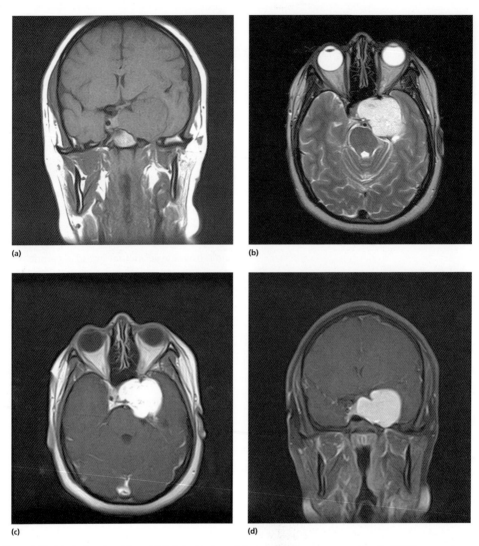

(a)

(b)

(c)

(d)

Figure 3.20 21 y/o female with multiple left-sided cranial neuropathies, most prominently CN III, worsening during pregnancy. Coronal T_1 MR (a) demonstrates a hypointense, well-defined, lobulated extra-axial supra-cellar mass. Axial T_2 MR (b) confirms a hyperintense supra-sellar extra-axial mass that is fairly homogenous in signal, though exerts region mass effect upon the pons and left cavernous sinus structures; post-contrast axial (c) and coronal (d) T_1 MR imaging demonstrates robust homogenous enhancement. Subsequent biopsy revealed a cavernous hemangioma. Reproduced from Reference 2 with permission of Elsevier.

mm), must be considered. When slow growing, medical therapy is an option, though surgical resection or debulking may be required in patients presenting with visual field abnormalities or symptoms relating to direct invasion of adjacent structures. Chiasmal compression, local invasion, and significant enlargement were found during pregnancy in up to 20% of pregnant patients with macroadenomas in one series (Figure 3.23). Microadenomas more frequently

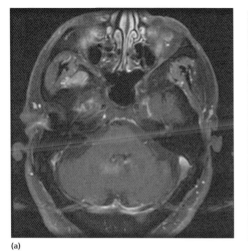 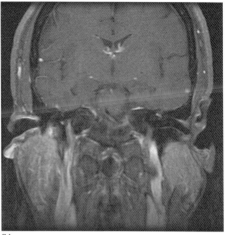

(a) (b)

Figure 3.21 Bell's palsy confirmed by contrast-enhanced T_1 MR with axial (a) and coronal (b) images demonstrate abnormal, asymmetric enhancement involving the labyrinthine facial nerve segment and geniculate ganglion. Reproduced from Reference 2 with permission of Elsevier.

have a benign course with up to 5% of pregnant patients reporting increases in headaches during pregnancy and only 1% presenting with visual fields deficits [123].

Other mass lesions of the parasellar region such as arachnoid cysts, Rathke's cleft cysts, and craniopharyngiomas may present during pregnancy. There are numerous reports on the puerperal presentation of craniopharyngiomas, often with visual symptoms due to chiasmal compression [124–128]. Hemodynamic changes of pregnancy can also lead to the presentation of vascular abnormalities, such as cavernous hemangiomas, including those involving the cavernous sinus as seen in Figure 3.16.

Lymphocytic hypophysitis

Lymphocytic hypophysitis is an immune-mediated condition that most commonly occurs in women late in pregnancy or during the peripartum period and may require biopsy for diagnosis. Lymphocytic infiltration of the adenohypophysis, neurohypophysis, and infundibular stalk causes abnormal enlargement, corresponding to the usual MRI findings (Figure 3.24). If the sella and lower infundibular stalk are primarily involved, there may be considerable overlap in the potential MRI appearance with that of a pituitary adenoma [129, 130]. Imaging features are based on evaluation of the pituitary stalk and usually require contrast administration for improved visualization.

Pituitary apoplexy/Sheehan's syndrome

Sheehan's syndrome describes the acute onset of pituitary hypothalamic dysfunction related to pituitary infarct and subsequent necrosis [6]. Maternal hypotension related to obstetric hemorrhage at or around the time of delivery, or any cause of hypotension or shock, may be a precipitating factor. Magnetic resonance evaluation at the time of the ischemic event demonstrates an enlarged pituitary gland without evidence of blood products. Over time, involution of the gland occurs and the sella may eventually exhibit a partially or completely "empty" appearance (Figure 3.25). Rarely, Sheehan's syndrome may present in a more chronic fashion during the postpartum period.

Pituitary apoplexy is characterized by an acute hemorrhagic infarction of the pituitary gland,

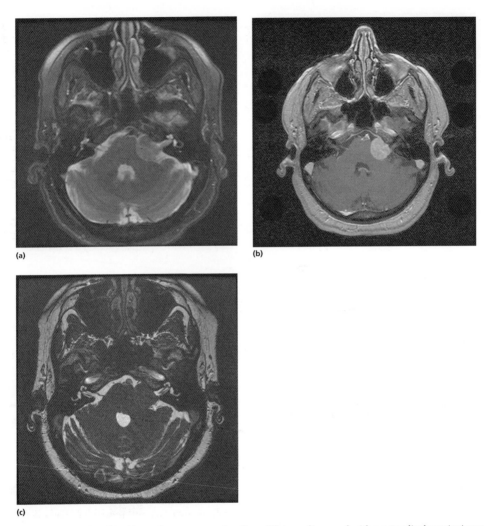

(a)

(b)

(c)

Figure 3.22 50 y/o female with persistent, progressive disequilibrium, diagnosed with a petroclival meningioma. Axial T_2 MR image through the level of the internal auditory canal (a) demonstrates a lobulated extra-axial cerebellopontine angle mass compressing the pons; contrast-enhanced T_1 MR image at the same level (b) demonstrates a homogenously enhancing mass with dural tail, a typical finding of meningioma; 3D gradient echo image (c) demonstrates the masses' proximity to the abducens nerve as well as the facial and vestibulocochlear nerve complex. Reproduced from Reference 2 with permission of Elsevier.

often into or involving an underlying adenoma (Figure 3.26) [6, 123]. Pituitary hemorrhage and rapid enlargement are associated with severe headache, nausea, vomiting, visual changes relating to upward mass effect on the optic chiasm and other cranial neuropathies. A non-contrast head CT will often be obtained

initially due to the acuity of clinical presentation, potentially demonstrating hemorrhage within an enlarged pituitary (Figure 3.27). If the clinical presentation suggests apoplexy, it is important to proceed with MRI despite a seemingly normal head CT. Contrast administration can be deferred as thin section evaluation will

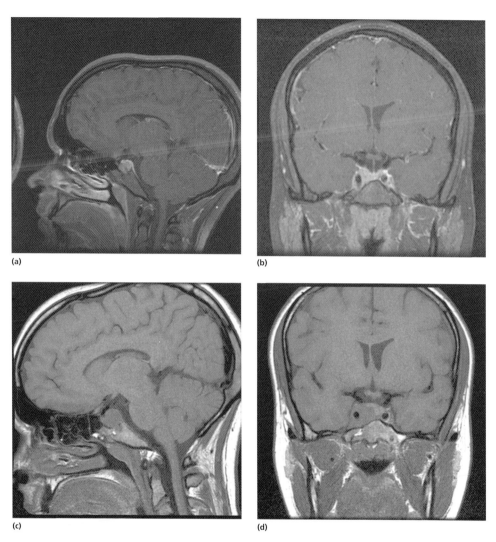

(a)

(b)

(c)

(d)

Figure 3.23 23 y/o with known prolactinoma, 25 weeks pregnant, presenting with persistent headaches and new left visual field disturbance. Magnetic resonance examination 10 months prior with post-contrast T_1 sagittal (a) and coronal (b) imaging demonstrates a lobulated, slightly hypo-enhancing and heterogeneous intra-pituitary lesion with partial encasement of the right cavernous carotid. Non-contrast imaging performed during pregnancy with sagittal (c) and coronal (d) T_1 MR images demonstrate marked enlargement of the sellar mass with circumferential encasement of the cavernous carotid. A 2-year postpartum MRI demonstrates marked size reduction of the pituitary lesion with less regional mass effect (e,f). Reproduced from Reference 2 with permission of Elsevier.

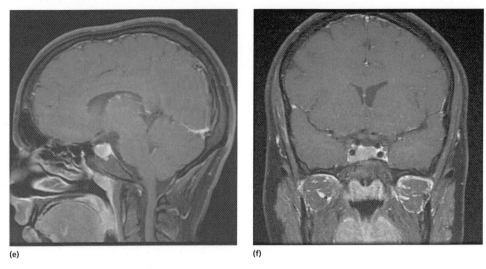

(e)   (f)

Figure 3.23 (*Continued*)

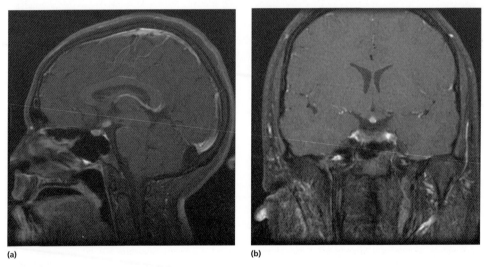

(a)   (b)

Figure 3.24 27 y/o female with diabetes insipidus and hypothyroidism. Contrast-enhanced sagittal (a) and coronal (b) T_1-weight images demonstrate abnormal enlargement and enhancement of the infundibulum and hypothalamus. Infectious causes were excluded and lumbar puncture was only significant for elevated protein. A presumptive diagnosis of hypophysitis was made and the patient improved with steroid therapy. Reproduced from Reference 2 with permission of Elsevier.

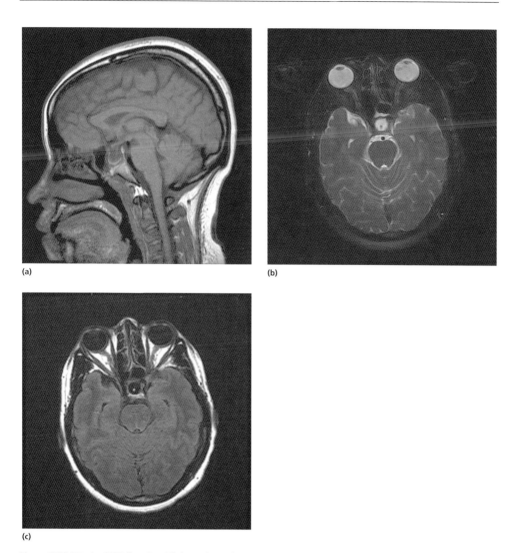

(a)

(b)

(c)

Figure 3.25 35 y/o G2P0 female with hypothyroidism, 31 weeks pregnant, presenting with worsening dizziness. Sagittal T_1 MR (a) demonstrates an empty or partially empty sella; in a 31-week pregnant female one would expect physiologic hypertrophy; T_2 (b) and FLAIR MR images (c) also demonstrate an empty sella with a "central dot" representing the non-displaced pituitary infundibulum. Imaging findings are consistent with the clinical diagnosis of Sheehan's. Reproduced from Reference 2 with permission of Elsevier.

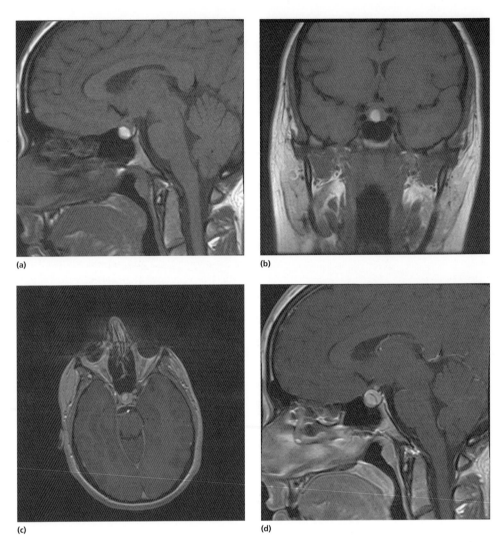

(a)

(b)

(c)

(d)

Figure 3.26 22 y/o female with history of infrequent and irregular menses and "pituitary tumor" presented to outside facility with headache, subsequently transferred for surgical management. Final pathology revealed a hemorrhagic adenoma. Sagittal (a) and coronal (b) non-contrast T_1 MR images demonstrate an intrinsically T_1 hyperintense lesion within the pituitary, consistent with acute blood products; post-contrast T_1 imaging (c–e) demonstrates appropriately enhancing pituitary parenchymal with a hypo-enhancing rim surrounding the region of hemorrhage presumably relate to the underlying adenoma. Reproduced from Reference 2 with permission of Elsevier.

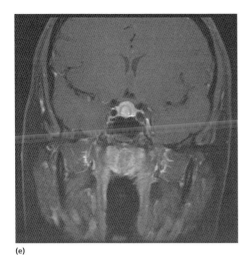

(e)

Figure 3.26 (*Continued*)

reveal sellar blood products and the mass effect due to gland enlargement. Rarely a fluid–fluid level may be seen (Figure 3.28).

Neoplasm: gestational trophoblastic disease

Choriocarcinoma is a malignant, aggressive, and highly vascular type of gestational trophoblastic disease. Rates of incidence vary and are generally 200 or less per 100,000 pregnancies [131]. Beyond local pelvic disease, brain, spinal, hepatic, and pulmonary metastases occur. Given the degree of vascularity, brain metastases may appear similar to other hypervascular metastatic lesions [132, 133]. A head CT may reveal parenchymal hyperdense lesions with surrounding edema or even areas of acute hemorrhage. Magnetic resonance imaging is more sensitive for the number and distribution of these parenchymal lesions, often with associated blood products demonstrating variable signal characteristics; often the degree of apparent enhancement may be quite subtle, in part masked by the increased intrinsic T_1 signal associated with blood products. Similar to the evaluation for other hemorrhagic metastases, blood product-sensitive sequences

may reveal tiny foci of disease that are relatively occult on other sequences due to their small size.

Back pain and cauda equina
Primary spinal pathology

Underlying causes of back pain during pregnancy range from benign conditions such as ligamentous laxity and uterine compression of the lumbosacral plexus to more serious conditions [134, 135]. Acute intervertebral disc herniation is reported to occur in approximately 1 in 10,000 pregnancies, with progression to cauda equina syndrome being rare [136, 137]. Tumors of the spinal canal and osseous vertebral column may also present with pain or a progressive neurologic syndrome. For instance, meningiomas, hemangiomas, and giant cell tumors are all reported during pregnancy as a cause of pain or neurologic impairment [138–140]. Spinal metastases related to gestational trophoblastic disease are also reported as a cause of progressive neurologic deficit [132]. Epidural hematomas may occur associated with pregnancy, spontaneously or related to spinal and/or epidural anesthesia [72, 141]. Likewise, epidural abscess formation may present spontaneously or related to instrumentation. Clinicians may also encounter pregnant, post-traumatic patients in which back pain or neurologic deficits are a finding.

In most cases, MRI should be the preferred method of evaluation, given the lack of ionizing radiation. As with the nonpregnant population, MR is the preferred method for evaluating any progressive neurologic syndrome. Though many etiologies may be excluded with non-contrast techniques, gadolinium-enhanced images may be required if inflammatory or demyelinating etiologies are suspected (Figure 3.29). While MRI may be used to assess bone marrow edema, significant back pain or neurological symptoms related to blunt trauma should still be evaluated with CT as the preferred modality for the detection of acute fracture.

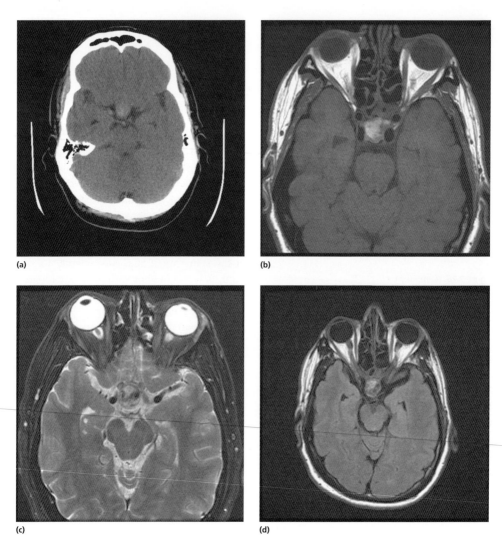

(a)   (b)

(c)   (d)

Figure 3.27 57 y/o male with 6 days of severe headache and third cranial nerve palsy. Axial non-enhanced CT (a) demonstrates hyperattenuating sellar soft tissue consistent with acute blood products. Axial pre-contrast T_1 (b), T_2 (c), and FLAIR (d) MR images demonstrate mixed-signal sellar material; axial susceptibility-weighted gradient echo image (e) demonstrates sellar blooming artifact; constellation of findings consistent with acute blood products. Post-contrast sagittal (f) and coronal (g) T_1 MR images demonstrate marked pituitary enlargement with heterogeneous enhancement; note mass effect upon the optic chiasm. Reproduced from Reference 2 with permission of Elsevier.

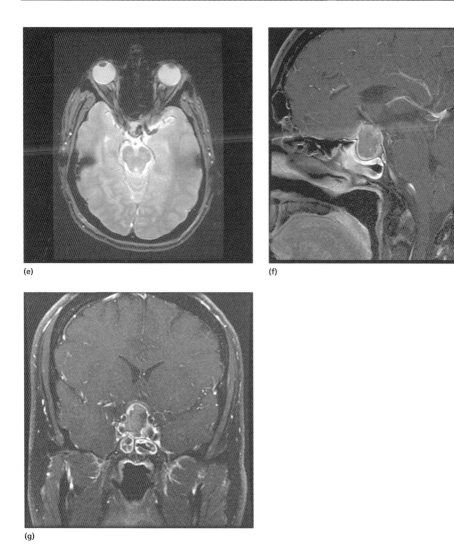

(e)

(f)

(g)

Figure 3.27 (*Continued*)

Following any imaging study in the patient with a progressive neurologic deficit, the key is correctly identifying the anatomic compartment involved by any abnormality noted, whether that is osseous, paraspinal, epidural, subdural, subarachnoid, or intramedullary. Appropriate anatomic localization is the first and usually most important step in arriving at a diagnosis for any imaging study, aiding in the rapid initiation of appropriate management.

Intracranial hypotension

Dural cerebrospinal fluid (CSF) leaks resulting in intracranial hypotension may occur following any dural puncture such as lumbar puncture, spinal surgery, spinal anesthesia, or related to epidural anesthesia with inadvertent dural puncture [142, 143]. Positional headaches relieved in the recumbent position are common, though symptoms and history may be varied, often causing difficulties in diagnosis

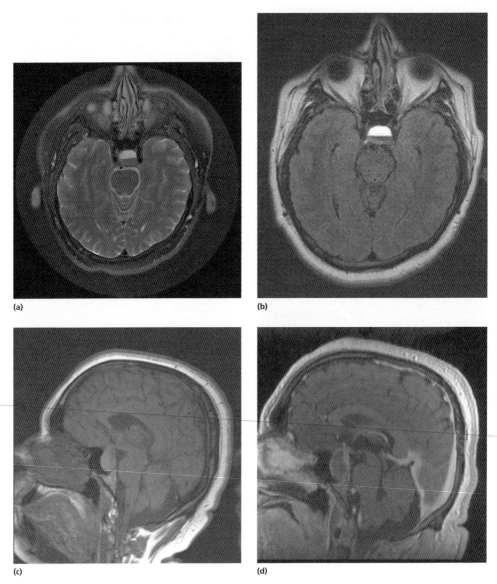

(a)

(b)

(c)

(d)

Figure 3.28 30 y/o male with "pituitary tumor" presenting with severe headaches. Axial T_2 (a) and FLAIR (b) MR images through the sella demonstrate a fluid–fluid level within the sella with T_2 hyperintense fluid layering non-dependently, consistent with acute hemorrhage; sagittal pre- (c) and post-contrast (d) T_1 MR images demonstrate intrinsically T_1-hyperintense non-dependent hemorrhagic fluid; note a normally enhancing pituitary gland displaced posteriorly. Reproduced from Reference 2 with permission of Elsevier.

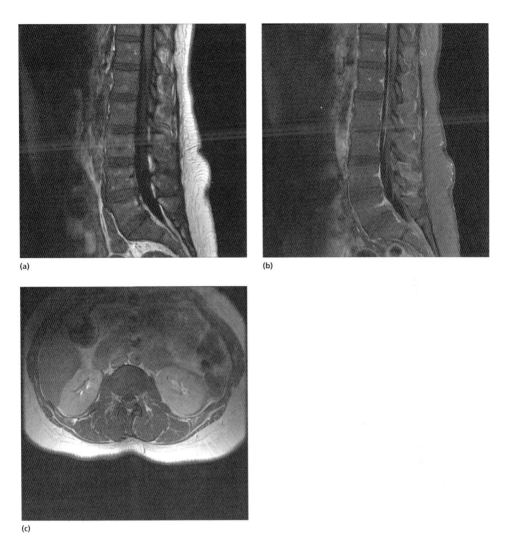

(a)

(b)

(c)

Figure 3.29 50 y/o female with migraines and progressive lower extremity weakness. Non-contrast sagittal (a) and contrast-enhanced sagittal (b) and axial (c) T_1 MR images demonstrate abnormal nerve root enhancement consistent with Guillain–Barre syndrome. Reproduced from Reference 2 with permission of Elsevier.

[144]. Radiologic findings are similarly varied, however, may include diffuse pachymeningeal enhancement, sagging of the brain, low-lying cerebellar tonsils, and thin, symmetric subdural collections (Figure 3.30) [116]. The cranial neuropathies reported in association with intracranial hypotension generally have no distinct imaging feature, rather are a clinical finding seen in the setting of the other imaging findings.

Conclusion

Diagnostic imaging will frequently be employed in the evaluation of the pregnant patient presenting with a neurologic sign or symptom. The underlying etiology may be benign and self-limited, a pathologic condition associated with pregnancy or a preexisting condition influenced by the various changes of pregnancy. We have

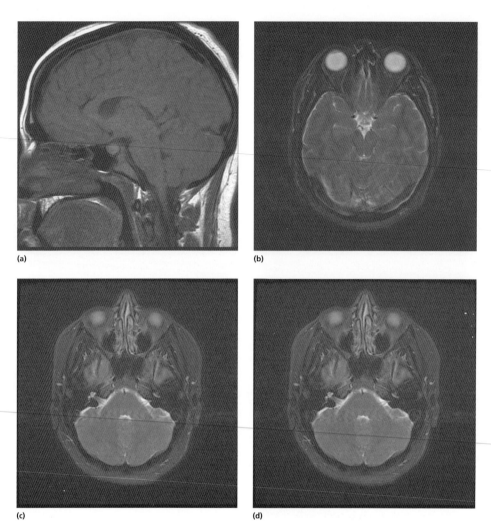

Figure 3.30 30 y/o female, 5 days postpartum, with persistent, severe headaches. Sagittal T_1 MR image (a) demonstrates subtle settling of the posterior fossa structures; axial T_2 images through the basal cisterns demonstrate effacement and crowding (b,c); axial T_2 (d) demonstrates thin, bi-hemispheric extra-axial CSF-equivalent collections; axial (e) and coronal (f) post-contrast T_1 MR images demonstrate smooth pachymeningeal enhancement. Constellation of findings are consistent with intracranial hypotension. Reproduced from Reference 2 with permission of Elsevier.

reviewed common strategies in selecting the most appropriate imaging studies in the evaluation of some common pregnancy-related conditions. Though a risk–benefit analysis involving radiation and intravenous contrast is prudent, these concerns should not hinder the execution of critical imaging examinations as the health of the mother is the single most important factor influencing the health of the fetus. With careful consideration, a variety of imaging modalities may be used safely, without sacrificing diagnostic power, allowing for prompt recognition of pathologic conditions and initiation of appropriate therapy.

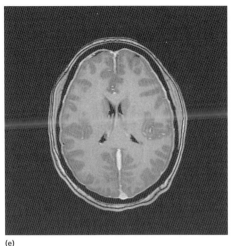

(e)

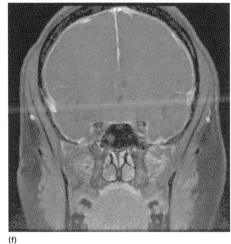

(f)

Figure 3.30 (*Continued*)

References

1 Hosley CM, McCullough LD. Acute neurological issues in pregnancy and the peripartum. *The Neurohospitalist.* 2011;1(2)104–116.

2 Delfyett WT, Fetzer DT. Imaging of neurologic conditions during pregnancy and the perinatal period. *Neurol Clin.* 2012;30(3):791–822.

3 Royek AB, Parisi VM. Maternal biological adaptations to pregnancy. In: HJ Reece EA, ed. *Medicine of the Fetus and Mother.* Philadelphia, PA: Lippincott-Raven, 1999; pp. 903–920.

4 Bentson J, Reza M, Winter J, Wilson G. Steroids and apparent cerebral atrophy on computed tomography scans. *J Comput Assist Tomogr.* 1978;2(1):16–23.

5 Oatridge A, Holdcroft A, Saeed N, et al. Change in brain size during and after pregnancy: study in healthy women and women with preeclampsia. *Am J Neuroradiol.* 2002;23(1):19–26.

6 Foyouzi N, Frisbaek Y, Norwitz ER. Pituitary gland and pregnancy. *Obstet Gynecol Clin North Am.* 2004;31(4):873–892, xi.

7 Karaca Z, Tanriverdi F, Unluhizarci K, Kelestimur F. Pregnancy and pituitary disorders. *Eur J Endocrinol.* 2010;162(3):453–475. doi: 10.1530/EJE-09-0923.

8 Dineen R, Banks A, Lenthall R. Imaging of acute neurological conditions in pregnancy and the puerpuerium. *Clin Radiol.* 2005;60(11):1156–1170.

9 Zak IT, Dulai HS, Kish KK. Imaging of neurologic disorders associated with pregnancy and postpartum period. *RadioGraphics.* 2007;27(1):95–108.

10 Claus EB, Park PJ, Carroll R, Chan J, Black PM. Specific genes expressed in association with progesterone receptors in meningioma. *Cancer Res.* 2008;68(1):314–322.

11 Krayenbühl N, Pravdenkova S, Al-Mefty O. De novo versus transformed atypical and anaplastic meningiomas: comparisons of clinical course, cytogenetics, cytokinetics, and outcome. *Neurosurgery.* 2007;61(3):495–503.

12 Pravdenkova S, Al-Mefty O, Sawyer J, Husain M. Progesterone and estrogen receptors: opposing prognostic indicators in meningiomas. *J Neurosurg.* 2006;105(2):163–173.

13 Leães CG, Meurer RT, Coutinho LB, Ferreira NP, Pereira-Lima JF, da Costa Oliveira M. Immunohistochemical expression of aromatase and estrogen, androgen and progesterone receptors in normal and neoplastic human meningeal cells. *Neuropathology.* 2010;30(1):44–49.

14 Patel AK, Alexander TH, Andalibi A, Ryan AF, Doherty JK. Vestibular schwannoma quantitative polymerase chain reaction expression of estrogen and progesterone receptors. *Laryngoscope.* 2008;118(8):1458–1463.

15 Vadivelu S, Sharer L, Schulder M. Regression of multiple intracranial meningiomas after cessation of long-term progesterone agonist therapy. *J Neurosurg.* 2010;112(5):920–924.

16 Brown CM, Ahmad ZK, Ryan AF, Doherty JK. Estrogen receptor expression in sporadic vestibular schwannomas. *Otol Neurotol.* 2011;32(1):158–162.

17 Jaiswal S, Agrawal V, Jaiswal AK, Pandey R, Mahapatra AK. Expression of estrogen and progesterone receptors in vestibular schwannomas and their clinical significance. *J Negat Results Biomed.* 2009;8:9.

18 Dalgorf DM, Rowsell C, Bilbao JM, Chen JM. Immunohistochemical investigation of hormone receptors and vascular endothelial growth factor concentration in vestibular schwannoma. *Skull Base.* 2008;18(6):377–384.

19 Beatty CW, Scheithauer BW, Katzmann JA, Roche PC, Kjeldahl KS, Ebersold MJ. Acoustic schwannoma and pregnancy: a DNA flow cytometric, steroid hormone receptor, and proliferation marker study. *Laryngoscope.* 1995;105(7 Pt 1):693–700.

20 Comeglio P, Fedi S, Liotta AA, et al. Blood clotting activation during normal pregnancy. *Thromb Res.* 1996;84(3):199–202.

21 Kotsenas AL, Roth TC, Hershey BL, Yi JK. Imaging neurologic complications of pregnancy and the puerperium. *Acad Radiol.* 1999;6(4):243–252.

22 Salonen Ros H, Lichtenstein P, Bellocco R, Petersson G, Cnattingius S. Increased risks of circulatory diseases in late pregnancy and puerperium. *Epidemiology.* 2001;12(4):456–460.

23 Bateman BT, Olbrecht VA, Berman MF, Minehart RD, Schwamm LH, Leffert LR. Peripartum subarachnoid hemorrhage: nationwide data and institutional experience. *Anesthesiology.* 2012;116(2):324–333.

24 Tiel Groenestege AT, Rinkel GJ, van der Bom JG, Algra A, Klijn CJ. The risk of aneurysmal subarachnoid hemorrhage during pregnancy, delivery, and the puerperium in the Utrecht population: case-crossover study and standardized incidence ratio estimation. *Stroke.* 2009;40(4):1148–1151.

25 AmericanPregnancy.org. (n.d.). Retrieved March 5, 2012. Available from http://www.americanpregnancy.org/main/statistics.html.

26 American College of Radiology. ACR Guidelines and Technical Standards. *ACR Practice Guideline for Imaging Pregnant or Potentially Pregnant Adolescents and Women with Ionizing Radiation.* Reston, VA: American College of Radiology, 2008.

27 American College of Obstetricians and Gynecologists. Committee on Obstetric Practice. *Guidelines for Diagnostic Imaging During Pregnancy.* Washington, DC: American College of Obstetricians and Gynecologists, 2004, reaffirmed 2009.

28 Webb JA, Thomsen HS, Morcos SK; Members of Contrast Media Safety Committee of European Society of Urogenital Radiology (ESUR). The use of iodinated and gadolinium contrast media during pregnancy and lactation. *Eur Radiol.* 2005;15(6):1234–1240.

29 Wang PI, Chong ST, Kielar AZ, Kelly AM, Knoepp UD, Mazza MB, Goodsitt MM. Imaging of pregnant and lactating patients: part 1, evidence-based review and recommendations. *AJR Am J Roentgenol.* 2012;198(4):778–784.

30 Cohnen M, Wittsack HJ, Assadi S, et al. Radiation exposure of patients in comprehensive computed tomography of the head in acute stroke. *AJNR Am J Neuroradiol.* 2006;27(8):1741–1745.

31 Imanishi Y, Fukui A, Niimi H, et al. Radiation-induced temporary hair loss as a radiation damage only occurring in patients who had the combination of MDCT and DSA. *Eur Radiol.* 2005;15(1):41–46.

32 Wagner BM. Genetics and the atomic bombs. *Hum Pathol.* 1985;16(2):101–102.

33 Wieseler KM, Bhargava P, Kanal KM, Vaidya S, Stewart BK, Dighe MK. Imaging in pregnant patients: examination appropriateness. *RadioGraphics.* 2010;30(5):1215–1229.

34 Goldberg-Stein SA, Liu B, Hahn PF, Lee SI. Radiation dose management: part 2, estimating fetal radiation risk from CT during pregnancy. *Am J Roentgenol.* 2012;198(4):W352–6. doi: 10.2214/AJR.11.7458.

35 Swartz HM, Reichling BA. Hazards of radiation exposure for pregnant women. *JAMA.* 1978;239(18):1907–1908.

36 Mole RH. Childhood cancer after prenatal exposure to diagnostic X-ray examinations in Britain. *Br J Cancer.* 1990;62:152–168.

37 Wakeford R, Little MP. Risk coefficients for childhood cancer after intrauterine irradiation. *Int J Radiat Biol.* 2003;79(5):293–309.

38 Wakeford R. Childhood leukaemia following medical diagnostic exposure to ionizing radiation in utero or after birth. *Radiat Prot Dosimetry.* 2008;132(2):166–174.

39 Little MP. Leukaemia following childhood radiation exposure in the Japanese atomic bomb survivors and in medically exposed groups. *Radiat Prot Dosimetry.* 2008;132(2):156–165. doi: 10.1093/rpd/ncn264.

40 Preston   DL, Cullings H, Suyama A, et al. Solid cancer incidence in atomic bomb survivors exposed in utero or as young children. *J Natl Cancer Inst.* 2008;100(6):428–436. doi: 10.1093/jnci/djn045.

41 Preston DL, Shimizu Y, Pierce DA, Suyama A, Mabuchi K. Studies of mortality of atomic bomb survivors. Report 13: Solid cancer and non-cancer disease mortality: 1950-1997. *Radiat Res.* 2003;160(4):381–407.

42 Preston DL, Ron E, Tokuoka S, et al. Solid cancer incidence in atomic bomb survivors: 1958-1998. *Radiat Res.* 2007;168(1):1–64.

43 Valentin J. Avoidance of radiation injuries from medical interventional procedures. *Ann ICRP.* 2000;30(2):7–67.

44 Stewart A, Kneale GW. Radiation dose effects in relation to obstetric x-rays and childhood cancers. *The Lancet.* 1970;295(7658):1185–1188.

45 Berlin L. Radiation exposure and the pregnant patient. *Am J Roentgenol.* 1996;167(6):1377–1379.

46 McCollough CH, Schueler Beth A, Atwell Thomas D, et al. Radiation exposure and pregnancy: when should we be concerned? *Radiographics.* 2007;27:909–918.

47 Van Unnik JG, Broerse JJ, Geleijns J, Jansen JT, Zoetelief J, Zweers D. Survey of CT techniques and absorbed dose in various Dutch hospitals. *Br J Radiol.* 1997;70(832):367–371.

48 Huda W, Randazzo W, Tipnis S, Frey GD, Mah E. Embryo dose estimates in body CT. *Am J Roentgenol.* 2010;194(4):874–880. doi: 10.2214/AJR.09.4032.

49 Shetty MK. Abdominal computed tomography during pregnancy: a review of indications and fetal radiation exposure issues. *Semin Ultrasound CT MR.* 2010;31(1):3–7. doi: 10.1053/j.sult.2009.09.001..

50 Hurwitz LM, Yoshizumi T, Reiman RE, et al. Radiation dose to the fetus from body MDCT during early gestation. *Am J Roentgenol.* 2006;186(3):871–876.

51 Damilakis J, Perisinakis K, Voloudaki A, Gourtsoyiannis N. Estimation of fetal radiation dose from computed tomography scanning in late pregnancy. *Invest Radiol.* 2000;35(9):527–533.

52 Angel E, Wellnitz CV, Goodsitt MM, et al. Radiation dose to the fetus for pregnant patients undergoing multidetector CT imaging: Monte Carlo simulations estimating fetal dose for a range of gestational age and patient size. *Radiology.* 2008;249(1):220–227. doi: 10.1148/radiol.2491071665.

53 McCollough CH, Bruesewitz MR, Kofler JM Jr. CT dose reduction and dose management tools: overview of available options. *Radiographics.* 2006;26(2):503–512.

54 Kaza RK, Platt JF, Al-Hawary MM, Wasnik A, Liu PS, Pandya A. CT enterography at 80 kVp with adaptive statistical iterative reconstruction versus at 120 kVp with standard reconstruction: image quality, diagnostic adequacy and dose reduction. *Am J Roentgenol.* 2012;198(5):1084–1092. doi: 10.2214/AJR.11.6597.

55 Desai GS, Uppot RN, Yu EW, Kambadakone AR, Sahani DV. Impact of iterative reconstruction on image quality and radiation dose in multidetector CT of large body size adults. *Eur Radiol.* 2012;22(8):1631–1640. doi: 10.1007/s00330-012-2424-3.

56 Singh   S, Kalra   MK, Shenoy-Bhangle AS, et al. Radiation dose reduction with hybrid iterative reconstruction for pediatric CT. *Radiology.* 2012;263(2):537–546. doi: 10.1148/radiol.12110268.

57 Lazarus E, Debenedectis C, North D, Spencer PK, Mayo-Smith WW. Utilization of imaging in pregnant patients: 10 year review of 5270 examinations in 3285 patients - 1997–2006. *Radiology.* 2009;251(2):517–524. doi: 10.1148/radiol.2512080736.

58 Helmrot E, Pettersson H, Sandborg M, Altén JN. Estimation of dose to the unborn child at diagnostic x-ray examinations based on data registered in RIS/PACS. *Eur Radiol.* 2007;17(1):205–209.

59 Kanal E, Barkovich AJ, Bell C, et al.; and the ACR Blue Ribbon Panel on MR Safety. ACR guidance document for safe MR practices 2007. *Am J Roentgenol.* 2007;188(6):1–27.

60 Grüters A, Krude H. Detection and Treatment of Congenital Hypothyroidism. *Nat. Rev. Endocrinol.* 2012;8:104–113.

61 American College of Radiology. *ACR Practice Guideline for the Use of Intravascular Contrast Media.* Reston, VA: American College of Radiology, 2007.

62 Marcus DA, Scharff L, Turk D. Longitudinal prospective study of headache during pregnancy and postpartum. *Headache.* 1999;39(9):625–632.

63 Marcus DA. Headache in pregnancy. *Curr Treat Options Neurol.* 2007;9(1):23–30.

64 Dixit A, Bhardwaj M, Sharma B. Headache in pregnancy: a nuisance or a new sense? *Obstet Gynecol Int.* 2012;2012:697697.

65 Lipton RB, Stewart WF, Scher AI. Epidemiology and economic impact of migraine. *Curr Med Res Opin.* 2001;17 Suppl 1:s4–s12.

66 Johannes CB, Linet MS, Stewart WF, Celentano DD, Lipton RB, Szklo M. Relationship of headache to phase of the menstrual cycle among young women: a daily diary study. *Neurology.* 1995;45(6):1076–1082.

67 Aube M. Migraine in Pregnancy. *Neurology.* 1999;53(4 suppl 1):S26–S28.

68 Sances G, Granella F, Nappi RE, et al. Course of migraine during pregnancy and postpartum: a prospective study. *Cephalalgia.* 2003;23(3):197–205.

69 Bartleson JD. When and how to investigate the patient with headache. *Semin Neurol.* 2006;26(2):163–170.

70 Detsky ME, McDonald DR, Baerlocher MO, Tomlinson GA, McCrory DC, Booth CM. Does this patient with headache have a migraine or need neuroimaging? *JAMA.* 2006;296(10):1274–1283.

71 De Luca GC, Bartleson JD. When and how to investigate the patient with headache. *Semin Neurol.* 2010;30:131–144.

72 Loo CC, Dahlgren G, Irestedt L. Neurological complications in obstetric regional anaesthesia. *Int J Obstet Anesth.* 2000;9(2):99–124.

73 Kriplani A, Relan S, Misra NK, Mehta VS, Takka D. Ruptured intracranial aneurysm complicating pregnancy. *Int J Gynaecol Obstet.* 1995;48(2):201–206.

74 Stoodley MA, Macdonald RL, Weir BK. Pregnancy and intracranial aneurysms. *Neurosurg Clin N Am.* 1998;9(3):549–556.

75 Kouskouras C, Charitanti A, Giavroglou C, et al. Intracranial aneurysms: evaluation using CTA and MRA. Correlation with DSA and intraoperative findings. *Neuroradiology.* 2004;46(10):842–850.

76 Villablanca JP, Rodriguez FJ, Stockman T, et al. MDCT angiography for detection and quantification of small intracranial arteries: comparison with conventional catheter angiography. *AJR Am J Roentgenol.* 2007;188(2):593–602.

77 Karamessini MT, Kagadis GC, Petsas T, et al. CT angiography with three-dimensional techniques for the early diagnosis of intracranial aneurysms. Comparison with intra-arterial DSA and the surgical findings. *Eur J Radiol.* 2004;49(3):212–223.

78 Shah AK. Non-aneurysmal primary subarachnoid hemorrhage in pregnancy-induced hypertension and eclampsia. *Neurology.* 2003;61(1):117–120.

79 Röther J, Waggie K, van Bruggen N, de Crespigny AJ, Moseley ME. Experimental cerebral venous thrombosis: evaluation using magnetic resonance imaging. *J Cereb Blood Flow Metab.* 1996;16(6):1353–1361.

80 Schaller B, Graf R, Sanada Y, et al. Hemodynamic changes after occlusion of the posterior superior sagittal sinus: and experimental PET study in cats. *Am J Neuroradiol.* 2003;24(9):1876–1880.

81 Yuh WT, Simonson TM, Wang AM, et al. Venous sinus occlusive disease: MR findings. *Am J Neuroradiol.* 1994;15(2):309–316.

82 Leach JL, Fortuna RB, Jones BV, Gaskill-Shipley MF. Imaging of cerebral venous thrombosis: current techniques, spectrum of findings, and diagnostic pitfalls. *RadioGraphics.* 2006;26:S19–S41.

83 Wetzel SG, Kirsch E, Stock KW, Kolbe M, Kaim A, Radue EW. Cerebral veins: comparative study of CT venography in intraarterial digital subtraction angiography. *Am J Neuroradiol.* 1999;20(2):249–255.

84 Renowden S. Cerebral venous sinus thrombosis. *Eur Radiol.* 2004;14:215–226.

85 Linn J, Michl S, Katja B, et al. Cortical vein thrombosis; the diagnostic value of different imaging modalities. *Neuroradiology.* 2010;52(10):899–911. doi: 10.1007/s00234-010-0654-0.

86 Simonds GR, Trewit CL. Anatomy of the cerebral vasculature. *Neuroimaging Clin N Am.* 1994;4(4):691–706.

87 Favrole P, Guichard JP, Crassard I, Bousser MG, Chabriat H. Diffusion weighted imaging of intravascular clots in cerebral venous thrombosis. *Stroke.* 2004;35(1):99–103.

88 Selim M, Fink J, Linfante I, Kumar S, Schlaug G, Caplan LR. Diagnosis of cerebral venous thrombosis with echo-planar T2* weighted magnetic resonance imaging. *Arch Neurol.* 2002;59(6):1021–1026.

89 Isensee C, Reul J, Thron A. Magnetic resonance imaging of thrombosed dural sinuses. *Stroke.* 1994;25(1):29–34.

90 Chu K, Kang DW, Yoon BW, Roh JK. Diffusion weighted magnetic resonance in cerebral venous

thrombosis. *Arch Neurol.* 2001;58(10):1569–76.

91 Lövblad KO, Bassetti C, Schneider J, et al. Diffusion weighted MR in cerebral venous thrombosis. *Cerebrovasc Dis.* 2001;11(3):169–176.

92 Ayanzen RH, Bird CR, Keller PJ, McCully FJ, Theobald MR, Heiserman JE. Cerebral MR venography: normal anatomy and potential diagnostic pitfalls. *Am J Neuroradiol.* 2000;21(1):74–78.

93 Gao K, Jiang H, Zhai RY, Wang JF, Wei BJ, Huang Q. Three-dimensional gadolinium enhanced MR venography to evaluate central venous steno-occlusive disease in hemodialysis patients. *Clin Radiol.* 2012;67(6):560–563. doi: 10.1016/j.crad.2011.11.010.

94 Lövblad KO, Schneider J, Bassetti C, et al. Fast contrast enhanced MR whole-brain venography. *Neuroradiology.* 2002;44(8):681–688.

95 Wetzel SG, Law M, Lee VS, Cha S, Johnson G, Nelson K. Imaging of the intracranial venous system with a contrast-enhanced volumetric interpolated examination. *Eur Radiol.* 2003;13(5):1010–1018.

96 Kaplan PW, Repke JT. Eclampsia. *Neurol Clin.* 1994;12:565–582.

97 Konstantinopoulos PA, Mousa S, Khairallah R, Mtanos G. Postpartum cerebral angiopathy: an important diagnostic consideration in the postpartum period. *Am J Obstet Gynecol.* 2004;191(1):375–377.

98 Geocadin RG, Razumovsky AY, Wityk RJ, Bhardwaj A, Ulatowski JAA. Intracerebral hemorrhage and postpartum vasculopathy. *J Neurol Sci.* 2002;205(1):29–34.

99 Chartier JP, Bousigue JY, Teisseyre A, Morel C, Delpuech-Formosa F. Postpartum cerebral angiopathy of iatrogenic origin. *Rev Neurol (Paris).* 1997;153(3):212–214.

100 Chiossi G, Neri I, Cavazzuti M, Basso G, Facchinetti F. Hyperemesis gravidarum complicated by Wernicke encephalopathy: background, case report, and review of the literature. *Obstet Gynecol Surv.* 2006;61(4):255–268.

101 Olafsson E, Hallgrimsson JT, Hauser WA, Ludvigsson P, Gudmundsson G. Pregnancies of women with epilepsy: a population based study in Iceland. *Epilepsia.* 1998;39(8):887–892.

102 Al Bunyan M, Abo-Talib Z. Outcome of pregnancies in epileptic women: a study in Saudi Arabia. *Seizure.* 1999;8(1):26–29.

103 Fairgrieve SD, Jackson M, Jonas P, et al. Population based, prospective study of the care of women with epilepsy in pregnancy. *BMJ.* 2000;321(7262):674–675.

104 Tomson T, Perucca E, Battino D. Navigating towards fetal and maternal health: the challenge of treating epilepsy in pregnancy. *Epilepsia* 2004;45(10):1171–1175.

105 Harden CL, Hopp J, Ting TY, et al.; American Academy of Neurology; American Epilepsy Society. Practice parameter update: management issues for women with epilepsy - focus on pregnancy (an evidence based review): teratogenesis and perinatal outcomes. *Neurology.* 2009;73(2):126–132. doi: 10.1212/WNL.0b013e3181a6b2f8.

106 Vajda FJE. Treatment options for pregnant women with epilepsy. *Expert Opin Pharmacother.* 2008;9(11):1859–1868. doi: 10.1517/14656566.9.11.1859.

107 Milazzo S, Mikou R, Berthout A, Bremond-Gignac D. Understanding refraction disorders and oculomotor problems during pregnancy. *J Fr Ophtalmol.* 2010;33(5):368–371.

108 Confavreux C, Hutchinson M, Hours MM, Cortinovis-Tourniaire P, Moreau T. Rate of pregnancy related relapse in multiple sclerosis. Pregnancy in Multiple Sclerosis Group. *N Engl J Med.* 1998;339:285–291.

109 Whitacre CC, Reingold SC, O'Looney PA. A gender gap in autoimmunity. *Science.* 1999;283(5406):1277–1278.

110 Voskuhl RR, Gold SM. Sex-related factors in multiple sclerosis susceptibility and progression. *Nat Rev Neurol.* 2012;8(5):255–263. doi: 10.1038/nrneurol.2012.43.

111 Vukusic S, Hutchinson M, Hours M, et al. Pregnancy and multiple sclerosis (the PRIMS study): clinical predictors of postpartum relapse. *Brain.* 2004;127(Pt 6):1353–1360. Epub 2004 May 6.

112 Kim W, Kim SH, Nakashima I. Influence of pregnancy on neuromyelitis optica spectrum disorder. *Neurology.* 2012;78(16):1264–1267.

113 Bourre B, Marignier R, Zéphir H. Neuromyelitis optica and pregnancy. *Neurology.* 2012;78(12):875–879.

114 Thurtell MJ, Sharp KL, Spies JM, Halmagyi GM. Isolated sixth cranial nerve palsy in preeclampsia. *J Neuroophthalmol.* 2006;26(4):296–298.

115 Barry-Kinsella C, Milner M, McCarthy N, Walshe J. Sixth nerve palsy: an unusual manifestation of

preeclampsia. *Obstet Gynecol.* 1994;83(5 Pt 2):849–851.

116 Schievink WI, Maya MM, Louy C, Moser FG, Tourje J. Diagnostic criteria for spontaneous spinal leaks and intracranial hypotension. *Am J Neuroradiol.* 2008;29(5):853–856. doi: 10.3174/ajnr.A0956.

117 Peitersen E. Bell's palsy: the spontaneous course of 2,500 peripheral facial nerve palsies of different etiologies. *Acta Otolaryngol Suppl.* 2002,(549):1–30.

118 Vrabec JT, Isaacson B, Van Hook JW. Bell's palsy and pregnancy. *Otolaryngol Head Neck Surg.* 2007;137(6):858–861.

119 Shmorgun D, Chan WS, Ray JG. Association between Bell's palsy in pregnancy and preeclampsia. *QJM.* 2002;95(6):359–362.

120 Alvis JS, Hicks RJ. Pregnancy-induced acute neurologic emergencies and neurologic conditions encountered in pregnancy. *Semin Ultrasound CT MR.* 2012;33(1):46–54.

121 Greenberg SA. Pearls: neuromuscular disorders. *Semin Neurol.* 2010;30(1):28–34.

122 Femia G, Parratt JD, Halmagyi GM. Isolated reversible hypoglossal nerve palsy as the initial manifestation of pre-eclampsia. *J Clin Neurosci.* 2012;19(4):602–603.

123 Motivala S, Gologorsky Y, Kostandinov J, Post KD. Pituitary disorders during pregnancy. *Endocrinol Metab Clin North Am.* 2011;40(4):827–836. doi: 10.1016/j.ecl.2011.08.007.

124 van der Wildt B, Drayer JI, Eskes TK. Diabetes insipidus in pregnancy as a first sign of a craniopharyngioma. *Eur J Obstet Gynecol Reprod Biol.* 1980;10(4):269–274.

125 Kodama T, Matsukado Y, Miura M, Takada A. Natural pregnancy and normal delivery after intracapsular irradiation for symptomatic craniopharyngioma–case report. *Neurol Med Chir (Tokyo).* 1986;26(1):40–43.

126 Johnson RJ Jr, Voorhies RM, Witkin M, Robichaux AG 3rd, Broussard WA Jr. Fertility following excision of a symptomatic craniopharyngioma during pregnancy: case report. *Surg Neurol.* 1993;39(4):257–262.

127 Maniker AH, Krieger AJ. Rapid recurrence of craniopharyngioma during pregnancy with recovery of vision: a case report. *Surg Neurol.* 1996;45(4):324–327.

128 Magge SN, Brunt M, Scott RM. Craniopharyngioma presenting during pregnancy 4 years after a normal magnetic resonance imaging scan:

case report. *Neurosurgery.* 2001;49(4):1014–1016; conclusion 1016-7.

129 Lupi I, Manetti L, Raffaelli V, et al. Diagnosis and treatment of autoimmune hypophysitis: a short review. *J Endocrinol Invest.* 2011;34(8):e245–e252.

130 Landek-Salgado MA, Gutenberg A, Lupi I, et al. Pregnancy, postpartum autoimmune thyroiditis, and autoimmune hypophysitis: intimate relationships. *Autoimmun Rev.* 2010;9(3):153–157.

131 Altieri A, Franceschi S, Ferlay J, Smith J, La Vecchia C. Epidemiology and aetiology of gestational trophoblastic diseases. *Lancet Oncol.* 2003;4(11):670–678.

132 Feng F, Xiang Y, Cao Y. Metastasis of gestational trophoblastic neoplasia to the spinal canal: a case report. *J Reprod Med.* 2009;54(9):576–578.

133 Huang CY, Chen CA, Hsieh CY, Cheng WF. Intracerebral hemorrhage as initial presentation of gestational choriocarcinoma: a case report and literature review. *Int J Gynecol Cancer.* 2007;17(5):1166–1171.

134 Chan YL, Lam WW, Lau TK, Metreweli C, Chan DP. Back pain in pregnancy: magnetic resonance imaging correlation. *Clin Radiol.* 2002;57(12):1109–1112.

135 Han IH. Pregnancy and spinal problems. *Curr Opin Obstet Gynecol.* 2010;22(6):477–481. doi: 10.1097/GCO.0b013e3283404ea1.

136 LaBan MM, Perrin JC, Latimer FR. Pregnancy and the herniated lumbar disc. *Arch Phys Med Rehabil.* 1983;64(7):319–321.

137 Mousavi SJ, Parnianpour M, Vleeming A. Pregnancy related pelvic girdle pain and low back pain in an Iranian population. *Spine (Phila Pa 1976).* 2007;32(3):E100–E104.

138 Kiroglu Y, Benek B, Yagci B, Cirak B, Tahta K. Spinal cord compression caused by vertebral hemangioma being symptomatic during pregnancy. *Surg Neurol.* 2009;71(4):487–492; discussion 492. doi: 10.1016/j.surneu.2007.09.025.

139 Kathiresan AS, Johnson JN, Hood BJ, Montoya SP, Vanni S, Gonzalez-Quintero VH. Giant cell tumor of the thoracic spine presenting in late pregnancy. *Obstet Gynecol.* 2011;118(2 Pt 2):428–431. doi: 10.1097/AOG.0b013e31821081a2.

140 Vijay K, Shetty AP, Rajasekaran S. Symptomatic vertebral hemangioma in pregnancy treated

antepartum. A case report with review of literature. *Eur Spine J.* 2008;17(Suppl 2):299–303. doi:10.1007/s00586-008-0592-2.

141 Case AS, Ramsey PS. Spontaneous epidural hematoma of the spine in pregnancy. *Am J Obstet Gyneco.* 2005;193:875–877.

142 Bell WE, Joynt RJ, Sahs AL. Low spinal fluid pressure syndrome. *Neurology.* 1960;10:512–521.

143 Rahman M, Bidari SS, Quisling RG, Friedman WA. Spontaneous intracranial hypotension: dilemmas in diagnosis. *Neurosurgery.* 2011;69(1):4–14; discussion 14. doi: 10.1227/NEU.0b013e3182134399.

144 Schievink WI. Spontaneous spinal cerebrospinal fluid leaks and intracranial hypotension. *JAMA.* 2006;295(19):2286–2296.

CHAPTER 4

Neurologic complications in the obstetrical anesthesia patient

Olajide Kowe[1] & Jonathan H. Waters[2]

[1] Yorktown Regional Hospital, Saskatchewan, Canada
[2] Magee Women's Hospital, University of Pittsburgh Medical Center, Pittsburgh, PA, USA

Neurologic deficits during or following labor and delivery can occur as a result of obstetric trauma. Anesthesia can also cause neurologic injury. Differentiation between the two mechanisms can present a diagnostic challenge. In addition, injury resulting from obstetric causes can present together with anesthesia-induced neurologic injury in the same patient. For this reason, a sound understanding of the kinds of neurologic injury that can occur and the mechanisms for these injuries is imperative when caring for this population of patients. This chapter will review presenting signs, diagnostic workup, and treatment of neurologic complications in the obstetrical anesthesia patient.

Anesthesia-related injury

Anesthesia-related injury can result from many causes as outlined in Table 4.1. Of all the neurologic problems, post-dural puncture headache is the most common neurologic problem associated with anesthesia care.

Post-dural puncture headache

Post-dural puncture headache (PDPH) can occur after epidural analgesia, which is used for labor pain management, or it can occur after spinal anesthesia, which is typically used for elective cesarean section. Anatomically, the epidural space is a narrow, crescent-shaped space superficial to the dura mater. When placing an epidural catheter for labor, a 17 gauge needle is passed into the space through which a 19 gauge catheter is passed. The catheter is used for continuous local anesthetic administration for labor or post-surgical analgesia. Given the narrowness of the epidural space, it is easy to inadvertently pass through the epidural space into the subarachnoid space, resulting in a dural puncture, or "wet tap." This complication occurs during placement of 1–3% of the epidurals used for labor analgesia [1–3].

Dural puncture headache is thought to be due to cerebrospinal fluid (CSF) leakage through the hole in the dural sac. As such, the size of the needle and the type of needle point influence the incidence and severity of the subsequent headache [4]. Needles used for epidural placement are typically larger than those used for spinal anesthesia because of the need to thread a catheter for continuous analgesia; whereas a spinal anesthetic is a one-time administration of a local anesthetic so a smaller needle can be used. Typically, needle size for a spinal needle is in the 24–25 gauge size. The gauge of a needle relates to how many needles laid side by side would equate 1 inch. So, 17 epidural needles would equal 24 spinal needles. Because of the larger size of the epidural needle, a bigger hole

Neurological Illness in Pregnancy: Principles and Practice, First Edition.
Edited by Autumn Klein, M. Angela O'Neal, Christina Scifres, Janet F. R. Waters and Jonathan H. Waters.

Table 4.1 Neuraxial-related injuries

Injury type	Causes/factors implicated
1. Spinal cord damage	
Direct injury	Unusually low conus medularis
	Traumatic catheterization
	High placement of needle
Indirect injury	Hematoma (epidural/spinal)
	Abscess (epidural/spinal)
2. Meningitis	
Infective	Bacterial, viral
	Aseptic
Non-infective	Chemical arachnoiditis
	Anterior spinal cord syndrome
3. Spinal cord ischemia	
4. Cauda equina syndrome	Intrathecal micro-catheter
	Intrathecal lidocaine (high concentration)
5. Others	Dural puncture and CSF leak (cranial nerve palsy)
	Total spinal block
	Back pain
	Seizures (systemic toxicity)
	Pneumocephalus

is made when passed into the dura. As a result, more CSF will leak through the hole, resulting in a higher incidence of dural puncture headache.

The point on the needle also influences the leakage. Classically, needles are hollow tubes cut at an angle to make a point. This type of needle is called a "cutting needle." Needles used for medication injection are of this type. If this type of needle is used for puncture of the dura, it will leave a well-described hole and allow for easy leakage of CSF. An epidural needle resembles a cutting needle except that the point has been dulled so that spinal ligaments are felt while it is passed into the epidural space. Needles used for spinal anesthesia are "pencil-point" needles with the point being in the shape of a pencil and the orifice of the needle being on the shaft of the needle. This type of needle leaves a hole that closes upon itself minimizing the leak of CSF. The incidence of PDPH is also higher in patients younger than 45 years and also in pregnant patients [5].

Symptoms usually occur within 24–48 hours after dural puncture. Headache resulting from CSF leak is bilateral, fronto-occipital, radiates to the neck, and worsens on standing or sitting upright. The headache is relieved by lying supine. The positional nature of the headache is thought to relate to traction on the meninges and meningeal vessels upon moving the head into an upright position [6].

Periodically, patients with a dural puncture headache will also experience diplopia and tinnitus. These symptoms are thought to result from traction on the sixth and eighth cranial nerves. Diplopia or tinnitus can be permanent so a prompt blood patch is indicated in this subset of patients.

Treatment of PDPH starts with conservative management. Conservative management involves bed rest for patients who do not tolerate ambulation, adequate rehydration, and analgesics. Intravenous (IV) or oral caffeine has been advocated to speed CSF production

[7]. Other conservative management that has been tried includes sumatriptan [8], adrenocorticotropic hormone, theophylline [9], and use of an abdominal binder.

If conservative management fails, an epidural blood patch can be performed. An epidural blood patch is performed by placing 15–20 mL of autologous blood into the epidural space. The blood acts as a patch over the dura hole. The volume of the blood is thought to push CSF back into the cranium thus resolving intracerebral hypotension. The effect is almost immediate upon placing the blood patch.

Before performing a blood patch, it is important to make sure that the patient is not septic, and that she does not have preeclampsia or other causes for her headache. Injection of blood should be stopped if the patient experiences back pain or neurologic symptoms in the lower limbs [10]. Epidural blood patch should be performed under strict aseptic conditions. The patient must be informed that the risk of performing a blood patch is the same as placement of the original neuraxial block. It is advisable to do an epidural blood patch at a level lower than the initial neuraxial block as 70% of the injected blood will spread cephalad. An epidural blood patch performed after 24 hours from the time of the wet tap has success rate of 70–97% [11]. In some circumstances, a second blood patch is needed for complete resolution of the headache.

For unknown reasons, a blood patch done less than 24 hours after the dural puncture has a high failure rate. In some circumstances, following a dural puncture, the anesthesiologist will place an epidural catheter at a different level than the wet tap. Some have advocated that following delivery, a prophylactic blood patch be performed in advance of symptoms. However, prophylactic blood patch has a high failure rate.

If two epidural blood patches have been performed, and the patient still complains of a headache, then other causes for the headache should be sought. A rare consequence of intracranial hypotension from dural puncture is

that the bridging veins which cross the subdural space will tear and lead to subdural hematoma. While most of these hematomas will resolve without intervention, some can increase intracerebral pressure and be life-threatening.

Direct spinal cord injury

Direct injury can result from failure to accurately determine the location of the lower end of the spinal cord before needle placement. In approximately 80% of the adult population, the spinal cord ends at the level of first lumbar vertebra while the remaining 20% have spinal cords which extend to the level of second lumbar vertebra [12]. Placement of neuraxial block, especially spinal anesthesia, at the level below the second lumbar vertebra reduces the risk of incidence of direct spinal cord injury [13–15].

When spinal cord trauma does occur, it results from either direct catheter injury or needle injury to the spinal cord, spinal nerve roots, conus medullaris, or intraneural injection of local anesthetics. Trauma to the spinal cord manifests as paresthesia or pain in the lower limbs which can be transient or persistent. If the patient experiences transient symptoms during the neuraxial block, the anesthesiologist may proceed with the procedure. If the paresthesia or pain persists in one or both limbs, then it is advisable to stop and reposition the needle or catheter. Local anesthetic injection into the epidural or intrathecal space should never be attempted in any patient who experiences persistent neurologic symptoms as sensory and motor block resulting from local anesthetics may mask the recognition of signs and symptoms of nerve injury.

Epidural hematoma

Epidural hematoma formation is a rare but serious complication of neuraxial anesthesia. Incidence varies from 1:200,000 after spinal anesthesia to 1:150,000 after epidural placement [16]. Epidural hematoma should be suspected in patients showing any of the following symptoms: epidural anesthesia persisting for more than the expected time of duration of action of the local anesthetic used, unusual back pain and local tenderness, persistent numbness or motor weakness, and sphincter dysfunction. Early diagnosis and management of an epidural hematoma is essential to prevent permanent neurologic injury. Urgent CT scan or MRI may be used to confirm the diagnosis of an epidural hematoma. Emergency surgical decompression within 6 hours of onset of signs and symptoms is necessary to avoid permanent neurologic dysfunction. Hematomas can occur with or without predisposing factors. Predisposing factors include gestational thrombocytopenia, preeclampsia/eclampsia, HELLP syndrome, and inherited or iatrogenic clotting dysfunctions. The most common factor associated with the formation of epidural hematoma is use of anticoagulants or antiplatelet agents. It is crucial to delay neuraxial anesthesia until the effect of the drug has subsided [17] (Table 4.2). Patients with any predisposing risk factor for bleeding should be investigated thoroughly before commencing with a neuraxial block. No patient should receive neuraxial anesthesia with full anticoagulation. It is important to carry out relevant laboratory investigations (e.g., platelet counts and coagulation profile) in patients with risk factors.

Table 4.2 Common anticoagulants and waiting period prior to a neuraxial procedure

Medication	Prior to neuraxial procedure
Unfractionated heparin, low dose	No time restrictions
Unfractionated heparin, high dose, IV continuous	When aPTT < 40 s
Enoxaparin (Lovenox), low dose	12 h
Enoxaparin (Lovenox), high dose	24 h
Fondaparinux (Arixtra)	72 h
Clopidogrel (Plavix)	48 h
Eptifibatide (Integrilin)	8 h
Abciximab (Reopro)	48 h
Tirofiban (Aggrastat)	8 h

aPTT, activated partial thromboplastin time.

The use of thromboelastography (TEG) in patients at risk of bleeding has been recommended if available [18]. Traditional laboratory testing measures a single component of the clotting system. For instance, a platelet count is just one component of a very complex clotting process. A prothrombin time (PT) simply measures the clotting factors of the extrinsic coagulation system. A platelet count or PT by itself neglects other changes in clotting function which occur during pregnancy. These changes include a doubling of fibrinogen concentration, an elevation in most other coagulation factors, and a reduction of fibrinolytic proteins, Protein C and Protein S. Differing from traditional clotting tests, the TEG measures all components of the clotting system together by evaluating the clotting of whole blood. Some obstetric patients with gestational thrombocytopenia, idiopathic thrombocytopenic purpura (ITP), or thrombocytopenia associated with preeclampsia may show normal TEG measurement. In these patients, the TEG has demonstrated that neuraxial block can be performed without complication despite low platelet counts.

Epidural abscess

Epidural abscess is an uncommon complication of neuraxial anesthetic techniques. Incidence in the general population varies from 1:1000–1:100,000 per of neuraxial blocks. In the obstetrical population, it is much rarer and is estimated to occur in 1:500,000 epidural blocks [19, 20]. Skin flora is usually the source of epidural abscess. *Staphylococcus aureus* is the most common underlying organism [21]. The risk of developing an abscess increases with prolonged duration of epidural catheterization. Most practitioners will limit the duration of the catheter to 3 days. Failure to adhere to aseptic condition while performing neuraxial block increase the risk of epidural abscess. Underlying depressed immunity in the patient may contribute to a higher incident of epidural hematoma. Clinical presentation includes fever, headache, back pain, malaise, and local tenderness. Nerve root pain develops within 3–5 days of the onset of back pain and this leads gradually to leg weakness, paraplegia, and bladder or bowel dysfunction. Urgent MRI with gadolinium should be done to confirm the diagnosis of epidural abscess in the postpartum patient. Aggressive antimicrobial therapy is the mainstay of treatment for epidural abscess. Surgical decompression is necessary if there are features of nerve root compression.

Meningitis

Meningeal infection is a rare complication of neuraxial block. The incidence has been estimated to be around 1:39,000 neuraxial procedures [22]. Incidence decreases with procedures done under strict aseptic condition (facemask, sterile gloves, and cap). Microbial contamination from the mouth and nose are the most common source of meningitis incurred after epidural or subarachnoid block. Most meningitis infections resulting from neuraxial procedures are due to *Streptococcus viridans*. Clinical manifestations of meningitis include fever, malaise, headache, irritability, altered consciousness level, and neck stiffness, Kernig's sign (when the examiner straightens the patients knees with the hips flexed, the patient has pain in the hamstrings) or Brudzinski's sign (when the examiner flexes the patients neck, the patient flexes her legs at the hip) may be present. Diagnostic investigation includes thorough physical examination, CBC, blood cultures, and CSF analysis. Treatment is aggressive antimicrobial therapy. Laboratory investigation must not delay commencement of antimicrobial therapy.

Chemical meningitis can also complicate epidural or spinal anesthesia. It occurs as a result of accidental injection of contaminated local anesthetics into the subarachnoid or epidural space. Chemical arachnoiditis can also result from traces of chlorhexidine-containing skin preparations being introduced into the subarachnoid space on a needle used for neuraxial procedure. Clinical features are difficult to differentiate from infective meningitis. It is a

diagnosis of exclusion. Chemical meningitis resolves spontaneously. Antimicrobial therapy is advised until infection is ruled out.

Anterior spinal artery syndrome (spinal cord ischemia)

This complication is extremely rare in obstetric anesthesia. The anterior two-thirds of the spinal cord are supplied by the anterior spinal artery. Vascular supply is reinforced by radicular arteries originating from the thoracolumbar aorta, the largest of which is the artery of Adamkiewicz. Anterior spinal artery syndrome may occur in the setting of severe, prolonged hypotension, arteriosclerosis, or surgery which interferes with blood flow to the arteries [23]. There has been a suggestion that epinephrine-containing local anesthetics may also predispose patients with vascular disease to this phenomena [24]. The most common causes for this syndrome relate to major spine instrumentation and thoracolumbar aneurysm repair [25]. This condition manifests as paraplegia, loss of pain and temperature sensation, and bladder and bowel incontinence. Sensations of proprioception, light touch, and vibration are all spared in this syndrome as they involve the posterior spinal column. Diffusion-weighted MRI can be used to confirm the diagnosis.

Cauda equina syndrome

This syndrome has been described after the use of lidocaine for spinal anesthesia. In the early 1990s, continuous intrathecal microcatheters were introduced. Shortly thereafter, reports of cauda equina syndrome surfaced [26,27]. Cauda equina syndrome is a dysfunction of nerve roots L2-S5. It manifests as burning low back pain, sphincter dysfunction, paraplegia, and sensory dysfunction in the perineum (saddle anesthesia). Pooling of local anesthetic, most specifically, lidocaine, was determined to be the causative agent. Lidocaine and to some extent tetracaine have the greatest potential to cause neurotoxicity. Patients with diabetic neuropathy have a higher risk of this complication.

Lidocaine is no longer favored as a spinal anesthetic agent.

Total spinal block

When performing an epidural block, from time to time, the epidural catheter will accidentally be threaded into the subarachnoid space. To test for this complication, a "test dose" of local anesthetic is given. This test dose involves injecting a small amount of local anesthetic which will result in a spinal block if the catheter is in the subarachnoid space. If the test dose is not performed, or if inadequate time is given between the test dose and the regular epidural dose, a total spinal block can occur. A total spinal block will occur if a large volume of local anesthetic, intended for the epidural space, is injected into the subarachnoid space. This can produce anesthesia of the entire spinal cord, cervical spinal nerves, and brainstem. The incidence of total spinal block is unknown.

When a total spinal block occurs, the symptoms are dramatic. First, the patient will mention that their lower extremities are paralyzed, followed by complaints of inability to breath. Respiratory arrest may follow shortly thereafter. Cardiovascular collapse can occur with profound hypotension and bradycardia.

Management of a total spinal block is mainly supportive. A high index of suspicion is important in early diagnosis and also in preventing irreversible organ damage in patients with total spinal block. Quick recognition of this condition is crucial to prevention of irreversible organ damage and fetal demise. Reverse Trendelenburg positioning may help to limit further cranial spread of local anesthetic. Hypotension should be treated with vasopressors or inotropes such as ephedrine, phenylephrine, epinephrine, or norepinephrine. Bradycardia can be treated with atropine or glycopyrolate. Respiratory collapse should be managed with 100% oxygen, positive pressure ventilation, and intubation.

There are several factors that may predispose a patient to a total spinal block. First, obese patients tend to have a reduced subarachnoid space which may favor cephalad spread of local anesthetics. Obesity also increases intra-abdominal pressure and may increase risk of high block. Pregnancy also may favor cephalad spread of local anesthetic in the subarachnoid space secondary to increased intra abdominal pressure. Fluid or local anesthetic in the epidural space may compress the subarachnoid space which may predispose these patients to total spinal block if such patient subsequently has a subarachnoid block. This typically occurs when an epidural has been deemed inadequate to perform a cesarean section.

Pharmacology of the local anesthetic can also influence spread of the drug. For instance, the baricity of the drug will change spread. Baricity is the specific gravity of the drug relative to the CSF. Hyperbaric drugs will sink in the subarachnoid space as the heavier drug displaces the lighter CSF. Hypobaric drugs will rise in the subarachnoid space. Most local anesthetics used for spinal anesthesia fall into the hyperbaric category. Local anesthetics used for epidural anesthesia are isobaric. In other words, their density is similar to that of CSF so they tend to stay in the location of their injection. Control of the spread of local anesthetic can be obtained by manipulating the patient's position. The dose and volume of local anesthetic will also determine the level of block.

Back pain

While back pain is a common complication of neuraxial block, most obstetrical patients will have some degree of back pain following delivery, regardless of whether they had a neuraxial block. The incidence of anesthesia-related back pain varies from 15% for spinal anesthesia to 30% for epidural anesthesia. Pain secondary to neuraxial block is largely self-limited. Patients complaining of unusual or severe back pain after neuraxial anesthesia should be thoroughly investigated.

Factors contributing to development of back pain after neuraxial anesthesia include multiple attempts, traumatic manipulation, ligamentous injury, periosteal trauma, and local inflammation. Management of post-neuraxial anesthesia back pain is conservative and most will resolve within few days to few weeks. Reassurance is all that is needed after excluding serious complications that might present with back pain. Analgesics such as nonsteroidal anti-inflammatory drugs or acetaminophen can be prescribed for severe and prolonged back pain.

Seizure from systemic toxicity of local anesthetics

This complication occurs after inadvertent intravascular injection of local anesthetic. It is extremely rare after spinal anesthesia due to the small volume and dose of local anesthetic required to achieve a good surgical block. Systemic toxicity can occur after obstetric epidural anesthesia or caudal block because larger volumes of local anesthetics are used for both procedures [28]. Toxicity mostly affects the central nervous system (CNS) and the cardiovascular system. Factors affecting patient response to inadvertent intravascular injection of local anesthetic include the type of local anesthetic used. Bupivacaine is the most toxic followed by ropivacaine, levobupivacaine, lidocaine, and chloroprocaine, respectively. The rate of the injection dictates the peak serum level so a faster injection will result in a quicker onset of systemic toxicity.

Local anesthetics act as membrane stabilizers by binding to sodium channels. The duration of the binding varies among different drugs. Bupivacaine binds almost irreversibly to sodium channel and thus has the highest toxicity of all the local anesthetics. Therefore, they alter the electrical activities of excitable tissues such as the neurons and cardiac muscles. The end result is CNS and cardiovascular system depression. Early signs and symptoms of systemic toxicity include agitation, metallic taste in the mouth, circumoral paresthesia, diplopia, tinnitus, and confusion. Later signs include seizures due to inhibition of inhibitory neurons in the CNS

and loss of consciousness. Further neurologic deterioration can result in cardiovascular collapse with hypotension, arrhythmias, and cardiac arrest.

It is very important to use preventive measures when administering local anesthetic drugs into the epidural space. Such techniques would include aspiration of the epidural catheter before giving a dose to exclude an intravascular catheter and dosing the epidural catheter with incremental doses of the drug rather than single large dose. The use of local anesthetic containing epinephrine can help to detect intravascular catheters as the patient will experience tachycardia.

Early recognition of signs and symptoms of systemic toxicity will help to expedite early management and prevent mobility and mortality. Hospitals administering neuraxial blocks for obstetric patients should have facilities available to manage toxicity incurred by local anesthetics. Lipid emulsion is the mainstay of treatment of local anesthetic toxicity [29]. A 20% intralipid should be given first as a 1.5 mL/kg IV bolus dose given over 60 seconds followed by a 0.25 mL/kg min^{-1} IV (400 mL) infusion over 30–40 minutes. The infusion of lipid should be maintained until a stable cardiovascular system exists. Cardiopulmonary bypass should be requested if available. It is important to continue cardiopulmonary resuscitation during lipid emulsion administration. Recovery from local anesthetic toxicity may take up to 2 hours.

Pneumocephalus

This condition is also referred to as intracerebral pneumatocele or aerocele. Pneumocephalus occurs when there is the presence of gas within the intracranial cavity (intraparenchymal, subarachnoid, intraventricular, epidural, and subdural). Pneumocephalus can occur after epidural anesthesia, caudal block, and spinal anesthesia [30]. When anesthesia is being administered, the epidural space is identified by a technique called "loss of resistance." An epidural needle is placed through the skin and subcutaneous fat, into one of the spinal ligaments. As the needle is advanced from the ligamentum flavum into the epidural space, a syringe containing air or saline is placed onto the needle. Pressure is applied on the barrel of the syringe as the needle is advanced. When the epidural space is entered, the air or saline is easily injected; whereas, while passing through the ligaments, it is not. If the epidural space is missed and the subarachnoid space is entered instead, the air or saline is injected into the CSF. Pneumocephalus is especially prominent with the use of air to find the loss of resistance; however, saline is never totally free of air when it is used. It has also been described after subarachnoid block.

Pneumocephalus presents with clinical features similar to those of post-dural puncture headache, meningitis, and chemical arachnoiditis. Therefore, this condition should be considered in any obstetric patient presenting with persistent headache. Pneumocephalus behaves like a space-occupying lesion in the rigid cranium and thus manifests signs and symptoms of raised intracranial pressure. Clinical manifestation of pneumocephalus include nausea, vomiting, headache, blurring of vision, tinnitus, dizziness, seizures, and may result in a depressed level of consciousness.

Diagnosis of intracranial aerocele can be made using CT scan of the brain which shows characteristic multiple small air bubbles in the cistern compressing the frontal lobe (Mount Fuji sign). This condition can also be diagnosed using plain x-ray. Management of pneumocephalus after obstetric neuraxial anesthesia is mainly conservative and involves patient reassurance, bed rest, and analgesics (acetaminophen, opioids, nonsteroidal anti-inflammatory drugs).

Obstetrical birth trauma

Peripheral nerve injury related to birth trauma is common. Obstetric factors that contribute to injuries during labor and delivery include instrumental delivery, short stature, prolonged labor, primiparous women, persistent transverse or posterior position of the fetal head and prolonged lithotomy position during pushing. Most of these injuries result from stretch or compression to a nerve. Epidural anesthesia has been associated with prolonged labor which may contribute to neurologic injury from these obstetrical causes [31]. The most commonly injured nerve is the lateral femoral cutaneous nerve [32]. It is important for the neurologist to understand the mechanism and presentation of these injuries (Table 4.3).

Lumbosacral plexus nerve injury

The lumbosacral plexus originates from nerve roots L_1, L_2, L_3, L_4, L_5, S_1, S_2, S_3, and S_4. Injury to the plexus can occur by compression of the fetal head against the posterior rim of the pelvic bone especially with forceps delivery. Injury to the lumbosacral plexus can be unilateral (75%) or bilateral (25%). Clinical manifestation is dependent upon the nerve roots involved.

Lateral femoral cutaneous nerve injury

This nerve originates from nerve root L2-L3 and passes beneath the inguinal ligament to

Table 4.3 Obstetric palsies

Obstetric palsy	Manifestations
Lumbosacral trunk	Quadriceps and hip adductor weakness, foot drop
Lateral femoral cutaneous nerve	Numbness of anterolateral thigh
Common peroneal nerve	Paresthesia on lateral calf and foot drop
Femoral nerve	Paresthesia of the thigh and calf, weak hip flexion, and weakness of quadriceps muscles
Obturator nerve	Paresthesia on medial side of the thigh and weakness of hip adduction

innervate the anterior thigh (sensory). It can be compressed during prolonged pushing in the lithotomy position or stirrups position. Injury to the lateral femoral cutaneous nerve manifests as numbness of the anterolateral thigh also known as *meralgia paresthetica*.

Common peroneal nerve injury

Common peroneal nerve originates from nerve roots L4-S2. This nerve can be injured as it winds around the head of the fibula where compression can occur especially in prolonged lithotomy or stirrups position. It manifest as paresthesia in the lateral calf and foot drop.

Femoral nerve injury

The femoral nerve originates from L2-L4 nerve root. It can be compressed along its route as it passes beneath the inguinal ligament lateral to the femoral artery. This happens during prolonged pushing with the hip excessively flexed. It manifest as paresthesia of the anterior thigh and medial calf, weak hip flexion, and weak knee extension.

Obturator nerve injury

The obturator nerve originates from nerve roots L2-L4 and passes through the obturator canal on the lateral pelvic wall where compression can occur by the fetal head or during forceps delivery. Injury to this nerve manifests as paresthesia in the medial aspect of the upper thigh and weakness of hip adduction.

Diagnosis and management of birth-trauma-related neuropathy

Patients presenting with neuropathy following labor and delivery should be thoroughly examined and investigated. The following questions will help in detecting the cause of the injury;
- What was the timing of onset of symptoms?
- What is the location and severity of the symptoms?
- Is symptom progressing or regressing?
- Does it radiate?
- Did the patient receive neuraxial anesthesia?
- Was there any paresthesia elicited during placement of neuraxial needle?
- If a paresthesia was elicited, what was its duration? Was it persistent or transient?
- Did the patient have full recovery from neuraxial anesthesia after delivery?
- What was the duration of labor?
- What was the position assumed by the patient during pushing and for how long?
- Was any instrumentation used for the delivery? (forceps)

Investigations that can help in diagnosing such injury include MRI, CT SCAN, electromyography, and nerve conduction studies. Nerve injuries secondary to birth trauma may take up to 10 weeks to resolve. Serial investigation, for example, nerve conduction studies may be needed to monitor recovery from the injury.

References

1 Berger CW, Crosby ET, Grodecki W. North American survey of the management of dural puncture occurring during labour epidural analgesia. *Can J Anaesth.* 1998;45:110–114.
2 Gleeson CM, Reynolds F. Accidental dural puncture rates in UK obstetric practice. *Int J Obstet Anesth.* 1998;7:242–246.
3 Sprigge JS, Harper SJ. Accidental dural puncture and post dural puncture headache in obstetric anaesthesia: presentation and management: a 23-year survey in a district general hospital. *Anaesthesia.* 2008;63:36–43.
4 Reynolds F. Damage to conus medularis after spinal anesthesia (case report). *Anesthesia.* 2001;56: 238–247.
5 Turnbull DK, Shepard DB. Post dural puncture headache: pathogenesis, prevention and treatment. *Brit J Anaesth.* 2003;91:718–729.
6 Turnbull DK, Shepherd DB. Post-dural puncture headache: pathogenesis, prevention and treatment. *Brit J Anaesth.* 2003;91:718–729.
7 Camann WR, Murray RS, Mushlin PS, Lambert DH. Effects of oral caffeine on postdural

puncture headache. A double-blind, placebo-controlled trial. *Anesth Analg.* 1990;70:181–184.

8 Carp H, Singh PJ, Vadhera R, Jayaram A. Effects of the serotonin receptor agonist sumatriptan on postdural puncture headache: report of six cases. *Anesth Analg.* 1994;79:180–182.

9 Schwalbe SS, Schiffmiller MW, Marx GF. Theophylline for post-dural puncture headache (abstract). *Anesthesiology.* 1991;75:A1082.

10 Abouleish E, Vega S, Blendinger I, Tio TO. Long term follow up of epidural blood patch. *Anesth Analg.* 1975;54:459–463.

11 Crawford JS. Experiences with epidural blood patch. *Anaesthesia.* 1980;35:513–515.

12 Broadbent CR, Maxwell WB, Ferrie R, et al. Ability of anaesthetists to identify a marked lumbar interspace. *Anaesthesia.* 2000;55:1122–1126.

13 Fettes PD, Wildsmith JA: Somebody else's nervous system. *Brit J Anaesth.* 2002;88:760–763.

14 Broadbent CR, Maxwell WB, Ferrie R, Wilson DJ, Gawne-Cain M, Russel R. Ability of anaesthetists to identify a marked lumbar interspace. *Anaesthesia.* 2000;55:1122–1126.

15 Reynolds F. Damage to the conus medullaris following spinal anaesthesia. *Anaesthesia.* 2001;56: 238–247.

16 Brooks H, May A. Neurological complications following regional anesthesia in obstetrics. *Brit J Anaesth CEPD Rev.* 2003;3:111–114.

17 Horlocker TT, Wedel DJ, Rowlingson JC, et al. Regional anesthesia in the patient receiving antithrombotic or thrombolytic therapy: American Society of Regional Anesthesia and Pain Medicine Evidence-Based Guidelines (Third Edition) *Reg Anesth Pain Med.* 2010;35:64–101.

18 Bigeleisen PE, Kang Y. Thrombelastography as an aid to regional anesthesia: preliminary communication. *Reg Anesth.* 1991;16:59–61.

19 Moen V, Dahlgren N, Irestedt L. Severe neurologic complications after central neuraxial blockades in Sweden 1990–1999. *Anesthesiology.* 2004;101:950–959.

20 Scott DB, Hibbard BM. Serious non-fatal complications associated with extradural block in obstetric practice. *Brit J Anaesth.* 1990;64:537–41.

21 Grewal S, Hocking G, Wildsmith JAW. Epidural abscesses. *Brit J Anaesth.* 2006;96:292–302.

22 Reynolds F. Neurological infections after neuraxial anesthesia. *Anesthesiol Clin.* 2008;26:23–52.

23 Eastwood DW. Anterior spinal artery syndrome after epidural anesthesia in a pregnant diabetic patient with scleroderma. *Anesth Analg.* 1991;73: 90–91.

24 Tetzlaff JE, Dilger J, Yap E, Smith MP, Schoenwald PK. Cauda equina syndrome after spinal anaesthesia in a patient with severe vascular disease. *Can J Anaesth.* 1998;45:667–669.

25 Zuber WF, Gaspar MR, Rothschild PD. The anterior spinal artery syndrome—a complication of abdominal aortic surgery: report of five cases and review of the literature. *Ann Surg.* 1970 November; 172(5):909–915.

26 Rigler ML, Drasner K, Krejcie TC, et al. Cauda equina syndrome after continuous spinal anesthesia. *Anesth Analg.* 1991;72:275–81.

27 Schell RM, Brauer FS, Cole DJ, et al. Persistent sacral nerve root deficits after continuous spinal anaesthesia. *Can J Anaesth.* 1991;38:908–911.

28 Dillane D, Finucane BT. Local anesthetic systemic toxicity. *Can J Anaesth.* 2010;57:368–380.

29 Brull SJ. Lipid emulsion for the treatment of local anesthetic toxicity: patient safety implications. *Anesth Analg.* 2008;106:1337–1339.

30 Roderick L, More DC, Artru AA. Pneumocephalus with headache during spinal anesthesia. *Anesthesiology.* 1985;62:690–692.

31 Alexander JM, Lucas MJ, Ramin SM, McIntire DD, Leveno KJ. The course of labor with and without epidural analgesia. *Am J Obstet Gynecol.* 1998;178: 516–520.

32 Dar AQ, Robinson APC, Lyons G. Postpartum neurologic symptoms following regional blockade: a prospective study with case controls. *Int J Obstet Anesth.* 2002;11:85–90.

CHAPTER 5

Headaches during pregnancy and peripartum

Huma Sheikh

Faulkner Headache Division, Brigham and Women's Hospital, Harvard Medical School, Boston, MA, USA

Women suffer headaches more frequently than men. Peak prevalence of headache in women occurs during childbearing years. In general, women experience improvement in frequency and intensity of headaches during later stages of pregnancy. Pregnancy is a prothrombotic state that puts women at risk for a number of potentially life-threatening conditions that can present with headache. Therefore, it is essential to differentiate secondary headaches from primary headache during pregnancy. This chapter focuses on the course of primary headache disorders, particularly migraine in pregnancy and peripartum period, and treatment options during both pregnancy and lactation. Secondary causes of headache including thrombosis, stroke, and preeclampsia are also discussed.

Migraine headaches

Migraine is three times more prevalent among women than men [1,2]. Peak prevalence occurs during the childbearing years, reaching about 40% in the third and fourth decades of life [3]. Data on migraine in pregnancy and peripartum have primarily come from retrospective studies [4–12], with few reports focusing on migraine in postpartum period. Prospective studies have generally been small [13, 14] and have focused on specific subpopulations [14,15].

Of note is the recent prospective study of pregnant women in Norway, MIGRA, that followed over 2000 women with daily diaries from the second trimester of pregnancy (18–20 weeks) until the first 2 months postpartum [16].

Overall, both retrospective and prospective studies suggest that migraine headaches improve during the course of pregnancy [4, 5, 7, 12, 13, 17–19]. About 50–80% of women experience a reduction or even complete remission of migraines during the second and third trimesters [8, 13, 16, 20, 21]. The effect is more pronounced as the pregnancy progresses with up to 87.2% of women experiencing improvement in the third trimester [17]. This improvement appears to be more pronounced in women who have migraine without aura compared with those with aura [17], but this effect has been inconsistent across studies [16]. Multiple studies have shown that women with a menstrual migraine component seem to experience the most benefit during pregnancy [4, 6, 7, 18]. Although some smaller studies have associated multiparity with worsening of migraine in the third trimester [13] and peripartum [22], the larger studies have not identified an association between headache frequency and parity [14, 16].

The first trimester generally presents the greatest challenge to women with migraine, in terms of headache frequency and intensity as

Neurological Illness in Pregnancy: Principles and Practice, First Edition.
Edited by Autumn Klein, M. Angela O'Neal, Christina Scifres, Janet F. R. Waters and Jonathan H. Waters.
© 2016 John Wiley & Sons, Ltd. Published 2016 by John Wiley & Sons, Ltd.

well as in treatment options. Studies of the first trimester are particularly challenging as headaches tend to be the worst during the first several weeks postconception, a period of time when women are often unaware that they are pregnant and may be experiencing other symptoms of pregnancy which can exacerbate migraine headaches.

New onset migraine occurs during the first trimester (12, 17) [12, 23] in about 3–6% of pregnant women [12, 16, 23, 24] and tends to be migraine with aura. Thankfully, less than 10% of women experience worsening of migraine during pregnancy. Interestingly, a recent prospective study of Japanese women did not identify any women with worsening headaches during pregnancy [25]. Limited data suggest that if migraines have not improved by the end of the first trimester, it is likely to continue through the rest of pregnancy with minimal improvement at best [14].

Postpartum headache occurs in about 30–40% of women overall [13,17,22]. Most women with a history of migraine experience a worsening in their headaches following delivery, though the headaches may have remitted during the final stage of pregnancy. There appears to be a sharp rise in migraine headaches within the first week of delivery [13,16] and a decrease in frequency at 5 weeks post-delivery noted by the recent large prospective study [16]. There may be a number of factors that play a role in the rapid rise in headaches post-delivery, including the precipitous drop in estrogen and other hormonal changes, effects of procedures (such as epidural and spinal anesthesia), and effects of medications (including anesthesia).

Lactation appears to mitigate the recurrence of postpartum headache, though data from studies have been mixed [13,14,16,17,25]. In general, breastfeeding has been associated with a protective effect on migraine headache thought to be due to suppression of ovulation in lactating women leading to relatively stable estrogen levels. Although the larger prospective studies have not been able to show significant difference between lactating and non-lactating women [16], likely due to small numbers of non-lactating women in the sample, the recent Japanese study evaluated women with migraine at 1, 3, 6, and 12 months postpartum, showing that up to 87.5% of women experienced recurrence in their headaches at the 12 month mark with the percentage of women steadily increasing over the course of the year [25]. Breast-feeding caused a delayed effect on migraine recurrence with lactating women having 50%, 65.8%, 71.1%, and 91.7% recurrence rates at 1, 3, 6, and 12 months, versus non-lactating women whose recurrence rates were 86.4%, 90.9%, 95.5%, and 81.3% respectively.

Pathophysiology of migraine in pregnancy and lactation

The effect of pregnancy on migraine is primarily mediated through female sex hormones. Migraine is impacted by female reproductive events including menarche, the menstrual cycle, use of oral contraceptives, pregnancy, and menopause [5, 6]. Estrogen withdrawal prior to menstruation has been linked to precipitation of menstrual migraine. It is reasonable to infer that the hormonal changes seen in the first trimester of pregnancy and postpartum would lead to unpredictable migraine patterns, whereas the steady rise in estrogen seen in second and third trimesters of pregnancy leads to migraine "stabilization" and even remission.

Effects of migraine on pregnancy

Migraine has been associated with increased risk of vascular disorders of pregnancy, particularly gestational hypertension and preeclampsia [26–29]. Women who have migraine with aura appear to be at higher risk for preeclampsia than those without aura (5.9% vs. 2.9%) [26], whereas the presence of aura appears to have no association with elevated risk of gestational hypertension. Furthermore, peripartum migraine has been associated with myocardial infarction, ischemic stroke, deep vein thrombosis, and thrombophilia [29]. Some researchers postulate that migraine presents a risk factor for reversible cerebral vasoconstriction syndrome (RCVS) as well as other cerebrovascular conditions, including sinus venous thrombosis and hemorrhagic stroke. A large Hungarian study of over 38,000 newborn infants did not find that migraine is related to unfavorable delivery outcomes or birth abnormalities [30]. A more recent study, however, found showed that women with migraine were more likely to have complications during pregnancy and premature birth [31].

Treatment of migraines during pregnancy and lactation

Both pregnancy and lactation complicate treatment options for women with migraine because of the risk of certain medications to the fetus and the nursing child.

There is no consensus on the best method for assessing the drug risk in pregnant women, but the two most widely used are the U.S. Food and Drug Administration (FDA) pregnancy risk rating system and the Teratogen Information Service (TERIS). The FDA assigns a drug to one of five categories. The TERIS classification assesses teratogenic risk rather than a balance between risk and benefit as in the FDA rating system. [32] During lactation, the guidelines of American Academy of Pediatrics [33, 34] and *LactMed* website are valuable resources that rate the safety of medications during breastfeeding. In order to avoid harm to the fetus, the best approach to treatment includes an integrative approach, using non-pharmacological methods in order to minimize the use of medications [35]. The addition of medications should be in a stepwise approach, starting with medications that have the longest history of safety. Table 5.1 provides

Table 5.1 FDA categories for migraine medication in pregnancy

			During pregnancy		
Class	**Abortives**	**Preventive**	**Class**	**Abortives**	**Preventives**
A	Magnesium	Magnesium	C	Triptans, Aspirin	Beta-blockers:taper in last weeks to avoid fetal bradycardia
	Opiates: without Codeine (possible risk of cleft malformations)	Riboflavin		Methadone/Meperidine	Calcium-channel Blockers
		Massage		Morphine-D in third trimester	Topamax
		Biofeedback		Prochlorperazine, Haldol, Promethazine	Gabapentin-concern for fetal bony growth plate
B	Acetaminophen			Isometheptene, Hydroxyzine	SSRIs
	NSAIDs PRN: up to 32 weeks			DHE, Chlorpromazine	Doxepin
	Butorphanol		D	Butalbital-in third semester due to risk of fetal dependence	TCAs
	Codeine, caffeine			Diazepam, Lorazepam	
	Metoclopramide			Pentobarbital	
	Ondansetron				
	Prednisone		X	Ergotamine	Phenytoin, Lithium

a breakdown of migraine acute and preventive treatments and their pregnancy risk rating.

Acute treatment

Women with mild headaches should be encouraged to get adequate rest, a regular sleep pattern, avoid skipping meals take regular exercise, drink plenty of fluids, and avoid caffeine, tobacco, and alcohol. Taking these steps may allow some women to avoid medication altogether. Treatment of acute migraine during pregnancy or lactation in the emergency room (ER) may be initiated with prochlorperazine 10 mg together with intravenous (IV) fluids [41]. Nonsteroidal anti-inflammatory drugs (NSAIDs) should be used cautiously while planning to conceive as they may affect implantation. They are contraindicated in the later stages of pregnancy as they may cause premature closure of fetal ductus arteriosus. Use of triptans is controversial [36–39]. A triptans registry started in 2006 includes 600 women who reported no structural malformations in their newborns after use of these medications during pregnancy. The low level of excretion of sumatriptan in breast milk suggests that breastfeeding following use is unlikely to pose a significant risk to the infant. Data on other triptans is insufficient [41]. Although acetaminophen has long been considered safe for use in pregnancy, a recent study has linked its use in pregnancy to risk of attention-deficit/hyperactivity disorder (ADHD). The effect appears to be related to the quantity of acetaminophen used [40]. Both NSAIDs and triptans are safe in lactation.

Although opiates are safe for treatment of pain during pregnancy, their use for migraine is inappropriate as they can increase nausea and can reduce gastric motility. Chronic use may cause neonatal withdrawal symptoms after delivery. They can be used during lactation but can be passed through breast milk to the infant causing sedation. Information on the safety of butalbital in pregnancy is limited. Phenobarbital is teratogenic and has been associated with hemorrhagic disease and withdrawal in the newborn. It is excreted in the breast milk and its use is not recommended during lactation. Ergots are contraindicated during pregnancy due to uterine hypertonicity and increased risk of miscarriage. Magnesium can be used as abortive treatment for acute migraine headache at a dose of 1 g IV over 15 minutes. A combination of IV prochlorperazine 10 mg every 8 hours and IV magnesium 1 g every 12 hours has been used effectively. Use of IV magnesium beyond 5 days should be avoided due to risk of maternal and fetal hypocalcemia. Metoclopramide, prochlorperazine, and promethazine have been widely used during pregnancy and lactation with no reports of adverse effects.

Preventive treatment

In patients with recurrent migraines, preventive therapy should be considered. Evidence supports the use of biofeedback [42]. This, however, can be very costly and requires considerable patient commitment. If this is not an option, first-line treatment is usually either magnesium or propranolol, although there is concern for intrauterine growth retardation (IUGR) with the beta-blocker, along with possible neonatal bradycardia and hypotension [32, 36]. Magnesium can be used daily as a preventive or in intravenous form as acute treatment in the emergency room. There is conflicting data regarding tricyclic antidepressants. They have been used without complications by numerous anecdotal reports, even though they are a Pregnancy Category D [43]. Low dose amitriptyline 10–25 mg daily has been used in some centers. Sodium valproate is associated with congenital malformations and should be avoided during pregnancy. Topamax is associated with increased risk of cleft palate and should be avoided as preventive therapy during pregnancy [41]. Preventive use in the lactation phase is dependent on the risk of the medication passing into breast milk. The Hales Lactation Rating and Briggs Category are useful resources when choosing therapies during this time. LactMed is an excellent resource provided by the National Library of Medicine's Drug and Lactation Database that is readily available to the public at http://toxnet.nlm.nih.gov/cgi-bin/sis/htmlgen?LACT.

Other primary headaches

In contrast with migraine, other primary headaches (tension and cluster headaches) have been little studied, while the rare primary headaches (hemicranias, other trigeminal autonomic cephalalgias (TACs), new daily persistent headache (NDPH)) have not been studied at all in pregnancy.

Tension-type headache

Tension-type headache is the most prevalent primary headache affecting over 80% of the population [9]. Compared to migraine, studies of tension-type headache during pregnancy have been greatly limited. The relationship between hormonal changes and tension-type headache has not been extensively studied although the possibility of "menstrual tension-type headache" has been suggested [44]. Limitations of studying tension-type headache include the relatively benign phenotype for which patients often do not seek help, and difficulty of diagnosis, especially via questionnaires in large population studies where migraine headaches can often be underdiagnosed as tension-type headaches. Furthermore, studying tension-type headache during pregnancy without the knowledge of prepregnancy diagnosis presents a challenge as migraine phenotype is known to improve in later stages of pregnancy and can therefore be misdiagnosed as tension-type headache.

A recent retrospective study from Turkey that evaluated the effect of sex hormones on migraine and tension-type headache circumvented a lot of these common challenges by performing a nationwide, community-based prevalence study with face-to-face physician interviews using a structured electronic questionnaire [45]. Interestingly, nearly twice the number of women with tension-type headache reported "pure menstrual headache" (defined as day −3 to +5 of menstruation) compared with those with migraine. Women with tension-type headache had fewer changes during pregnancy than those with migraine, with about 20% of women improving versus only 2% worsening [45]. These findings are supported by other studies that have found tension-type headache to be less affected by pregnancy than migraine [9,46]. A relationship of non-migraine headache with parity has been suggested by the Norwegian population-based Head-HUNT study, where the association between headache and pregnancy was significant for women pregnant with their first child, but not for multiparous women [21].

Tension headaches have not been demonstrated to cause adverse effects in pregnancy. Treatment of tension-type headache is often not needed as symptoms tend to be mild or easily treated with routine over-the-counter medications. In the case of severe tension-type headache, acute and preventive treatment used in migraine can be applied, as outlined earlier and in Table 5.1.

Cluster headaches

Cluster headaches are typically more prevalent in men. Therefore, data about the prevalence or impact of cluster headaches on pregnancy are limited. Unlike migraine, cluster headaches do not seem to be affected by hormonal fluctuations during the menstrual cycle [47]. It has also been reported that cluster migraine may be associated with hypofertility possibly due to severe pain experienced by sufferers.

The approach to cluster headaches during pregnancy is similar to that of migraine, with the goal being as conservative as possible to avoid harm to the fetus. Non-pharmacological approaches should be tried first. In cluster headaches, extra consideration should be taken to encourage women who use tobacco or alcohol to abstain during pregnancy because it can lower the risk of cluster outbreaks. It may be useful to screen for sleep apnea as it can increase the risk of complications during pregnancy, including preeclampsia, as well as the episodes of cluster attacks and migraine frequency [48]. The first line of abortive treatment is high-flow oxygen. Although sumatriptan is rated as category C during pregnancy, it may be a reasonable choice given the severe intensity of pain during a cluster attack [49]. The nasal formulation may be tried first before advancing to the injectable form. Occipital nerve blocks can be tried as well as they may break a cluster cycle. Another abortive option could be intranasal lidocaine which is category B. If abortive treatment is not sufficient, preventive therapy may be required. The most frequently used preventive therapy for cluster headache, Verapamil, is a category C medication. Steroids, which are relatively safe in pregnancy, can also be used in attempt to break a cluster cycle [49]. A dose of 60 mg for 2 days, then 40 mg for 2 days, then 20 mg for 2 days is recommended.

Aside from the above discussed primary headaches, very little is known about the course of other primary headaches during pregnancy. Anecdotal reports suggest that primary headaches that are not hormonally regulated (such as tension-type headache) are likely to stay the same or worsen during pregnancy.

Secondary headaches

The major concern with women who complain of headaches during their pregnancy or postpartum period is that they could be having a complication with a secondary cause for their headache that may bring harm to the mother or her developing child. For the most part, the cause of headaches in pregnant women may be similar to nonpregnant women. The evaluation is also similar, including examination for signs and symptoms that may point toward a secondary cause. This is even more pertinent in a woman who complains of first-time headaches during pregnancy, in which case, it is crucial to do a thorough evaluation. Treatment is then based on the postulated underlying etiology. The evaluation of headache begins with a thorough history and physical examination [50]. Important elements of the history include previous history of headaches, especially possible primary headache, as well as a detailed history of the characteristics of their current headache [51]. Important characteristics include location (unilateral vs. bilateral), associated symptoms (nausea, sensitivity to light or sound, change in headache with position, presence of tinnitus, visual or other focal neurological symptoms like numbness or weakness) [51, 52]. The patient's family, medical, and medication use history should also be sought out. Specific answers should alert the clinician about possible red flags or elements of the history that implicate a secondary cause.

Some important red flags to be aware of include sudden onset of a severe headache or the "worst headache," which can raise concern for an intracranial hemorrhage, including ruptured aneurysm. Headaches that are associated with visual changes or pulsatile tinnitus may point to disorders causing increased intracranial pressure. Headaches that are strictly unilateral or "side-locked," or awaken someone overnight are also worrisome. Focal deficits that may alert the clinician to a diagnosis of stroke or mass lesions. Even in patients with a prior history of primary headaches, worsening of the severity or frequency, or change in their previous pattern of headaches can be a sign of a secondary cause. Patients with a previous or current malignancy or an immunosuppressed state, such as human immunodeficiency virus (HIV) also merit further testing. A complete neurological examination, including an ophthalmoscopic examination to look for papilledema, is an essential element of the evaluation.

For the most part, the work-up of headache in pregnant women is similar to that of nonpregnant women, with some specific considerations. If imaging is required, MRI is preferred over CT scan to avoid risk of radiation to the fetus. Iodinated contrast can potentially decrease thyroid function, and if used, thyroid function should be checked in the first week after birth in the infant [53]. While use of MRI is preferred over use of CT, gadolinium contrast is FDA class C and should be avoided during pregnancy if possible. In animal studies, maternal exposure to gadolinium leads to higher rates of developmental abnormalities and fetal loss. Non-contrast MR angiogram and MR venogram can be done with time of flight sequences. If gadolinium is necessary to guide treatment, the mother may be counselled on potential risks to the fetus. There is no contraindication to use of gadolinium after delivery in breastfeeding mothers [54]. Some obstetricians advocate a 24-hour pump and dump period after administration of gadolinium [55]. Because this represents a time of quickly shifting hormones, many of the secondary conditions may also occur during the peri- and postpartum period. Migraines that had improved during pregnancy may also return during this time. Up to 75% of headaches in the postpartum period are due to primary headaches, with the majority related to migraine, but it is crucial to exclude secondary headaches with more ominous prognoses [56].

Preeclampsia and Eclampsia

Preeclampsia and eclampsia occur in 2–8% of pregnancies. They may present after weeks 20 (most commonly after week 28) until 8 weeks postpartum. Preeclampsia presents with hypertension, proteinuria, peripheral edema, and often with headaches. When these symptoms present with seizures, a diagnoses of eclampsia is established. Risk is elevated in women with primiparity, advanced maternal age, multiparity, history of preeclampsia, history of hypertension, DM, kidney failure, and systemic lupus erythematosus [57].

HELLP syndrome

The HELLP syndrome is associated with hemolysis, elevated liver enzymes, and low platelet count. It occurs in 10–20% of women with severe eclampsia. In addition to hypertension and headaches, women with HELLP will often complain of abdominal pain, malaise, nausea and vomiting, confusion, blurred vision, scintillating scotoma, paresthesias, and photophobia. Neurologic examination reveals hyperreflexia. Severe cases may be complicated by acute renal failure, pulmonary edema, and disseminated intravascular coagulation. Eclampsia occurs in 1–2% of patients with severe preeclampsia and presents with generalized tonic–clonic seizures as a result of cerebral involvement. It carries a mortality rate of up to 14%. One-third of patients who present with eclampsia do not have associated proteinuria nor hypertension. Delivery of the placenta is curative. Seizures are controlled until delivery with administration of magnesium [41].

Post-dural headaches

Post-dural headache can be a complication of epidural or spinal anesthesia. These low pressure headaches can be distinguished from other types of headache as they worsen with upright position and improve with lying flat. There may also be associated pulsatile tinnitus, diplopia, or hypacusia, symptoms usually not seen in primary headache disorders [55]. The mechanism is thought to be an unintended dural puncture, but can occur with spontaneous leakage of CSF during labor. They usually present early in the same day but have been reported days or weeks after the epidural or labor, therefore should be considered with any positional headache and a history of pregnancy. In some reports, incidence is as high as 16% [58]. If mild, initial treatment may be conservative including caffeine and fluids, generally leading to resolution of the headache within a few days. If severe or persistent, placement of a blood patch should be considered. There should be a low threshold for imaging with MRI or MRV to rule out other possible causes including sinus venous thrombosis [55].

Sheehan's syndrome

This is a syndrome of pituitary insufficiency usually due to postpartum pituitary hemorrhage. A retrospective study showed that most patients presented with symptoms of hypopituitarism, which in some cases can be subtle [59]. Headache may be a presenting symptom as well, although it is usually overshadowed by other signs, including the inability to lactate as the most common [59].

Other secondary headaches

Other secondary causes of headaches that can occur in pregnant women include stroke, sinus venous thrombosis, and RCVS. Aura is an important symptom to look for as it can present for the first time during pregnancy, but also can be a symptom of a vascular etiology, including carotid dissection, thrombocytopenia or imminent eclampsia. Migraine has been associated with increased risk of hypertensive disorders of pregnancy, which can lead to other complications during this time [26, 56].

Reversible cerebral vasoconstriction syndrome/postpartum angiopathy

Reversible cerebral vasoconstriction syndrome (RCVS) is an important cause of morbidity during pregnancy. Precipitating factors include medications such as SSRIs, ergot alkaloids, and sympathomimetics. Uncontrolled hypertension and endocrine dysfunction have also been recognized as triggering factors. In the pregnant and postpartum population, RCVS is felt to be a manifestation of eclampsia/preeclampsia, but may present in the absence of hypertension

and proteinuria. It is most common in the first four weeks of the postpartum period. Affected patients complain of acute onset of severe thunderclap headaches, photophobia, nausea, and vomiting. Focal neurologic deficits, confusion, and seizures may also occur [60]. Brain MRI/MRA is abnormal in 80% of patients. MRI may demonstrate patchy foci of abnormal T_2 hyperintensity in the white matter and watershed regions. Acute ischemic infarction and hemorrhage may be associated. The MRA/CTA or angiogram reveals multifocal and scattered constriction and post-stenotic dilation of arteries in a "string of beads" pattern. Treatment includes calcium channel blockers including verapamil [41].

Posterior reversible encephelopathy syndrome

Posterior reversible encephalopathy syndrome (PRES) was first described in 1996 [61]. It is seen in clinical conditions that increase the permeability of the blood–brain barrier, especially vulnerable in the posterior regions of the brain. Although the presenting symptoms can be vague, acute headache, and cortical visual symptoms are common, along with seizures or encephalopathy. There have been case reports of preeclampsia and eclampsia that are complicated by PRES. The MRI will reveal hyperintensities in the posterior regions, including the occipital and parietal lobes, although frontal abnormalities are occasionally seen.

Stroke—Ischemic/hemorrhagic

Women with migraine are at a higher risk of stroke during pregnancy and peripartum. Women are hypercoagulable during pregnancy and postpartum thereby increasing the risk of clotting diseases [62]. The incidence of stroke during this time is 11–26 per 100,000 deliveries, with a mortality of 10–13% [63, 64]. Although headache can be a presenting symptom of either type of stroke, it is more common with hemorrhage than ischemic stroke. There will usually be other presenting symptoms, including focal neurological deficits or elevated blood pressure. The headache is usually acute in onset. Most strokes occur in the third trimester or postpartum because this is when peak hypercoagulability occurs [55]; MRI is usually diagnostic. Treatment of acute ischemic stroke can be difficult as tPa has not been tested in pregnant women.

Sinus venous thrombosis

Sinus venous thrombosis is another potential complication during pregnancy due to the hypercoagulable state. One large retrospective study showed that the rate of SVT during pregnancy and puerperum was 0.15% with almost three-fourth of that during the peripartum period [65]. In another study, the prevalence of SVT was about 11.6 cases per 100,000 deliveries. Headache was a frequent presenting symptom, present in almost all of the patients followed by nausea, vomiting, and blurred vision. The most frequent associated factor is any type of congenital thrombophilia, while pregnancy is also a known risk factor, due to fluctuating intracranial pressure and hypercoaguability during this time. Although most cases will present acutely, at times patients can complain of a moderate to severe subacute headache ongoing for a few weeks up to a month. The headache is usually diffuse and progressive, although there are case reports of it presenting as "thunderclap," as well. Other reported symptoms include papilledema and sixth nerve palsies, for which increased intracranial pressure is in the differential. Venous infarcts may occur and can present with focal deficits or seizures. The diagnosis is made with imaging of the sinuses with noncontrast MR venogram. Treatment with low-molecular-weight heparin is indicated [66].

Pregnancy and the peripartum period pose particular challenges for women with preexisting history of headache due to the limitations of treatment options in these periods. Fortunately, headache in general and migraine in particular tend to improve as pregnancy progresses. Challenge is presented by the recurrence of headache postpartum and the need to treat headache in lactating women, though breastfeeding (vs. bottle-feeding) itself is also protective.

Treatment of severe headache and in particular migraine which peaks during childbearing age is often limited by plans of conception. Childbearing potential and family planning need to be considered in treatment of all premenopausal women with headache. Migraine is significantly affected by fluctuating sex hormones and is furthermore associated with gestational hypertension and preeclampsia of pregnancy. Both women with and without preexisting history of primary headache can develop secondary headaches during pregnancy. The diagnostic workup of these headaches is somewhat "challenging given" the risk of some tests and procedures in pregnancy. However, as pregnancy is a prothrombotic state, a high index of suspicion needs to be present in the evaluation of any new or changed headache during this time.

References

1 Macgregor EA, Rosenberg JD, Kurth T. Sex-related differences in epidemiological and clinic-based headache studies. *Headache*. 2011;51(6): 843–859.

2 Victor TW, Hu X, Campbell JC, Buse DC, Lipton RB. Migraine prevalence by age and sex in the United States: a life-span study. *Cephalalgia*. 2010;30(9):1065–1072.

3 Stewart WF, Lipton RB, Celentano DD, Reed ML. Prevalence of migraine headache in the United States. Relation to age, income, race, and other sociodemographic factors. *JAMA*. 1992;267(1): 64–69.

4 Lance JW, Anthony M. Some clinical aspects of migraine. A prospective survey of 500 patients. *Arch. Neurol*. 1966;15(4):356–361.

5 Granella F, Sances G, Zanferrari C, Costa A, Martignoni E, Manzoni GC. Migraine without aura and reproductive life events: a clinical epidemiological study in 1300 women. *Headache*. 1993; 33(7): 385–389.

6 Cupini LM, Matteis M, Troisi E, Calabresi P, Bernardi G, Silvestrini M. Sex-hormone-related events in migrainous females. A clinical comparative study between migraine with aura and migraine without aura. *Cephalalgia*. 1995;15(2): 140–144.

7 Granella F, Sances G, Pucci E, Nappi RE, Ghiotto N, Napp G. Migraine with aura and reproductive life events: a case control study. *Cephalalgia*. 2000; 20(8):701–707.

8 Mattsson P. Migraine headache and obesity in women aged 40–74 years: a population-based study. *Cephalalgia*. 2007;27(8):877–880.

9 Rasmussen BK. Migraine and tension-type headache in a general population: precipitating factors, female hormones, sleep pattern and relation to lifestyle. *Pain*. 1993;53(1):65–72.

10 Epstein MT, Hockaday JM, Hockaday TD. Migraine and reproductive hormones throughout the menstrual cycle. *Lancet*. 1975;1(7906):543–548.

11 Callaghan N. The migraine syndrome in pregnancy. *Neurology*. 1968;18(2):197–199 (passim).

12 Somerville BW. A study of migraine in pregnancy. *Neurology*. 1972;22(8):824–828.

13 Scharff L, Marcus DA, Turk DC. Headache during pregnancy and in the postpartum: a prospective study. *Headache*. 1997;37(4):203–210.

14 Marcus DA, Scharff L, Turk D. Longitudinal prospective study of headache during pregnancy and postpartum. *Headache*. 1999;39(9): 625–632.

15 Chen TC, Leviton A. Headache recurrence in pregnant women with migraine. *Headache*. 1994; 34(2):107–110.

16 Kvisvik EV, Stovner LJ, Helde G, Bovim G, Linde M. Headache and migraine during pregnancy and puerperium: the MIGRA-study. *J Headache Pain*. 2011;12(4):443–451.

17 Sances G, Granella F, Nappi RE, et al. Course of migraine during pregnancy and postpartum: a prospective study. *Cephalalgia*. 2003;23(3):197–205.

18 Melhado E, Maciel JA, Guerreiro CAM. Headaches during pregnancy in women with a prior history of menstrual headaches. *Arq Neuropsiquiatr*. 2005;63(4):934–940.

19 Mattsson P. Hormonal factors in migraine: a population-based study of women aged 40 to 74 years. *Headache*. 2003;43(1):27–35.

20 Maggioni F, Alessi C, Maggino T, Zanchin G. Headache during pregnancy. *Cephalalgia*. 1997;17(7):765–769.

21 Aegidius K, Zwart J-A, Hagen K, Stovner L. The effect of pregnancy and parity on headache prevalence: the Head-HUNT study. *Headache*. 2009;49(6):851–859.

22 Stein G, Morton J, Marsh A, et al. Headaches after childbirth. *Acta Neurol Scand*. 1984;69(2): 74–79.

23 Wright GD, Patel MK. Focal migraine and pregnancy. *Br Med J (Clin Res Ed)*. 1986;293(6561): 1557–1558.

24 Aubé M. Migraine in pregnancy. *Neurology*. 1999;53(4 Suppl 1):S26–S28.

25 Hoshiyama E, Tatsumoto M, Iwanami H, et al. Postpartum migraines: a long-term prospective study. *Intern Med*. 2012;51(22):3119–3123.

26 Facchinetti F, Allais G, Nappi RE, et al. Migraine is a risk factor for hypertensive disorders in pregnancy: a prospective cohort study. *Cephalalgia*. 2009;29(3):286–292.

27 Facchinetti F, Allais G, D'Amico R, Benedetto C, Volpe A. The relationship between headache and preeclampsia: a case-control study. *Eur J Obstet Gynecol Reprod Biol*. 2005;121(2):143–148.

28 Sanchez SE, Qiu C, Williams MA, Lam N, Sorensen TK. Headaches and migraines are associated with an increased risk of preeclampsia in Peruvian women. *Am J Hypertens*. 2008;21(3):360–364.

29 Bushnell CD, Jamison M, James AH. Migraines during pregnancy linked to stroke and vascular diseases: US population based case-control study. *BMJ*. 2009;338:b664.

30 Bánhidy F, Acs N, Horváth-Puhó E, Czeizel AE. Maternal severe migraine and risk of congenital limb deficiencies. *Birth Defects Res A Clin Mol Teratol*. 2006;76(8):592–601.

31 Marozio L, Facchinetti F, Allais G, et al. Headache and adverse pregnancy outcomes: a prospective study. *Eur J Obstet Gynecol Reprod Biol*. 2012;161(2): 140–143.

32 Lucas S. Medication use in the treatment of migraine during pregnancy and lactation. *Curr Pain Headache Rep*. 2009;13(5):392–398.

33 Transfer of drugs and other chemicals into human milk. *Pediatrics*. 2001;108(3):776–789.

34 Sachs HC. The transfer of drugs and therapeutics into human breast milk: an update on selected topics. *Pediatrics*. 2013;132(3):e796–809.

35 Nezvalová-Henriksen K, Spigset O, Nordeng H. Maternal characteristics and migraine pharmacotherapy during pregnancy: cross-sectional analysis of data from a large cohort study. *Cephalalgia*. 2009;29(12):1267–1276.

36 Pfaffenrath V, Rehm M. Migraine in pregnancy: what are the safest treatment options? *Drug Saf.* 1998;19(5):383–388.

37 Evers S, Afra J, Frese A, et al. EFNS guideline on the drug treatment of migraine–revised report of an EFNS task force. *Eur J Neurol.* 2009;16(9):968–981.

38 Loder E. Safety of sumatriptan in pregnancy: a review of the data so far. *CNS Drugs.* 2003;17(1):1–7.

39 Hutchinson S, Marmura MJ, Calhoun A, Lucas S, Silberstein S, Peterlin BL. Use of common migraine treatments in breast-feeding women: a summary of recommendations. *Headache.* 2013;53(4):614–627.

40 Liew Z, Ritz B, Rebordosa C, Lee P-C, Olsen J. Acetaminophen use during pregnancy, behavioral problems, and hyperkinetic disorders. *JAMA Pediatr.* 2014;168(4):313–320.

41 MacGregor EA. Headache in Pregnancy. *Continuum.* 2014;20(1):128–147.

42 Airola G, Allais G, Castagnoli Gabellari I, Rolando S, Mana O, Benedetto C. Non-pharmacological management of migraine during pregnancy. *Neurol Sci.* 2010;31(Suppl 1):S63–S65.

43 Brandes JL. Headache related to pregnancy: management of migraine and migraine headache in pregnancy. *Curr Treat Options Neurol.* 2008;10(1):12–19

44 Arjona A, Rubi-Callejon J, Guardado-Santervas P, Serrano-Castro P, Olivares J. Menstrual tension-type headache: evidence for its existence. *Headache.* 2007;47(1):100–103.

45 Karlı N, Baykan B, Ertaş M, et al. Impact of sex hormonal changes on tension-type headache and migraine: a cross-sectional population-based survey in 2,600 women. *J Headache Pain.* 2012;13(7):557–565.

46 Ertresvåg JM, Zwart J-A, Helde G, Johnsen H-J, Bovim G. Headache and transient focal neurological symptoms during pregnancy, a prospective cohort. *Acta Neurol Scand.* 2005;111(4):233–237.

47 Manzoni GC, Micieli G, Granella F, Martignoni E, Farina S, Nappi G. Cluster headache in women: clinical findings and relationship with reproductive life. *Cephalalgia.* 1988;8(1):37–44.

48 Graff-Radford SB, Newman A. Obstructive sleep apnea and cluster headache. *Headache.* 2004;44(6):607–610.

49 Calhoun AH, Peterlin BL. Treatment of cluster headache in pregnancy and lactation. *Curr Pain Headache Rep.* 2010;14(2):164–173.

50 Von Wald T, Walling AD. Headache during pregnancy. *Obstet Gynecol Surv.* 2002;57(3):179–185.

51 Digre KB. Headaches during pregnancy. *Clin Obstet Gynecol.* 2013;56(2):317–329.

52 Mandel S. Hemiplegic migraine in pregnancy. *Headache.* 1988;28(6):414–416.

53 Webb JAW, Thomsen HS. Gadolinium contrast media during pregnancy and lactation. *Acta Radiol.* 2013;54(6):599–600.

54 ACOG Committee Opinion. Guidelines for diagnostic imaging during pregnancy. Number 299, September 2004 (replaces No. 158, September 1995). *Obstet Gynecol.* 2004;104(3):647–651.

55 430Bove RM, Klein JP. Neuroradiology in women of childbearing age. *Continuum.* 2014;20(1):23–41.

56 Klein AM, Loder E. Postpartum headache. *Int J Obstet Anesth.* 2010;19(4):422–

57 Adeney KL, Williams MA, Miller RS, Frederick IO, Sorensen TK, Luthy DA. Risk of preeclampsia in relation to maternal history of migraine headaches. *J Matern Fetal Neonatal Med.* 2005; 18(3):167–172.

58 Goldszmidt E, Kern R, Chaput A, Macarthur A. The incidence and etiology of postpartum headaches: a prospective cohort study. *Can J Anaesth.* 2005;52(9):971–977.

59 Sanyal D, Raychaudhuri M. Varied presentations of Sheehan's syndrome at diagnosis: A review of 18 patients. *Indian J Endocrinol Metab.* 2012; 16(Suppl 2):S300–S301.

60 Sheikh HU, Mathew PG. Reversible cerebral vasoconstriction syndrome: updates and new perspectives. *Curr Pain Headache Rep.* 2014;18(5):414.

61 Krishnamoorthy U, Sarkar PK, Nakhuda Y, Mullins PD. Posterior reversible encephalopathy syndrome (PRES) in pregnancy: a diagnostic challenge to obstetricians. *J Obstet Gynaecol.* 2009;29(3):192–194.

62 Wickström K, Edelstam G, Löwbeer CH, Hansson LO, Siegbahn A. Reference intervals for plasma levels of fibronectin, von Willebrand factor, free protein S and antithrombin during third-trimester pregnancy. *Scand J Clin Lab Invest.* 2004;64(1):31–40.

63 Kittner SJ, Stern BJ, Feeser BR, et al. Pregnancy and the risk of stroke. *N Engl J Med.* 1996; 335(11):768–774.

64 Sharshar T, Lamy C, Mas JL. Incidence and causes of strokes associated with pregnancy and

puerperium. A study in public hospitals of Ile de France. Stroke in Pregnancy Study Group. *Stroke.* 1995;26(6):930–936.

65 Zhou Q, Wang F, Zhang P, Long X, Sun X, Liu T. Clinical characteristics and outcomes of cerebral venous sinus thrombosis during pregnancy and puerperium. *Zhonghua Fu Chan Ke Za Zhi.* 2010;45(5):358–362.

66 Wittmann M, Dewald D, Urbach H, et al. Sinus venous thrombosis: a differential diagnosis of postpartum headache. *Arch Gynecol Obstet.* 2012; 285(1):93–97.

CHAPTER 6

Stroke in pregnancy and the puerperium

Louis R. Caplan[1] & Diogo C. Haussen[2]

[1] Beth Israel Deaconess Medical Center, Harvard Medical School, Boston, MA, USA
[2] Emory University School of Medicine, Atlanta, GA, USA

Introduction

Pregnancy and the puerperium (period of 6 weeks postpartum) are times of important physiological changes in the mother. These adaptive changes impact cerebrovascular homeostasis and lead to an increased risk for strokes and other vascular changes. Some cerebrovascular complications involve circumstances related to pregnancy and the postpartum period while others are maternal conditions that preceded pregnancy and might have occurred at any time. Despite ischemic or hemorrhagic strokes being uncommon during this period, they constitute a challenging diagnostic complication that often leads to therapeutic dilemmas and to significant morbidity and mortality. Herein we emphasize those conditions that are unique to pregnancy and the puerperium or occur much more frequent during these times. Causes of stroke that are unrelated to pregnancy are covered in much more detail elsewhere [1].

Physiological changes that affect blood vessels and blood flow

Endocrinological

Steroid hormones generate changes in glucose metabolism that can lead to elevated gestational glycemia and contribute to an enhanced risk of stroke [2].

Progesterone levels increase during pregnancy and drop after delivery. The increased progesterone levels at the end of pregnancy is posited to cause increased venous distensibility, which could in part explain varicose veins and a susceptibility for thrombotic events [2]. Estrogen levels rise during pregnancy and become much more important in proportion to progesterone levels by the end of gestation; this has been posited to increase the production of clotting factors in the liver [2].

Hematological

Variance analyses show an increase of procoagulant factors with advancing gestational age: fibrinogen increases, natural anticoagulants (protein C and S) decrease, and prothrombin fragments increase. In regard to the fibrinolytic system, an increase both for type 1 plasminogen activator inhibitor activity and tissue plasminogen activator (tPA) antigen have been described [3]. This explains why there is an increased tendency of developing thromboembolic events in the third trimester of pregnancy [2]. Inherited and acquired thrombophilias confer an increased risk of venous thromboembolic events during pregnancy, as well as arterial events in the case of the antiphospholipid antibody syndrome [2].

Neurological Illness in Pregnancy: Principles and Practice, First Edition.
Edited by Autumn Klein, M. Angela O'Neal, Christina Scifres, Janet F. R. Waters and Jonathan H. Waters.
© 2016 John Wiley & Sons, Ltd. Published 2016 by John Wiley & Sons, Ltd.

Cardiovascular

In the early months of pregnancy, the body retains water and cardiac output substantially increases. Cardiac output continues to increase until mid-pregnancy, and then remains stable afterward. Blood pressure decreases during early pregnancy, reaches a nadir in mid pregnancy, and returns to baseline at term. During labor, both cardiac output and blood pressure increase. After birth, cardiac output begins to decrease within the first hour to reach baseline 2 weeks postpartum [4].

Epidemiology

Despite the general understanding that pregnancy and the postpartum period are associated with an increased risk of stroke, the quantitative data supporting this assumption is not sufficient for precise conclusions [5]. In many studies all strokes are considered together and are not separated into ischemic or hemorrhagic strokes or into subtypes of these two polar opposites.

In a nationwide Swedish registry evaluation, the frequency of thromboembolic conditions per 100,000 pregnancies during pregnancy and the postpartum period were 92.3 for venous thrombosis, 17.0 for pulmonary embolism, 4.0 for cerebral infarction, 3.8 for intracerebral hemorrhage (ICH), 2.4 for subarachnoid hemorrhage (SAH), and 0.6 for acute myocardial infarction [6].

The spectrum of cerebrovascular disease associated with pregnancy and the puerperium was characterized in a study that reviewed the medical records of a single institution during a 17-year period [7]. Among more than 50,000 deliveries at this tertiary referral center, 34 strokes were identified; 21 (62%) were ischemic (13 arterial and 8 venous) and 13 (38%) were hemorrhagic (7 subarachnoid and 6 intracerebral) [7]. They estimated that among 100,000 deliveries there might be 67 cerebrovascular events (41 infarctions and 26 hemorrhages).

The overall risk of pregnancy-related stroke in a U.S. Nationwide Inpatient Sample was less than that reported above, being 34.2 per 100,000 deliveries (ischemic, hemorrhagic, or cerebral venous thrombosis (CVT)) [8].

Another study was conducted in 63 public maternity centers in a well defined geographic area in France (which should have minimized selection bias related to single-tertiary center referrals). The authors estimated the frequencies per 100,000 deliveries as approximately 4 ischemic strokes (including postpartum angiopathy, dissections, etc.) and 4 hemorrhagic strokes (including malformations, aneurysms) [9].

In a study of hemorrhagic strokes over a 10-year representative sample of the entire U.S. obstetrical population through the Nationwide Inpatient Sample, the rate of pregnancy-related ICH was 6.1 per 100,000 deliveries [10].

The frequencies of eclampsia and preeclampsia and their relation to strokes are not reliable since definitions vary especially regarding puerperal eclampsia. Information available is cited in the section of the chapter on eclampsia. Knowledge about the reversible cerebral vasoconstriction syndrome (RCVS) and technology to document its presence are quite recent so that there are very scant data about the frequency of this syndrome and its relation to stroke. Imaging able to document occlusion of the draining brain dural sinuses and veins is also relatively new so that data about the occurrence of venous occlusion-related infarcts and hemorrhages is also scanty.

A precise incidence of cerebrovascular diseases is difficult to ascertain due to heterogeneous definitions, due to the retrospective nature of the majority of the studies, and due to selection bias. Multiple studies used discharge coding for detection of cases. Nevertheless, in contrast to a preponderance of ischemic strokes in the nonpregnant population, there is a clear relative increased risk of intracranial hemorrhages during pregnancy and the postpartum period [5, 9].

In contradistinction to the numbers cited above, a retrospective study done in a large health maintenance organizations (HMOs) population defined the incidence of stroke in nonpregnant women aged 15–44 years as just slightly higher than cases related to pregnancies within the same studied population. The incidence for nonpregnant women was 10.7/100,000 women-years compared with 5.6 per 100,000 deliveries in pregnant women [11].

The risk of stroke according to race indicates that African-American women might have a higher risk of stroke compared with Hispanic or White women [8]. There is scant epidemiological data for the Asians [12].

Timing of ischemic strokes according to the pregnancy stage or puerperium

A large retrospective single-institutional review from Canada investigated the timing of different subtypes of strokes according to the trimester of pregnancy or puerperal period [7]. The authors reported that most arterial ischemic strokes presented in the third trimester and puerperium, and that all but one venous infarction presented in the puerperium [7]. A multicenter regional hospital-based registry (Baltimore–Washington Cooperative Young Stroke Study) corroborated these findings and described that the risk of ischemic stroke is greatest during the postpartum period, the third trimester being the second most important time [5].

In a multicenter study from Ile de France involving more than 60 maternity centers, the incidence of ischemic stroke was found to increase progressively from the first trimester to the third, supporting the suggestion that the peak incidence is reached in the puerperium [9].

Of note, only one case of ischemic stroke was related to CVT in the Baltimore–Washington population, and CVTs were excluded from the French study. Therefore, the puerperal predominance of ischemic strokes is likely truly related to a higher frequency of arterial ischemic strokes in this period, and not explained by the admixing of CVT cases.

Timing of hemorrhagic strokes according to the pregnancy stage or puerperium

The timing of intracranial hemorrhages is less clearly defined. A French study reported a peak of hemorrhagic strokes in the third trimester, but this population had a high frequency of eclampsia (44%) [9]. A recent study from the United States showed that the most common period was the puerperium [10]. The Baltimore–Washington Cooperative Study also suggested that postpartum was the most common period. The second peak was in the second trimester. Most occurrences during the second trimester were related to bleeding from arteriovenous malformations (AVM) [5].

In a Canadian study, patients were divided into patients with ICH and patients with SAH; these two groups presented very similarly regarding the timing, with a peak in the second trimester followed by a second peak in the puerperium [7]. Among patients with intracranial bleeds with determined etiology, aneurysm-related bleeds presented during pregnancy in all trimesters but not in the puerperium. The AVM-related bleeds occurred most commonly in the second trimester, but also in the third trimester and puerperium. Coagulopathy-related bleeds all occurred during the postpartum period [7].

These population and registry-derived studies have limitations. The risk of ischemic or hemorrhagic events seems to be more prominent in the end of the third trimester and in the ultra-early puerperium. One study reported the risk to be the highest within the period of 2 days before and 1 day after delivery [6].

Pregnancy-related conditions

Preeclampsia and eclampsia

Preeclampsia refers to the development of new-onset hypertension (>140/90 mmHg) and proteinuria after 20 weeks of gestation in a previously normal woman, although it may arise during the postpartum period [13]. If a grand-mal seizure develops, the classification becomes eclampsia. The PE/E are important variables that impact not only on general maternal morbidity and mortality, but also the tendency of strokes to occur in the end of pregnancy and postpartum period [2, 9]. The HELLP syndrome (Hemolysis, Elevated Liver enzymes, Low Platelets) represents a severe form of preeclampsia; however, the syndrome may develop independently.

The pathophysiology of PE/E is posited to relate to an inadequate secondary trophoblastic placental invasion with abnormal development of spiral arteries; this leads to placental ischemia and consequent multiorgan disorder associated with diffuse endothelial dysfunction [14]. The PE/E is characterized by widespread dysfunction of the maternal endothelium that results in enhanced formation of endothelin and thromboxane (a platelet-derived vasoconstrictor and stimulant of platelet aggregation), increased vascular sensitivity to angiotensin II, and decreased formation of vasodilators (nitrous oxide (NO) and prostacyclin) [14, 15]. The endothelial injury may provoke hypertension, vasoconstriction with consequent ischemia, and development of thrombosis. Treating physicians must pay special attention to elevations of blood pressure compared to the pressures earlier during pregnancy. In a woman whose blood pressures averaged 100/60 during pregnancy, a blood pressure of 140/90 along with pedal edema and proteinuria is diagnostic of PE and the blood pressure must be urgently reduced.

Abnormal vascular autoregulation might lead to vasoconstriction and consequent distal ischemia, potentially leading to brain infarction. Patients with PE/E might develop exhaustion of the cerebral vasomotor reactivity, leading to vasoplegia, loosening of the blood–brain barrier tight junctions, and extravasation of plasma into the parenchymal interstitium. Hyperactivity and exaggerated deep tendon reflexes and pedal edema are important signs of early preeclampsia. This process can cause brain swelling and potentially hemorrhagic changes,

leading to a non-rare complication of eclampsia: the posterior reversible encephalopathy syndrome (PRES) (which is discussed later in this chapter).

Eclampsia has been related to almost half of the strokes during pregnancy, accounting for 47% of cases of ischemic and 44% of ICH patients in one study [9]. In the Baltimore–Washington Cooperative Young Stroke Study, 38% of brain infarctions were attributable to eclampsia and angiographically defined central nervous system vasculopathy [5]. Eclampsia was correlated with 15% of the cases of ICH [5].

A detailed description of the treatment strategies for PE/E treatment is beyond the scope of this chapter. Low dose aspirin has been observed to have moderate benefits when used for prevention and treatment of preeclampsia in a meta-analysis [16]. Lowering of blood pressure is imperative for the prevention of PE/E complications. Magnesium sulfate has been shown to reduce the frequency of seizures but does not effectively reduce blood pressure. Antihypertensive agents are essential to normalize blood pressure. Nevertheless, delivery of the baby is the only effective treatment of PE/E during the last trimester [2].

Posterior reversible encephalopathy syndrome

The PRES is a clinicoradiographic entity that includes headaches, confusion, seizures, visual loss, and stereotypical radiological findings. The neuroimaging findings are characterized by vasogenic subcortical white matter edema (although the cerebral cortex is also sometimes involved), most often in the posterior regions of the cerebral hemispheres [17–19]. Characteristically, the paramedian striate cortex is spared on both sides, differentiating the imaging findings from embolic infarction of the bilateral posterior cerebral artery supplied occipital and temporal lobes (Figure 6.1). The edema can also involve the frontal lobes and occasionally the brain stem and/or cerebellum.

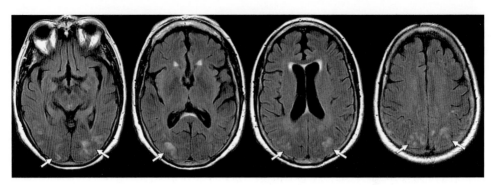

Figure 6.1 Illustrative case posterior reversible encephalopathy syndrome. FLAIR MR sequence with axial cuts. Arrows indicate vasogenic edema predominantly affecting the posterior cerebral regions with sparing of the paramedian occipital cortex.

The PRES has been described in association with multiple conditions, including hypertensive emergencies, cytotoxic/immunosuppressant drugs, acute renal disease, acute porphyria, toxic/systemic conditions, and dialysis [19, 20].

This syndrome is believed to be a capillary leak syndrome, related to increased body fluid retention and endothelial injury [2]. There is no definitive explanation for the predominant involvement of the posterior circulation supplied territories. The posterior circulation has been posited to have less important sympathetic innervation, which could potentially make it more prone to loss of autoregulation [21]. A loss of vascular reactivity has been demonstrated by the finding of impaired vasomotor responses as measured by transcranial Doppler [22]. The PRES is classically a transitory disorder that resolves once the offending mechanism is treated.

The MRI imaging is the most appropriate diagnostic test. In one study, MR was performed in 30 patients with preeclampsia and 9 with eclampsia, being normal in 21 of them. In 18 patients, cortical–subcortical lesions (iso/hypointense on T_1W and hyperintense on T_2W/FLAIR images) were detected in the occipital lobes of all patients. Lesions in the parietal, frontal, and temporal lobes, and basal ganglia and pons were also detected, as well as changes in the watershed distribution in 13 patients [23].

The MRI is very sensitive to ischemia and to blood products, which are occasionally detected in addition to the vasogenic edema. The PRES patients show areas of diffusion-weighted imaging (DWI) hyperintensity in 17–27% [24, 25]. Intracranial hemorrhage (parenchymal hematoma or isolated sulcal/subarachnoid blood) has been described in approximately 17% of PRES patients [25]. The treatment of PRES in the setting of PE/E is mainly controlling blood pressure and treating seizures.

Reversible cerebral vasoconstriction syndrome

Reversible cerebral vasoconstriction syndrome constitutes a very important and underrecognized cause of strokes in the pregnancy and puerperium. It is a group of disorders characterized by the development of a sudden and very severe headache ("thunderclap headache") associated with prolonged but reversible segmental narrowing (or "beading") in medium and large intracranial arteries. The arteries typically affected are the internal carotid, middle cerebral, anterior cerebral, vertebral, basilar, posterior cerebral, and/or superior/anterior inferior/posterior inferior cerebellar arteries (Figure 6.2) [2, 26].

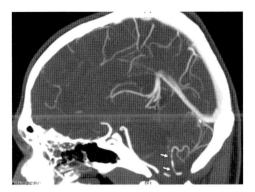

Figure 6.2 Illustrative case of reversible cerebral vasoconstriction syndrome. Sagital CT angiogram (maximum intensity projection images). Arrows indicate segments of constriction and dilatation ("beading") of the left posterior inferior cerebellar artery.

The RCVS is associated with many different conditions and has been labeled over the last decades with different names, including Call–Fleming syndrome, benign angiopathy of the central nervous system, thunderclap headache with reversible vasospasm, migrainous vasospasm (or migraine angiitis), drug-induced cerebral angiopathy (consequence of exposure to vasoactive drugs such as stimulants, serotonin reuptake inhibitor antidepressants, marijuana splurges, nasal decongestants, cocaine and amphetamines, etc.), and postpartum angiopathy [26]. Of note, some posit a history of migraines before pregnancy might predispose to RCVS. Only recently physicians have recognized that these entities represent one condition collectively called RCVS [2, 26].

In a seminal report published in 1988, Gregory Call, Marie Fleming and colleagues described 7 patients from their institution with "reversible cerebral arterial segmental vasoconstriction" and collected another 12 cases reported from the literature. Among the 19 patients, 6 were in the puerperium. There was an overall noticeable female preponderance, and patients were young, and typically had acute and severe headache and normal CSF

studies. The RCVS is occasionally still referred as Call–Fleming syndrome [27].

Reversible cerebral vasoconstriction syndrome can occur in late pregnancy, early puerperium and can be associated with PE/E [26, 28, 29]. Most patients with RCVS presenting in the puerperium have had an uncomplicated pregnancy, labor, and delivery. One suggested pathophysiological mechanism include the rapid fall of progesterone (which acts as a vasodilator) contributing to constriction. Other possibility is related to stress in "predisposed-to-hyperactivity" cranial vessels due to changes in blood volume, blood pressure, and blood flow in the end of pregnancy and the puerperium [2].

In a recent retrospective series of 18 patients with postpartum angiopathy, neurological symptoms began on average on day 5 postpartum and included headache (89%), focal deficit (50%), visual disturbance (44%), encephalopathy (33%), and seizures (28%), commonly in combination [30]. Two-thirds had a history of a prior uneventful pregnancy [30]. The headache is usually diffuse or occipital, severe in intensity, typically throbbing, and may be accompanied by nausea, vomiting, and photosensitivity [26]. The cephalalgia might be recurrent and may present with or without neurological findings. The most important elements for diagnosis are described in Table 6.1. The findings described

Table 6.1 Important elements for the diagnosis of Reversible Cerebral Vasoconstriction Syndrome [26].

1 Segmental cerebral artery vasoconstriction (by TCD, conventional angiogram, CTA, or MRA)
2 Absence of aneurysmal subarachnoid hemorrhage
3 Normal/near-normal CSF analysis (protein <80 mg%, leukocytes <10 mm³, normal glucose)
4 Severe and acute and recurrent headache(s)
5 Reversibility of angiographic abnormalities within 3 months after onset

TCD: transcranial Doppler; MRA: magnetic resonance angiogram; CTA: computed tomography angiogram; CSF: cerebrospinal fluid.

in the table may or may not be associated with focal neurologic symptoms or signs [26].

The vasoconstriction is transient but may persist for days and sometimes weeks [2]. The greatest concern related to the development of RCVS is that it might lead not only to severe headaches, but to PRES, to ischemia (which may progress to infarction) and/or to hemorrhagic strokes (intracerebral or subarachnoid) [2]. In one case series, brain imaging was abnormal in 72% of patients—intracranial hemorrhage (39%), vasogenic edema (35%), and infarction (35%) [30]. Infarcts most often involve watershed areas, presumably due to hypoperfusion distal to constricted arteries [26]. Some parenchymal hemorrhages are related to reperfusion injury [26]. Some patients have bleeding on brain imaging characteristically located within convexal sulci on the brain surface.

The methods of choice for monitoring the vasoconstriction are CT angiogram (CTA) and MR angiogram (MRA). Transcranial Doppler might be also used. In a literature review that included 152 patients with vasoconstriction (>25% were pregnant), 87% had segmental constriction and 91% showed resolution of vasoconstriction [31].

Vasculitis, the diagnosis often proffered by radiologists, is extremely rare and is <1000 times less common than pregnancy-related RCVS. The clinical picture is completely different: RCVS begins abruptly with headache while vasculitis is subacute and present with progressing neurological signs and high CSF protein.

We advocate treatment of hypertension with calcium channel blockers, like long-acting verapamil. Nimodipine and nicardipine have shorter half-lives but are also useful [2, 26]. Magnesium and glucocorticoids have also been used and might be considered [28, 32].

This disorder has been considered to be relatively benign and self-limited, but some patients have a severe course with significant disability and even death. Outcomes vary substantially in different reports. A recently published series described poor outcomes in a large proportion of cases: full recovery occurred in 9 of 18 patients (50%), residual deficits in 5 of 18 (28%), and a fulminant course leading to death in 4 of 18 (22%) [30]. The proportion of non-benign outcomes was substantial and contrasted with prior studies. It becomes clear, therefore, that early recognition and treatment are paramount. Some patients seen by one of the authors (LRC) have had residual cognitive dysfunction after self-limited PE/E and/or RCVS; they may be unable to regain the previous level of proficiency and executive function. There are few detailed neuropsychological studies of patients who have recovered from RCVS. We favor aggressive management of hypertension and vasoconstriction, watchfully to avoid hypoperfusion of ischemic territories.

Cerebral venous thrombosis

The pathophysiology of CVT involves thrombosis of cerebral dural sinuses, leading to abnormal venous drainage with potential elevation of intracranial pressures. Cortical veins that drain into the sinuses might occlude as a progression of the sinus thrombosis or as an isolated phenomenon. Cortical vein thrombosis can cause symptoms related to brain edema, infarction, or hemorrhage in brain tissue drained by the occluded venous structures. The first description of CVT associated with pregnancy was made by Abercrombie in 1828 [33]. The CVT is now known to be one of the commonest causes of stroke during pregnancy and puerperium. In the multicenter prospective International Study on Cerebral Venous and dural sinus Thrombosis (ISCVT), 17% of the patients were women in pregnancy or who had recently given birth [34].

A retrospective review of a cohort composed of 73 patients (67 in the puerperium, 1 after abortion, and 5 during pregnancy) revealed that CVT occurred 13 times more often during puerperium than during pregnancy [35]. Cases during pregnancy occurred in any trimester (1 in the first, 2 in the second, and 2 in the third trimester). In relation to puerperal cases, 34.4% occurred during the first week after delivery (almost half of these within first 48 hours) and 59% during weeks 2–3 postpartum [35].

The known risk factors are anemia, dehydration, and hypercoagulability. The clinical presentation is similar from CVTs in nonpregnant patients, with headaches, confusion, focal neurological signs, and seizures. Some patients have symptoms of increased intracranial pressure without neurological signs. Patients develop symptoms more commonly in a sub-acute manner (50%), but headaches and neurological symptoms/signs can develop acutely (30%) or chronically (20%) [36].

D-dimer levels are usually elevated. The diagnosis is made with neuroimaging. A CT is typically the initial study and may show the empty delta-sign. This finding might be observed after intravenous (IV) contrast administration and consists of a triangular area of enhancement with a relatively low-attenuating center (representing the clot) on contiguous transverse CT images in the region of the superior sagittal sinus or torcula [37]. Indirect signs such as hypodensities (resultant from ischemia) and hyperdensities (from hemorrhage or from hemorrhagic infarction) are more common. The frequency of parenchymal lesions has been reported to be as high as 70% (including venous infarcts and ICHs) [35]. Both CT and MR venograms are essential imaging modalities and may show a lack of flow in sinuses and/or cortical veins. The MRI may show not only parenchymal changes (infarct or hemorrhage) but also reveal the presence of the clot present by hypointensity in GRE/T_2*-weighted scans, hyperintensity on DWI (depending on the stage), or isointensity in T_1-weighted scans [2, 38, 39].

The optimal timing to perform the thrombophilia screening and which specific laboratory tests to request is a matter of debate. Diverse laboratory values are transiently affected by multiple factors, including antithrombotic treatment, pregnancy, acute thrombotic events, etc [40, 41]. Screening should be done at least 6 weeks postpartum or 4 weeks after discontinuation of anticoagulation (due to the effects on coagulation factors) [12]. Some advocate performing a baseline test (prior to the institution of heparin) [40].

In a study evaluating the prevalence of thrombophilias in 16 CVT patients, one was pregnant and 3 were in the postpartum period. The overall mean delay between discontinuation of oral anticoagulation and screening was 7 months, and the laboratory screening revealed a prothrombotic condition in 75%. Of the 3 postpartum patients, one patient had protein S deficiency, another had a heterozygous Leiden mutation of factor V gene and protein C deficiency, and the remaining patient had a high factor VIII level. The pregnant patient was heterozygous Leiden mutation of factor V gene and had hyperhomocysteinemia [42]. This contrasts with a prior series of 40 patients that demonstrated a lower frequency of thrombophilia (15%); however, of the 8 cases that developed in the postpartum period, only one had a congenital thrombophilia [43]. In India and Mexico, multiparous women, especially vegetarians, often have anemia and high homocysteine levels; the latter causes increased coagulability.

Therapy with anticoagulation for the treatment of CVT is safe and is associated with a potentially important reduction in the risk of death or dependency [44]. The use of anticoagulation and thrombolytics during pregnancy and puerperium will be discussed in more depth later in this chapter. A recent study randomized 66 patients with CVT, 14 of whom were either pregnant or taking oral contraceptives, to either low-molecular-weight heparin (LMWH) or unfractionated heparin (UFH) for 14 days before starting warfarin. The LMWH was safer and associated with lower in-hospital mortality. Only 3 extracranial bleeds developed (1 gum and 2 vaginal—not specified if in the pregnant patients), all in the UFH group [45].

As in non-obstetric CVT patients, the presence of a concomitant hemorrhagic infarction is not a contraindication for anticoagulation therapy. The duration of the treatment is unclear in pregnant and puerperal women. If evaluation shows that the only risk factor is the puerperium *per se*, a 3-month duration anticoagulation treatment is reasonable [12].

Heparin should be discontinued if uterine contractions begin, if membranes rupture, or the evening before planned induction of labor or cesarean section. Full heparinization is safe after 24 hours from delivery, and warfarin could be started 2–3 days after birth [12].

Thrombolysis for venous occlusions is quite different from that applied to arterial occlusions. Usually a catheter is placed within the thrombosed sinus and high dose of tPA is slowly infused. The dural sinuses have many fronds and septate regions so that mechanical device removal of thrombi is difficult. Thrombolysis in dural sinus occlusions probably should be limited to patients with multiple sinus occlusions who have increased intracranial pressure. These patients have a very poor prognosis unless some venous drainage is obtained. The published experience with local endovascular thrombolysis for CVT includes some good maternal outcomes [46, 47]. In the thrombolysis or anticoagulation for cerebral venous thrombosis trial (TO-ACT trial), patients will be randomized to standard treatment (anticoagulation) versus endovascular intervention. Although pregnancy is an exclusion criteria, postpartum patients will be included [48].

Choriocarcinoma

Choriocarcinoma is a tumor generated by malignant transformation of the trophoblast. It usually occurs following a molar pregnancy but also can follow a term delivery, abortion, or an ectopic pregnancy. Brain metastasis develops in approximately 20% of choriocarcinoma patients. Trophoblasts can invade the brain's blood vessels (in the same manner as in the uterus), damaging the blood vessels and leading to thrombosis and potential embolism [2]. Neoplastic vascular invasion can also generate aneurysms or varicosities, which can rupture and bleed. Metastases are usually hemorrhagic; bleeding may occur into the tumor mass, in the

brain parenchyma surrounding the tumor, or in the subarachnoid space [12, 49].

Amniotic fluid embolism

Amniotic fluid embolism is a rare but severe complication of pregnancy, estimated to occur every 13,000–56,000 deliveries [2]. It tends to affect multiparous women older than 30 years and is associated with the use of forceps, vacuum-assisted deliveries, cesarean sections, placenta previa, placental abruption, eclampsia, and fetal distress [2]. It typically develops during labor, presenting as sudden dyspnea, cyanosis, hypotension, and can be potentially followed by cardiorespiratory arrest. Although focal deficits are possible, the presentation rarely suggests an acute stroke.

The pathophysiological basis is unclear. The mechanism for amniotic embolism is posited to relate to amniotic fluid reaching the maternal venous circulation at the site of trauma or placental attachment due to pressure gradients during labor or at the time of uterine involution [2]. Paradoxical cerebral amniotic fluid emboli might occur and coagulopathy might play a role in vessel thrombosis [49].

Peripartum cardiomyopathy

In this uncommon condition, congestive heart failure due to a dilated cardiomyopathy develops in the last month of pregnancy or within 5 months after delivery, in the absence of a preexisting heart condition. It more commonly affects older, black, and multiparous women. The heart size normalizes in more than 50% of patients, but can recur in subsequent pregnancies. About 5% of affected patients develop brain infarction mostly due to embolism from the malfunctioning heart [49].

Ischemic stroke

The etiology of ischemic strokes during pregnancy and the puerperium is widely varied. Physicians should not only consider the few pregnancy-specific causes described earlier, but also other causes of stroke in the young, since some might require specific management [49].

The etiology of ischemic strokes during pregnancy and puerperium might relate to arteriopathies that might lead to embolic/thromboembolic events or to hypoperfusion. These conditions might affect the extracranial large vessels (premature atherosclerosis, dissections, radiation vasculopathy, fibromuscular dysplasia, or vasculitis—Takayasu's), or the intracranial vasculature (Table 6.2).

Increased age, African-American race, hypertension, diabetes, smoking, valvular heart disease (infective endocarditis and rheumatic disease), cardiomyopathies, arrhythmias, and hyperemesis gravidarum (dehydration) might

Table 6.2 Intracranial arteriopathies during pregnancy and the puerperium

Large-vessel arteriopathies

Noninflammatory vasculitis
   RCVS (migraine, drug-induced, postpartum, etc)
   Moyamoya
Infectious vasculitis
   Varicella-zoster virus
   HIV
   Hepatitis B and C
   Epstein–Barr virus
   Cytomegalovirus
Inflammatory vasculitis
   Isolated CNS vasculitis
   Necrotizing vasculitis
   Hypersensitivity angiitis/connective tissue disease
Behçet's
Dissections
   Traumatic
   Spontaneous
Premature atherosclerosis
Fibromuscular dysplasia
Radiation vasculopathy

Small-vessel arteriopathies

Lipohyalinosis
Vasculitis (Varicella-Zoster, Cryoglobulin-related, Henoch–
   Schonlein purpura)

predispose to embolic, thrombotic, or thromboembolic events. Hematological disorders, such as disseminated intravascular coagulation, sickle cell disease, thrombophilias might be observed [2, 8, 10, 12, 50–52]. Up to 25% of the patients with thrombotic thrombocytopenic purpura are pregnant or in the postpartum and might present with strokes [12].

Some obstetric variables have been correlated with ischemic stroke, but the presence of possible confounders blurs the association. Cesarean deliveries were associated with stroke; however, this might have been observed because of concomitant pregnancy-related conditions (like preeclampsia) [12, 53]. Blood transfusions correlate with development of strokes, but this may relate to the presence of underlying anemia or postpartum hemorrhage [12].

The most common treatments for ischemic strokes are antiplatelets, anticoagulants, and thrombolytics (including intra-arterial treatment).

Antiplatelets

Aspirin is the most frequently prescribed agent for ischemic stroke treatment, and is used for primary and secondary prevention. The potential adverse reactions associated with aspirin use during pregnancy constitute the main concern. Risks include fetal and maternal hemorrhage, premature closure of the ductus arteriosus, and the possibility of prolonging labor.

In preeclampsia, the activation of platelets and the clotting system may occur early in the course of the disease, even before clinical symptoms develop [54]. Low-dose aspirin (<150 mg) has been studied as a potential preventive treatment for this complication. These publications provide good-quality data regarding the effects/safety of low dose aspirin in the second and third trimesters of pregnancy.

In a large trial evaluating aspirin in preeclampsia, there was no significant increase in placental hemorrhages or bleeding during epidural anesthesia, despite a correlation with a slight increased use of blood transfusion after delivery. Low-dose aspirin was considered safe for the fetus and newborn infant, with no evidence of increased risks of bleeding [55]. A Cochrane meta-analysis of antiplatelets for preeclampsia revealed that, compared to placebo, there were no significant benefits regarding the risk of eclampsia, maternal death, cesarean section, induction of labor, antenatal admission, low birth-weight, admission to special care baby units, intraventricular hemorrhage or other neonatal bleeding. Aspirin alone was the therapy in >90% of the included studies, and seemed safe [16].

The safety of higher doses of aspirin or aspirin administration during the first trimester remains unclear [56]. The safety profile of clopidogrel and dipyridamole during pregnancy is not clear [2].

Anticoagulants

Anticoagulation is indicated during pregnancy for treatment of certain stroke subtypes. Heparin does not cross the placenta and is not found in breast milk. It is considered safe since it does not have the potential of causing fetal hemorrhage or teratogenicity. There is a risk of bleeding at the uteroplacental junction, which can indirectly harm the fetus. The development of heparin-induced thrombocytopenia, although uncommon (especially with the use of LMWH instead of UFH [57]), can develop and warrants close monitoring. The LMWH is effective in the treatment of acute venous thromboembolism during pregnancy and is not associated with an increased risk of severe peripartum bleeding [58, 59].

In contrast, coumarin derivatives cross the placenta and can cause both fetal bleeding and teratogenicity. Coumarin derivatives can cause an embryopathy (nasal hypoplasia and/or stippled epiphyses) if exposure occurs during the first trimester of pregnancy. Warfarin is likely safe during the first 6 weeks of gestation, but carries a risk of embryopathy if taken between 6 and 12 weeks. A small proportion (3%) of liveborn infants exposed to coumarin derivatives during pregnancy was found to have central nervous system abnormalities (e.g., agenesis of the corpus callosum, Dandy–Walker malformation, mid-line cerebellar atrophy). These central nervous system anomalies may occur after exposure to such drugs during any trimester [56, 60].

Different approaches to anticoagulation regimen might be taken according to the context (e.g., treatment of acute thromboembolism during pregnancy vs. prevention of thromboembolic events) [56]. Options include either LMWH or UFH between 6 and 12 weeks and close to term (with warfarin at other times), or dose-adjusted UFH or LMWH throughout the pregnancy [12]. Heparin (LMWH and UFH) as well as warfarin is safe for nursing mothers: breastfeeding is encouraged [56]. Full heparinization was deemed safe to be started 24 hours after birth, which can be switched to warfarin 2–3 days after delivery [12].

Thrombolytics

Alteplase (rt-PA) does not cross the placenta and was not found to be teratogenic in rats and rabbits [61]. The main concern regarding the use of thrombolytics during pregnancy is related to the potential effect on the placenta: premature labor, placental abruption, or fetal demise. The first report of use of fibrinolytic during pregnancy was made in 1962 with streptokinase [62], and multiple cases and case series describing experiences with thrombolytic agents for diverse clinical indications have accrued since. Thrombolysis has been described for pulmonary embolism with no adverse events to mother and delivery. Alteplase has been reported multiple times in the setting of ischemic stroke. Reports include exposure during different stages of pregnancy (including within the first trimester [inadvertently] and in the immediate postpartum), and through IV or intra-arterial routes [46, 63–67].

In a review that analyzed off-label uses of rt-PA for stroke, 11 pregnant women were identified. Nine patients were treated in the first trimester and 2 in the third; 5 patients received IV administration and 6 intra-arterial. Among the 11 fetuses, 5 were delivered at term and 6 died: 1 died at the mother's death, 3 because the mothers elected induced abortion, and the other 2 were miscarriages after urokinase administration (one had a lethal chromosomal anomaly at autopsy) [68].

A review of 172 pregnant women treated with thrombolytic agents for various thromboembolic conditions (mainly deep venous thrombosis; only 1 stroke) found maternal hemorrhagic complications in 8% of patients. Hemorrhages occurred most often with the use of streptokinase, most likely related to the greater number of patients treated with this agent. The type of hemorrhagic complications included 1 spontaneous abortion, 5 instances of minor vaginal bleeding, 1 of spontaneous hematomas in the inguinal and axillary region requiring transfusion, 1 fatal abruptio placenta with fetal death, 4 instances of uterine bleeding resulting in emergent cesarean delivery, and 2 postpartum hemorrhages requiring transfusion [62].

A literature review of 28 reported cases of rt-PA thrombolysis during pregnancy included treatment for pulmonary embolism, deep venous thrombosis, thrombotic complications related to cardiac valve prosthesis, myocardial infarction, and for acute stroke ($n = 10$). Although the safety for pregnant patients and their unborn children cannot be attested, it is likely not justified to withhold thrombolytic therapy from pregnant patients if effective alternatives are lacking [61].

Murugappan reported 8 patients who received thrombolytic therapy for acute stroke during pregnancy. Three were treated with IV tPA, 1 with intra-arterial tPA, 2 with intra-arterial urokinase, and 2 received local urokinase (cerebral sinus thrombosis). No patient given IV tPA had a major hemorrhagic complication, and there were no symptomatic ICHs. Hemorrhagic adverse outcomes in these 8 women included 1 intrauterine hematoma,

1 buttock hematoma, 2 asymptomatic small intracranial hemorrhages (both after urokinase) [46].

These case reports demonstrate that thrombolysis for acute ischemic stroke during pregnancy may result in favorable maternal outcomes [69]. Complication rates appear similar compared with nonpregnant patients [70], but no clear conclusions can be drawn considering the different stroke etiologies and clinical characteristics. The effects on fetal outcomes remain uncertain. Risks and benefits to mother and fetus must be cautiously weighted prior to deciding for thrombolysis, and notification of such cases in an international registry would be a useful initiative [12, 69].

Hemorrhagic strokes

Intracranial hemorrhage is estimated to account for 2–7% of instances of neurological dysfunction during pregnancy [12].

In one series, among 50,700 admissions for delivery, 34 patients with a diagnosis of stroke were identified; 38% of strokes were hemorrhagic [7]. In another report, 45% of 31 pregnancy-related strokes were hemorrhagic [5]. The proportion of pregnancy-related hemorrhagic strokes is higher than in the general population, where approximately 20% of strokes are intracranial hemorrhages [1].

Preeclampsia or eclampsia accounts for 15–44% of the pregnancy-related intracranial hemorrhages. Among 154 pregnant patients with intracranial hemorrhage from an identified intracranial lesion, 77% were secondary to aneurysmal rupture and 23% were due to AVMs [71].

In a study that evaluated the relative frequency of AVMs and aneurysms, nonpregnant young women had many more bleeds from aneurysms than from AVMs. During pregnancy and postpartum, a more even split between these two causes of hemorrhage was reported and attributed to a greater proportional risk of AVM rupture during pregnancy/postpartum [72].

Diagnosis is based on neuroimaging and CT scans are sensitive enough to detect intra-parenchymal hemorrhage and SAHs. The MRI is performed to better evaluate for an underlying cause for bleeding. According to the presentation and CT appearance, contrast-enhanced studies (CT with iodine or MRI with gadolinium) can be used to exclude vascular malformations, neoplasms, or other causative processes. Vascular imaging with CTA or MRA is essential for evaluating for aneurysms and is useful for assessment of carotid-cavernous fistulas.

Subarachnoid hemorrhage

Similarly to the general population, aneurysms diagnosed during pregnancy involve predominantly the arteries of circle of Willis and are multiple in up to 20% of patients [73]. Hemodynamic stress that occurs during pregnancy might contribute to the growth and development of aneurysms [74,75]. Pregnancy does not seem to alter significantly the risk of aneurysmal rupture [12].

The indication for elective treatment of aneurysms during pregnancy is debated, but bleeding aneurysms should be secured [12]. One study showed that surgical management of aneurysms during pregnancy in patients that presented with hemorrhage was associated with significantly lower maternal and fetal mortality [71]. Endovascular intervention with coiling might be associated with less complications than clipping [12, 73, 76].

In the situations where there is family history of aneurysms, it may be important to perform aneurysm screening before pregnancy. Optimal management of women with a known aneurysm who become pregnant is not clearly established [77].

Subarachnoid hemorrhage (SAH) has been reported in patients that had a dural puncture; the suggestion is that the resulting decrement in cerebrospinal fluid volume leads to a relative hypotension and might increase the aneurysm transmural pressure. Epidural anesthesia should be cautiously performed or avoided in patients with known aneurysms [12].

Arteriovenous malformations

Cerebrovascular malformation are noted in 7.1% patients who have pregnancy-related hemorrhages [10]. The risk of AVM hemorrhage is not significantly increased during pregnancy; the bleeding frequency is similar during pregnancy for women with an unruptured AVM (3.5% per person-year) compared with nonpregnant women of childbearing age with an unruptured AVM (3.1%). These calculations assumed that there was no selection bias, which certainly cannot be excluded [78].

In a series of 100 consecutive supratentorial AVM hemorrhages in a referral hospital, only 1 patient was pregnant at the time of hemorrhage, while 9 already had uncomplicated previous pregnancies. The authors stated that their series contradicted the suggestion of others of a high incidence of bleeding from these lesions during pregnancy [79]. This impression of a small risk of AVM bleeding related to pregnancy was corroborated by a review of 70 cases over 20 years, where only 1 pregnant patient bled (first trimester of the third pregnancy), while 10 that had children presented outside of pregnancy or the puerperium with a rupture [80].

Most reported patients with hemorrhage from AVM during pregnancy or the puerperium present in the second trimester [7, 72]. Although it is rational to avoid a difficult labor to minimize hypertension and an adrenergic state, it is unclear if epidural anesthesia to minimize pain or cesarean section are indicated in patients with untreated malformations [71].

Although treatment for an AVM that has not hemorrhaged should be deferred until after delivery [12], the decision analysis for patients that bleed during pregnancy is more complex. A retrospective analysis of published cases revealed that surgical management of AVMs may not result in lower maternal and fetal mortality [71]. Endovascular techniques have not been evaluated in a structured manner but might have an impact.

Safety and use of radiological studies during pregnancy

Computed tomography

Cranial CT is usually the first-line study for the evaluation of maternal cerebrovascular complications. It exposes the fetus to radiation. Fortunately, the exposure is likely minimal/trivial if abdominal shields are used [49]. Guidelines for diagnostic imaging during pregnancy affirmed that exposures of less than 5 rads have not been correlated with fetal anomalies; head CT scans are relatively safe since they expose the fetus to only 1 rad [2, 81]. The use of contrast is frequently important for the evaluation of the vascular anatomy (performed through a CTA) or for assessment of potential vascular malformations, infectious, inflammatory, or tumoral changes (through a contrast enhanced CT). Despite the fear that the use of iodine contrast during pregnancy might generate thyroid dysfunction in the fetus, a recent study showed that a single high dose is unlikely to be significant. It is prudent to check thyroid function in the neonate in the first week of life if contrast was given during pregnancy [2, 82].

Magnetic resonance imaging and angiography

Although animal studies raised the potential of teratogenicity in early pregnancy, MRI does not seem to generate short-term changes and is the preferred imaging method [12, 49]. Mothers need to be informed that adverse events have not been described, and that MRI may be performed regardless of the trimester in case the treating physician considers that the results might affect maternal care; oral and written informed consent are wise [83]. The MRI safety data during pregnancy originates from 1.5 Tesla studies, while the profile of 3.0 Tesla MRI remains to be determined [84]. The

safety of gadolinium administration has been debated since some animal studies have shown growth retardation while no controlled studies in humans have corroborated this finding [84]. The MRA should be performed without contrast to evaluate the intracranial vasculature. The use of time-of-flight (non-contrast) neck MRA usually shows the extracranial carotids and vertebral arteries well.

Catheter-based angiography

Cerebral angiography exposes the fetus to radiation, which can be minimized with the use of lead aprons. The risks related to iodinated contrast administration were discussed previously. Due to its invasiveness, this test is reserved for special circumstances during pregnancy.

Maternal and fetal prognosis

In one review, the overall maternal case fatality rate for ischemic and hemorrhagic strokes was 4.1%, while the mortality rate was 1.4 per 100,000 deliveries [8]. The case fatality seemed low when compared to non-obstetric populations; this might, in part, be explained by the fact that pregnant women are usually younger, healthier and that late deaths might have been missed due to the coding system used by this study.

The study from Ile de France provides good quality data, reporting no maternal deaths secondary to ischemic stroke, and minimal or a moderate residual deficits in half of women; maternal mortality following hemorrhagic stroke was of 25% [9]. In another study, more than one-fifth of women with pregnancy-related ICH died [10].

In a series of 34 patients with a diagnosis of stroke (21 infarctions and 13 hemorrhages), all patients with infarction survived and 3 of 13 patients with hemorrhage died during hospitalization (1 due to an AVM and 2 of unknown etiology) [7].

The reported mortality rates related to CVT in pregnant or puerperal varies from 4% to 36% [85]. Interestingly, one study reported a mortality rate of 9% for patients with obstetric causes for CVT versus 33% for non-obstetric causes [35].

A previous ischemic stroke is not a contraindication to subsequent pregnancy [86]. A multicenter retrospective study of 489 consecutive women aged 15–40 years with a first-ever arterial ischemic stroke or CVT showed that the risk of recurrent stroke in women with a history of an ischemic stroke is low. Only 13 recurrent strokes were detected and only 2 during a subsequent pregnancy. The calculated overall risk of recurrence was 1% within 1 year and 2.3% within 5 years [86].

Fetal prognosis is harder to estimate due to scarce literature. The study from Ile de France reported a fetal death rate of 12% [9]. In another series of patients with strokes during pregnancy, 6 presented with ischemic strokes: 3 live deliveries, 1 miscarriage, and a pregnancy termination. The outcome of the other 3 pregnancies was not available [7]. Nine patients presented with hemorrhagic strokes before delivery: 5 live deliveries, 3 fetal deaths due to maternal death, and 1 due to termination [7].

References

1 Caplan LR. *Caplan's Stroke: A Clinical Approach.* 4th ed. Philadelphia, PA: Saunders, 2009.

2 Sidorov EV, Feng W, Caplan LR. Stroke in pregnant and postpartum women. *Expert Rev Cardiovasc Ther.* 9:1235–1247.

3 Cerneca F, Ricci G, Simeone R, et al. Coagulation and fibrinolysis changes in normal pregnancy. Increased levels of procoagulants and reduced levels of inhibitors during pregnancy induce a hypercoagulable state, combined with a reactive fibrinolysis. *Eur J Obstet Gynecol Reprod Biol.* 1997;73: 31–36.

4 Duvekot JJ, Peeters LL. Maternal cardiovascular hemodynamic adaptation to pregnancy. *Obstet Gynecol Surv.* 1994;49:S1–14.

5 Kittner SJ, Stern BJ, Feeser BR, et al. Pregnancy and the risk of stroke. *N Engl J Med.* 1996;335: 768–774.

6 Salonen Ros H, Lichtenstein P, Bellocco R, et al. Increased risks of circulatory diseases in late pregnancy and puerperium. *Epidemiology.* 2001;12:456–460.

7 Jaigobin C, Silver FL. Stroke and pregnancy. *Stroke.* 2000;31:2948–2951.

8 James AH, Bushnell CD, Jamison MG, et al. Incidence and risk factors for stroke in pregnancy and the puerperium. *Obstet Gynecol.* 2005;106: 509–516.

9 Sharshar T, Lamy C, Mas JL. Incidence and causes of strokes associated with pregnancy and puerperium. A study in public hospitals of Ile de France. Stroke in Pregnancy Study Group. *Stroke.* 1995;26:930–936.

10 Bateman BT, Schumacher HC, Bushnell CD, et al. Intracerebral hemorrhage in pregnancy: frequency, risk factors, and outcome. *Neurology.* 2006;67:424–429.

11 Petitti DB, Sidney S, Quesenberry CP Jr, et al. Incidence of stroke and myocardial infarction in women of reproductive age. *Stroke.* 1997;28: 280–283.

12 Davie CA, O'Brien P. Stroke and pregnancy. *J Neurol Neurosurg Psychiatry.* 2008;79:240–245.

13 ACOG practice bulletin. Diagnosis and management of preeclampsia and eclampsia. Number 33, January 2002. American College of Obstetricians and Gynecologists. *Int J Gynaecol Obstet.* 2002;77:67–75.

14 Granger JP, Alexander BT, Llinas MT, et al. Pathophysiology of hypertension during preeclampsia linking placental ischemia with endothelial dysfunction. *Hypertension.* 2001;38:718–722.

15 Bussolino F, Benedetto C, Massobrio M, et al. Maternal vascular prostacyclin activity in preeclampsia. *Lancet.* 1980;2:702.

16 Duley L, Henderson-Smart DJ, Meher S, et al. Antiplatelet agents for preventing pre-eclampsia and its complications. *Cochrane Database Syst Rev.* 2007;CD004659.

17 Hinchey J, Chaves C, Appignani B, et al. A reversible posterior leukoencephalopathy syndrome. *N Engl J Med.* 1996;334:494–500.

18 Hinchey JA. Reversible posterior leukoencephalopathy syndrome: what have we learned in the last 10 years? *Arch Neurol.* 2008;65:175–176.

19 Lee VH, Wijdicks EF, Manno EM, et al. Clinical spectrum of reversible posterior

leukoencephalopathy syndrome. *Arch Neurol.* 2008;65:205–210.

20 Bartynski WS. Posterior reversible encephalopathy syndrome, part 2: controversies surrounding pathophysiology of vasogenic edema. *AJNR Am J Neuroradiol.* 2008;29:1043–1049.

21 Edvinsson L. Neurogenic mechanisms in the cerebrovascular bed. Autonomic nerves, amine receptors and their effects on cerebral blood flow. *Acta Physiol Scand Suppl.* 1975;427:1–35.

22 Forteza AM, Echeverria Y, Haussen DC, Gutierrez J, Wiley E, Gusmao CM. Cerebral vasomotor reactivity monitoring in posterior reversible encephalopathy syndrome. *BMJ Case Reports.* 2010; doi:10.1136/bcr.10.2009.2345

23 Demirtas O, Gelal F, Vidinli BD, et al. Cranial MR imaging with clinical correlation in preeclampsia and eclampsia. *Diagn Interv Radiol.* 2005;11: 189–194.

24 Covarrubias DJ, Luetmer PH, Campeau NG. Posterior reversible encephalopathy syndrome: prognostic utility of quantitative diffusion-weighted MR images. *AJNR Am J Neuroradiol.* 2002;23: 1038–1048.

25 McKinney AM, Short J, Truwit CL, et al. Posterior reversible encephalopathy syndrome: incidence of atypical regions of involvement and imaging findings. *AJR Am J Roentgenol.* 2007;189:904–912.

26 Calabrese LH, Dodick DW, Schwedt TJ, et al. Narrative review: reversible cerebral vasoconstriction syndromes. *Ann Intern Med.* 2007;146:34–44.

27 Call GK, Fleming MC, Sealfon S, et al. Reversible cerebral segmental vasoconstriction. *Stroke.* 1988; 19:1159–1170.

28 Singhal AB. Postpartum angiopathy with reversible posterior leukoencephalopathy. *Arch Neurol.* 2004;61:411–416.

29 Trommer BL, Homer D, Mikhael MA. Cerebral vasospasm and eclampsia. *Stroke.* 1988;19:326–329.

30 Fugate JE, Ameriso SF, Ortiz G, et al. Variable presentations of postpartum angiopathy. *Stroke.* 2012;43:670–676.

31 Singhal AB. Cerebral vasoconstriction without subarachnoid blood: associated conditions, clinical and neuroimaging characteristics. *Ann Neurol.* 2002;52:59–60.

32 Hajj-Ali RA, Furlan A, Abou-Chebel A, et al. Benign angiopathy of the central nervous system: cohort of 16 patients with clinical course and long-term followup. *Arthritis Rheum.* 2002;47: 662–669.

33 Abercrombie J. *Pathological and Practical Researches on Disease of Brain and Spinal Cord.* Waugh and Innes; 1828.

34 Coutinho JM, Ferro JM, Canhao P, et al. Cerebral venous and sinus thrombosis in women. *Stroke.* 2009;40:2356–2361.

35 Cantu C, Barinagarrementeria F. Cerebral venous thrombosis associated with pregnancy and puerperium. Review of 67 cases. *Stroke.* 1993;24:1880–1884.

36 Bousser MG. Cerebral venous thrombosis: diagnosis and management. *J Neurol.* 2000;247:252–258.

37 Lee EJ. The empty delta sign. *Radiology.* 2002;224:788–789.

38 Chu K, Kang DW, Yoon BW, et al. Diffusion-weighted magnetic resonance in cerebral venous thrombosis. *Arch Neurol.* 2001;58:1569–1576.

39 Selim M, Fink J, Linfante I, et al. Diagnosis of cerebral venous thrombosis with echo-planar T2*-weighted magnetic resonance imaging. *Arch Neurol.* 2002;59:1021–1026.

40 Deschiens MA, Conard J, Horellou MH, et al. Coagulation studies, factor V Leiden, and anticardiolipin antibodies in 40 cases of cerebral venous thrombosis. *Stroke.* 1996;27:1724–1730.

41 Cumming AM, Tait RC, Fildes S, et al. Development of resistance to activated protein C during pregnancy. *Br J Haematol.* 1995;90: 725–727.

42 Cakmak S, Derex L, Berruyer M, et al. Cerebral venous thrombosis: clinical outcome and systematic screening of prothrombotic factors. *Neurology.* 2003;60:1175–1178.

43 Martinelli I, Sacchi E, Landi G, et al. High risk of cerebral-vein thrombosis in carriers of a prothrombin-gene mutation and in users of oral contraceptives. *N Engl J Med.* 1998;338:1793–1797.

44 Coutinho J, de Bruijn SF, Deveber G, et al. Anticoagulation for cerebral venous sinus thrombosis. *Cochrane Database Syst Rev.* CD002005.

45 Misra UK, Kalita J, Chandra S, et al. Low molecular weight heparin versus unfractionated heparin in cerebral venous sinus thrombosis: a randomized controlled trial. *Eur J Neurol.* 2012;19:1030–1036.

46 Murugappan A, Coplin WM, Al-Sadat AN, et al. Thrombolytic therapy of acute ischemic stroke during pregnancy. *Neurology.* 2006;66:768–770.

47 Weatherby SJ, Edwards NC, West R, et al. Good outcome in early pregnancy following direct thrombolysis for cerebral venous sinus thrombosis. *J Neurol.* 2003;250:1372–1373.

48 Coutinho JM, Ferro JM, Zuurbier SM, et al. Thrombolysis or anticoagulation for cerebral venous thrombosis: rationale and design of the TO-ACT trial. *Int J Stroke.* 2013;8:135–140.

49 Mas JL, Lamy C. Stroke in pregnancy and the puerperium. *J Neurol.* 1998;245:305–313.

50 Schoenberg BS, Whisnant JP, Taylor WF, et al. Strokes in women of childbearing age. A population study. *Neurology.* 1970;20:181–189.

51 Wiebers DO, Mokri B. Internal carotid artery dissection after childbirth. *Stroke.* 1985;16:956–959.

52 Oehler J, Lichy C, Gandjour J, et al. Dissection of four cerebral arteries after protracted birth. *Nervenarzt.* 2003;74:366–369.

53 Lanska DJ, Kryscio RJ. Risk factors for peripartum and postpartum stroke and intracranial venous thrombosis. *Stroke.* 2000;31:1274–1282.

54 Janes SL, Kyle PM, Redman C, et al. Flow cytometric detection of activated platelets in pregnant women prior to the development of pre-eclampsia. *Thromb Haemost.* 1995;74:1059–1063.

55 CLASP: a randomised trial of low-dose aspirin for the prevention and treatment of pre-eclampsia among 9364 pregnant women. CLASP (Collaborative Low-dose Aspirin Study in Pregnancy) Collaborative Group. *Lancet.* 1994;343:619–629.

56 Bates SM, Greer IA, Hirsh J, et al. Use of antithrombotic agents during pregnancy: the Seventh ACCP Conference on Antithrombotic and Thrombolytic Therapy. *Chest.* 2004;126:627S-44S.

57 Warkentin TE, Levine MN, Hirsh J, et al. Heparin-induced thrombocytopenia in patients treated with low-molecular-weight heparin or unfractionated heparin. *N Engl J Med.* 1995;332:1330–1335.

58 Greer IA, Nelson-Piercy C. Low-molecular-weight heparins for thromboprophylaxis and treatment of venous thromboembolism in pregnancy: a systematic review of safety and efficacy. *Blood.* 2005;106:401–407.

59 Roshani S, Cohn DM, Stehouwer AC, et al. Incidence of postpartum haemorrhage in women receiving therapeutic doses of low-molecular-weight heparin: results of a retrospective cohort study. *BMJ Open.* 1:e000257.

60 Hall JG, Pauli RM, Wilson KM. Maternal and fetal sequelae of anticoagulation during pregnancy. *Am J Med.* 1980;68:122–140.

61 Leonhardt G, Gaul C, Nietsch HH, et al. Thrombolytic therapy in pregnancy. *J Thromb Thrombolysis.* 2006;21:271–276.

62 Turrentine MA, Braems G, Ramirez MM. Use of thrombolytics for the treatment of thromboembolic disease during pregnancy. *Obstet Gynecol Surv.* 1995;50:534–541.

63 Li Y, Margraf J, Kluck B, et al. Thrombolytic therapy for ischemic stroke secondary to paradoxical embolism in pregnancy: a case report and literature review. *Neurologist.* 18:44–48.

64 Wiese KM, Talkad A, Mathews M, et al. Intravenous recombinant tissue plasminogen activator in a pregnant woman with cardioembolic stroke. *Stroke.* 2006;37:2168–2169.

65 Mendez JC, Masjuan J, Garcia N, et al. Successful intra-arterial thrombolysis for acute ischemic stroke in the immediate postpartum period: case report. *Cardiovasc Intervent Radiol.* 2008;31:193–195.

66 Fasullo S, Scalzo S, Maringhini G, et al. Thrombolysis for massive pulmonary embolism in pregnancy: a case report. *Am J Emerg Med.* 29:698 e1–4.

67 Holden EL, Ranu H, Sheth A, et al. Thrombolysis for massive pulmonary embolism in pregnancy–a report of three cases and follow up over a two year period. *Thromb Res.* 127:58–59.

68 Aleu A, Mellado P, Lichy C, et al. Hemorrhagic complications after off-label thrombolysis for ischemic stroke. *Stroke.* 2007;38:417–422.

69 Cronin CA, Weisman CJ, Llinas RH. Stroke treatment: beyond the three-hour window and in the pregnant patient. *Ann N Y Acad Sci.* 2008;1142:159–178.

70 De Keyser J, Gdovinova Z, Uyttenboogaart M, et al. Intravenous alteplase for stroke: beyond the guidelines and in particular clinical situations. *Stroke.* 2007;38:2612–2618.

71 Dias MS, Sekhar LN. Intracranial hemorrhage from aneurysms and arteriovenous malformations during pregnancy and the puerperium. *Neurosurgery.* 1990;27:855–865; discussion 65–6.

72 Robinson JL, Hall CS, Sedzimir CB. Arteriovenous malformations, aneurysms, and pregnancy. *J Neurosurg.* 1974;41:63–70.

73 Meyers PM, Halbach VV, Malek AM, et al. Endovascular treatment of cerebral artery aneurysms during pregnancy: report of three cases. *AJNR Am J Neuroradiol.* 2000;21:1306–1311.

74 Fox MW, Harms RW, Davis DH. Selected neurologic complications of pregnancy. *Mayo Clin Proc.* 1990;65:1595–1618.

75 Simolke GA, Cox SM, Cunningham FG. Cerebrovascular accidents complicating pregnancy and the puerperium. *Obstet Gynecol.* 1991;78:37–42.

76 Piotin M, de Souza Filho CB, Kothimbakam R, et al. Endovascular treatment of acutely ruptured intracranial aneurysms in pregnancy. *Am J Obstet Gynecol*. 2001;185:1261–1262.

77 Grosset DG, Ebrahim S, Bone I, et al. Stroke in pregnancy and the puerperium: what magnitude of risk? *J Neurol Neurosurg Psychiatry*. 1995;58:129–131.

78 Horton JC, Chambers WA, Lyons SL, et al. Pregnancy and the risk of hemorrhage from cerebral arteriovenous malformations. *Neurosurgery*. 1990;27:867–871; discussion 71–2.

79 Parkinson D, Bachers G. Arteriovenous malformations. Summary of 100 consecutive supratentorial cases. *J Neurosurg*. 1980;53: 285–299.

80 Kelly DL Jr, Alexander E Jr, Davis CH Jr, et al. Intracranial arteriovenous malformations: clinical review and evaluation of brain scans. *J Neurosurg*. 1969;31:422–428.

81 Guidelines for diagnostic imaging during pregnancy. The American College of Obstetricians and Gynecologists. *Int J Gynaecol Obstet*. 1995;51: 288–291.

82 Webb JA, Thomsen HS, Morcos SK. The use of iodinated and gadolinium contrast media during pregnancy and lactation. *Eur Radiol*. 2005;15: 1234–1240.

83 Shellock FG, Crues JV. MR procedures: biologic effects, safety, and patient care. *Radiology*. 2004;232:635–652.

84 Levine D, Obstetric MRI. *J Magn Reson Imaging*. 2006;24:1–15.

85 Canhao P, Ferro JM, Lindgren AG, et al. Causes and predictors of death in cerebral venous thrombosis. *Stroke*. 2005;36:1720–1725.

86 Lamy C, Hamon JB, Coste J, et al. Ischemic stroke in young women: risk of recurrence during subsequent pregnancies. French Study Group on Stroke in Pregnancy. *Neurology*. 2000;55:269–274.

CHAPTER 7

Selecting contraception for women treated with antiepileptic drugs

Page B. Pennell[1] & Anne Davis[2]

[1] *Department of Neurology, Brigham and Women's Hospital, Harvard Medical School, Boston, MA, USA*
[2] *Department of Obstetrics and Gynecology, Columbia University Medical Center, New York, NY, USA*

Introduction

Effective and safe contraceptive options are important for all women but are arguably even more essential, and more complicated, for women on antiepileptic drugs (AEDs). Many of the studies that report on contraceptive failures with concomitant AEDs as well as adverse pregnancy outcomes are primarily in women with epilepsy (WWE). However, the same principles can be applied to women of childbearing age on AEDs for a variety of neuropsychiatric and other indications, including bipolar disorder, migraine headaches, other pain syndromes, drug abuse treatment, and even obesity. Recent studies have shed new light on the enormous magnitude of this issue [1, 2].

Millions of women are treated with AEDs in the United States alone and the numbers are increasing. Adedinsewo, et al. examined individual prescriptions for reproductive-age adolescent girls and adult women ages 15–44 years in the United States, using de-identified data from the National Hospital and Ambulatory Medical Care Surveys (1996–2007) [1]. They used ICD-9 diagnosis codes to classify subjects as WWE and women without epilepsy (WWoE). They estimated that approximately 4.3 million AED prescriptions were issued to reproductive-aged WWoE per year. Moreover, the prevalence of AED prescriptions for reproductive-aged WWoE tripled during the study periods from 10.3 (1996–1998) to 34.9 per 1000 patient visits (2005–2007). Of these prescriptions, approximately 17% were for valproic acid, the AED that consistently demonstrates the greatest risk for MCMs and for adverse neurodevelopmental outcomes [3, 4]. Another study analyzed data from the Medication Exposure in Pregnancy Risk Evaluation Program (MEPREP) database from 2001 to 2007, with selection specifically for pregnancy exposures to AEDs from liveborn deliveries [2]. The prevalence of AED use during pregnancy increased from 15.7 per 1000 deliveries in 2001 to 21.9 per 1000 deliveries in 2007; 13% of deliveries were on AED polytherapy. Psychiatric disorders were the most common diagnoses followed by epilepsy and pain disorders. At the time of publication of this chapter, the numbers are likely substantially even higher.

Avoiding unplanned pregnancies is a key cornerstone to improving outcomes for children of women treated with AEDs. Using an AED with a favorable risk profile for structural and neurodevelopmental teratogenicity, at the lowest effective dose for that patient, good disease control for the prior 9 months, and use of periconceptional supplemental folic acid optimize pregnancy outcomes [3–5]. When a pregnancy

Neurological Illness in Pregnancy: Principles and Practice, First Edition.
Edited by Autumn Klein, M. Angela O'Neal, Christina Scifres, Janet F. R. Waters and Jonathan H. Waters.
© 2016 John Wiley & Sons, Ltd. Published 2016 by John Wiley & Sons, Ltd.

is unplanned, women on AEDs can miss the opportunity to benefit from these modifiable aspects of care.

The average woman, assuming she has two children, will require some form of contraception for at least three decades during her child-bearing years. In the United States, of the 43 million fertile and sexually active women not seeking pregnancy, 89% use contraception [6]. Nationally representative surveys in the United States show that 63% of those who use contraception rely on reversible methods, most often the oral contraceptive pill and male condom, whereas 37% rely on the permanent methods of tubal sterilization or vasectomy [6]. Notably, use of long-acting reversible methods in the United States (IUD or implant) increased to 8.5% by 2009 but remains relatively uncommon compared to European countries where sterilization is much less common and use of the IUD is widespread.

Contraceptive use in women treated with AEDs

Data from existing, large contraception surveys cannot be used to estimate contraception use among women on AEDs for different indications, or even WWE because such surveys do not collect information on co-existent chronic illness. Data from small samples of women suggest contraception remains a challenge for WWE, despite published guidelines [7]. One questionnaire study at an urban medical center queried 145 WWE regarding current sexual activity and contraception use [8]. Only 53% of those at risk of unplanned pregnancy used methods with typical pregnancy rates of ≤10% in the first year of use; most often sterilization or oral contraceptives. The rest relied on condoms, spermicide, natural family planning (timed intercourse) or withdrawal, alone or in combination. These methods have typical failure rates between 10% and 20% per year. Not surprisingly, half of their 181 pregnancies were unplanned. Poor, Hispanic WWE were more vulnerable; they experienced more unplanned pregnancies than Caucasian women of higher socioeconomic status. This disparity mirrors the U.S. population overall.

Healthy women face barriers to access effective contraception including prohibitive cost and misperceptions regarding efficacy and safety. Women on AEDs face another barrier; physicians responsible for contraceptive counseling are often not adequately knowledgeable about this complicated topic. Although performed almost two decades ago, a national survey of U.S. obstetricians and neurologists highlighted this gap in the treating physicians' knowledge. The 1996 survey queried U.S. obstetricians and neurologists about interactions between oral contraceptives and AEDS [9]. Approximately a quarter in both groups reported awareness of contraceptive failures in their patients taking AEDs and oral contraceptives. They were asked if they knew the interactions between oral contraceptives and the six most common AEDs at that time (phenytoin, carbamazepine, valproic acid, phenobarbital, primidone, and ethosuximide). The average percentage correct for the neurologists' knowledge of oral contraceptive (OC) interactions was $61\% \pm 2.2\%$ and for obstetricians' knowledge was $37.8 \pm 1.9\%$. Only 4% of the neurologists and none of the obstetricians answered correctly for all six AEDs. Since this survey was published, the subject has gotten even more complicated with new AEDs and contraceptives. Like many healthcare providers, women also experience confusion about AEDs and contraception. In their questionnaire study of WWE, Pack and Davis found that among the 66 women currently using enzyme-inducing AEDs (EIAEDs), 65% did not know whether or not their AED changed the effectiveness of OCs [10].

Contraception methods

For all women, efficacy and safety are primary considerations when selecting a contraceptive method. Pregnancy rates are less than

Table 7.1 Contraceptives available in the United States

Method	Efficacy[a]	Reversibility	Effect on bleeding	Duration of use	Ovulation inhibition?
Oral contraceptive pill	88–94%	Immediate	Decreased, regular	Daily	Yes
Transdermal patch	88–94%	Immediate	Decreased, regular	Weekly	Yes
Vaginal ring	88–94%	Immediate	Decreased, regular	Monthly	Yes
Depot Medroxyprogesterone acetate (DMPA)	88–94%	Delayed[b]	Initially irregular, amenorrhea likely with continuation	Every 3 months	Yes
Subdermal implant	>99%	Immediate	Decreased, irregular	3 years	Yes
Levonorgestrel IUD	>99%	Immediate	Decreased, initially irregular	5 years	Sometimes
Copper IUD	>99%	Immediate	Sometimes increased, regular	10 years	No

[a]With typical use, per year assuming no drug interaction present.
[b]Median return to ovulation >6 months from time of last injection.

1% per year for highly effective methods and these should be considered first-line or top-tier (Table 7.1). Highly effective methods include permanent contraception via tubal ligation or vasectomy and long-acting reversible contraception (LARC) methods of intrauterine devices (IUDs) and the single-rod, 3-year contraceptive implant. A recent large, prospective cohort study demonstrated that unplanned pregnancy was 20 times more likely among users of short-term hormonal methods such as OCs compared to LARC [11].

Long-acting reversible contraception

The progestin (levonorgestrel (LNG)) releasing and the copper T 380A IUDs are widely used around the world (Figures 7.1 and 7.2). The LNG IUD is approved for 5 years of use by the U.S. FDA; the non-hormonal copper device for 10 years. Both IUDs primarily prevent pregnancy by pre-fertilization mechanisms of interference with sperm transport and function [12]. The IUD is an appropriate choice for women and adolescents who have never been pregnant as well as women who have children [13]. Recent data clearly demonstrate excellent safety and efficacy for nulliparous women [11]. Neither IUD increases rates of pelvic infection or associated infertility. Both IUDs are completely reversible; fertility quickly and completely returns after removal.

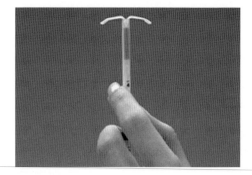

Figure 7.1 Progestin-releasing intrauterine device, containing levonorgestrel. Courtesy of Association of Reproductive Health Professionals (AHRP). Reproduced under the Creative Commons License: http://creativecommons.org/licenses/by/3.0/

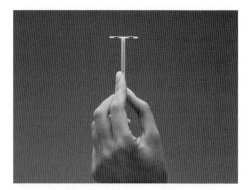

Figure 7.2 Copper T 380A Intrauterine Device. Courtesy of Association of Reproductive Health Professionals (AHRP). Reproduced under the Creative Commons License: http://creativecommons.org/licenses/by/3.0/

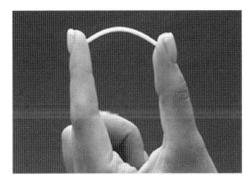

Figure 7.3 The contraceptive implant elutes etonogestrel. Courtesy of Association of Reproductive Health Professionals (AHRP). Reproduced under the Creative Commons License: http://creativecommons .org/licenses/by/3.0/

The contraceptive implant is a 3 cm soft, flexible single rod placed sub-dermally in the upper arm (Figure 7.3). The device continuously elutes the contraceptive progestin etonogestrel and is approved for 3 years of use. A trained provider can place the implant in a few minutes after administering a small amount of local anesthesia. Implant use may be complicated by difficult removal due to deep insertion. Implant use is not associated with weight gain. Neither IUD nor the implant contain estrogenic components and therefore do not increase the risk of thrombosis.

Long-acting reversible methods have different effects on menstrual bleeding. Copper IUD users experience no change in cycle length; however, menstrual flow and cramping may increase. The LNG IUD causes irregular bleeding during the first months after insertion. Thereafter, menstrual bleeding becomes regular and decreases markedly for most women; 20% develop amenorrhea after 1 year. The LNG IUD is approved for the treatment of heavy menstrual bleeding in the United States. Bleeding is irregular during use of the contraceptive implant, users may experience more or fewer episodes of bleeding than during spontaneous menstrual cycles. The implant is the only top-tier method which reliably inhibits ovulation.

Intramuscular depo-medroxy progesterone acetate (DMPA) is also a highly effective method with a failure rate comparable to the IUD or implant. Unlike those methods, however, the high efficacy of DMPA depends on re-injection every 3 months thus placing it overall efficacy in the 88–94% range for all users. Like the contraceptive implant, DMPA reliably inhibits ovulation. Bleeding with DMPA is irregular but decreases greatly over time. After 1 year, 75% of users experience amenorrhea. Unlike the IUD and all other hormonal methods, DMPA is not immediately reversible. Return to full fertility may be delayed up to 18 months. Overall, intramuscular DMPA is relatively safe; like other progestin-only methods, DMPA does not increase the risk of thrombosis. However, DMPA does cause modest decreases in bone mineral density. Compared to the contraceptive implant, DMPA has more profound inhibition of the hypothalamic–pituitary–ovarian axis. The stronger inhibition of follicle-stimulating hormone (FSH) production reduces endogenous estradiol production, leading to bone changes. With the contraceptive implant, FSH is produced and endogenous estradiol levels remain in the physiologic range. In healthy women receiving DMPA, these bone mineral density changes are reversible and do not appear to increase the risk of fracture in the short or long term [14]; therefore, no routine bone density screening is recommended. The U.S. Center for Disease Control Medical Eligibility Criteria (CDC MEC) guidelines for contraception recommend caution (risk may outweigh benefits) when using DMPA in women with other risk factors for osteoporosis such as chronic steroid use [15]. Since some AEDs may decrease bone density, use of DMPA with these AEDs should be individualized.

Oral contraceptives

Many OCs are available. Combined oral contraceptives (COCs) contain an estrogen (usually ethinyl estradiol (EE)) and a synthetic progestin, which differ from natural progesterone. Early progestins include norethindrone and LNG, whereas newer progestins include desogestrel, norgestimate, and drospirenone. The progestins differ in half-life, potency, and bioavailability. Norethindrone has the shortest half-life, drospirenone the longest. In one large study, pregnancy rates were lower among women using an EE and drospirenone-containing OC than among users of a pill with a comparable EE dose and a shorter-acting progestin [16]. The majority of available OCs contain EE as the estrogenic component, and some newer formulations have estradiol valerate. For non-contraceptive indications, most of these differences do not directly impact choice of an OC because few head-to-head comparisons guide pill choice. Acne and heavy menstrual bleeding are expected to improve on all combined OCs; some OCs have FDA approval for those indications. When choosing a pill for a woman treated with a strong enzyme-inducing AED, a pill with highest doses should be chosen. A formulation with 50 μg of EE and relatively high doses of progestin is best; however, these pills are not widely available. While practical and often suggested in the clinical literature, this strategy is unsupported by data proving efficacy. Any woman treated with a strong inducer using an OC should use another method, such as condoms, as well.

The progestin-only pill (POP) formulation available in the United States is a very low dose pill; it is taken continuously and does not reliably inhibit ovulation. Its primary mechanism is thickening of cervical mucous. Additionally, it is difficult to use, as it must be taken at the same time of day since the progestin dose is low and has a short half-life. Prescription of the POP in the United States is generally limited to women who are breastfeeding or have other contraindications to use of EE. Higher dose progestin-only OCs are available in other parts of the world.

In addition to COCs, which are taken daily, other combined hormonal methods include a transdermal patch and a vaginal ring. These are administered weekly and for 3 weeks, respectively. These methods inhibit ovulation and have non-contraceptive benefits of regular and decreased menstrual bleeding. Oral contraceptive use improves acne and prevents ovarian cysts, and if sustained, greatly decreases the risk of ovarian cancer and uterine cancer. The estrogenic component of combined methods is associated with an increased risk for thrombosis; however, the absolute risk of venous thrombosis for a healthy woman using these methods is very low, about one in 1000 users. Women with risk factors for thrombosis, stroke, or myocardial infarction should not use combined hormonal contraception, including migraine with aura and even migraine without aura if the woman is >35 years old. For smokers older than 35 years, OC use is contraindicated because of an increased risk of myocardial infarction and stroke [15].

Traditional OC formulations as well as the patch and ring are used for 3 weeks then stopped for 1 week to allow for a menstrual withdrawal bleed. Newer OC formulations shorten the time off (pill-free interval) to 4 days monthly, or 1 week every 3 months or eliminate the pill-free interval completely. Some of these methods results in very short, infrequent menses or induce complete amenorrhea. This is safe for women; the amenorrhea is due to reversible endometrial thinning and does not impact fertility after discontinuation. Breakthrough bleeding may occur with these extended regimens. Studies of continuous OC use up to 1 year show excellent safety and return to fertility. Longer studies are lacking but data from long-term use of traditionally administered OCs are reassuring.

Dual method contraception

The term dual method use usually refers to a male barrier method combined with some other method. Most often, in healthy women, this strategy is recommended for pregnancy prevention and sexual transmitted infection (STI) prevention, especially for adolescents. In the context of women treated with AEDs, the usual STI prevention recommendations would apply for those at risk, but condoms could also be recommended as a "backup" method to reduce the risk of pregnancy in the context of a drug interaction. If STI prevention is not a concern, dual method use is not a first-choice strategy for contraception because adherence becomes more complex. Dual method use would be recommended for strong inducer AEDs co-administered with oral contraceptives, ring patch, or implant. Dual method use would not improve efficacy in a clinically meaningful way for either IUD or DMPA.

Bidirectional interactions of hormonal contraceptives and AEDs

Effects of antiepileptic drugs on reproductive hormones

Oral contraceptives were the first effective reversible method of contraception and became available in the 1960s. Shortly after their introduction, clinicians caring for WWE observed pregnancies during co-administration of certain AEDS, despite the high doses of contraceptive steroids in these early formulations [17]. Since those early observations, AEDS have been systematically studied for how they impact the pharmacokinetic (PK) properties of EE and various contraceptive ingredients and grouped as enzyme-inducing or non-enzyme inducing. Unfortunately, these groupings based on PK changes do not clearly and directly relate to the risk of ovulation or pregnancy.

Antiepileptic drugs may impact contraceptive PK by several mechanisms. Some induce the hepatic cytochrome P-450 system, and specifically Cyp3A4, the primary metabolic pathway of EE and progestins. Some AEDs also enhance glucuronidation, another hepatic elimination pathway for these sex steroid hormones. More rapid clearance of the sex steroid hormones may allow ovulation in women using hormonal contraceptive agents [18]. In general, AEDs that induce hepatic metabolic enzymes are labeled EIAEDs and directly alter reproductive hormone levels (Table 7.2). These AEDs

Table 7.2 Antiepileptic drugs: degree of induction of metabolism of hormonal contraceptive agents

Strong inducers[a]	Weak inducers[b]	Non-inducers
Phenobarbital	Topiramate	Ethosuximide
Phenytoin	Lamotrigine	Valproate
Carbamazepine	Felbamate	Gabapentin
Primidone	Rufinamide	Clonazepam
Oxcarbazepine	Clobazam	Tiagabine
Perampanel	Eslicarbazepine	Levetiracetam
		Zonisamide
		Pregabalin
		Vigabatrin
		Lacosamide
		Ezogabine

[a] Avoid concomitant use with the lowest dose oral contraceptive pills.

also induce production of sex hormone binding globulin (SHBG), thereby reducing biologically active (free) reproductive hormone serum levels [19].

Hormonal contraceptives work by inhibiting ovulation and changes in cervical mucous. Ovulation inhibition depends largely on the contraceptive progestin via inhibition of LH production. This is a threshold effect. If the progestin component remains above the level at which ovulation is inhibited, the contraceptive effect should be preserved even if enzyme induction occurs. Prescribers of hormonal contraception for women on AEDs should be aware that efficacy also depends on adherence. Missed pills, late patches, or rings decrease contraceptive effectiveness. These adherence challenges are very common in typical users of short-acting hormonal contraception.

Pharmacokinetic studies have been performed with many specific AEDs and various formulations of hormonal contraceptives. No clear data identify which PK parameters relate to pregnancy risk; trough progestin levels are likely to be critical. Only one study has extended PK changes to a true pharmacodynamics study of pregnancy risk, and this study was for the commonly prescribed AED carbamazepine [20].

Categorization of the AEDs and recommendations in this chapter were developed with the best available information at this time despite the limitations of the study designs and the data available.

Older AEDs

Phenobarbital: A prospective study of the effect of phenobarbital (PB) on OC hormonal levels was performed in four women [21]. In this very small study, all four women used an OC with 50 mcg of EE, in three cases with norethindrone, and in one case norgestrel. Hormone levels were measured for one cycle prior to PB administration, and then for 2 months with PB 30 mg BID. Significant falls in the peak plasma EE concentrations occurred in two women (from 104.8 ± 13.4 to 37.7 ± 2.0 pg/mL and from 125.6 ± 23.8 to 34.8 ± 6.7 pg/mL), and they experienced breakthrough bleeding. No changes occurred in progesterone, norethindrone, norgestrel, or FSH levels. A significant increase in SHBG capacity occurred (100.7 ± 5.8 to 133.3 ± 1.2 nmoles per liter.

Primidone: Primidone is metabolized to PB, and therefore, the same principles should be applied for interactions with hormonal contraceptives. Previous reports included primidone as polytherapy and unexpected pregnancies occurred.

Phenytoin and carbamazepine: An early study directly examined the effects of phenytoin (PHT) ($n = 6$) and carbamazepine (CBZ) ($n = 4$) on the PK parameters of a single dose of a combined oral contraceptive containing 50 mcg of EE and 250 mcg of LNG [22]. Initial evaluation was prior to beginning the AED and compared to findings of the single-dose study after 8–12 weeks of treatment of PHT or CBZ. The area under the plasma concentration–time curve (AUC) was measured over a 24-hour period. Significant reductions were seen with both AEDs. With chronic PHT use, the AUC for EE was reduced from 806 ± 50 (mean $\pm$ SD) to 411 ± 132 pg mL per hour ($P < 0.05$) and for LNG from 33.6 ± 7.8 to 19.5 ± 3.8 ng mL per hour ($P < 0.05$). With chronic CBZ use, the AUC for EE was reduced from 1163 ± 466 to 672 ± 211 pg mL per hour ($P < 0.05$) and for LNG from 22.9 ± 9.4 to 13.8 ± 5.8 ng mL per hour ($P < 0.05$).

Carbamazepine: Only one enzyme-inducing AED, CBZ, has been adequately studied to determine whether changes in EE and the progestin LNG permitted ovulation [20]. In that study, 10 healthy women took 600 mg of CBZ or a placebo daily for 2 months with a low-dose oral contraceptive (EE 20 and LNG 150 mcg). Ovulation was detected by twice weekly sonography to identify developing dominant follicles and repeated progesterone assays. Compared to placebo, dramatic changes in EE and LNG occurred during CBZ use. Importantly, the trough level of LNG during CBZ use was very low, even undetectable. This large decrease in progestin levels was associated with ovulation in half of the CBZ cycles and an increase in breakthrough bleeding. Results demonstrate clearly that CBZ at 600 mg daily can lead to low-dose OC failure.

Newer AEDs

Reports and recommendations regarding many of the second-generation AEDs have been conflicting and incongruous.

Oxcarbazepine: A randomized, double-blind cross-over study of oxcarbazepine (OXC), (1200 mg/day) in 16 healthy women and on an OC with 50 mcg of EE and 250 mcg of LNG demonstrated a decrease in EE AUC by 47%, Cmax by 35%, and LNG AUC by 46% and Cmax by 24%, compared with the cycle with no OXC intake [23]. Many experts now include OXC in the strong inducer category for effects on hormonal contraceptive agents.

Felbamate: A randomized, placebo-controlled trial of 30 healthy women reported that with felbamate and a low-dose OC, there was minor 13% decline in EE AUC, but a larger decline in the progestin gestodene AUC by 42%, compared with placebo. Despite this, there was no evidence of ovulation in either group by progesterone and LH levels [24]. Felbamate is considered a weak inducer (Table 7.2).

Topiramate: A study of 12 WWE with topiramate (TPM) 200–800 mg/day and OCs (35 mcg EE/1 mg norethisterone) demonstrated that EE mean AUC values significantly declined 18–30% compared to baseline, in a dose-dependent manner. However, no changes in norethisterone occurred [25]. A randomized trial in healthy women using lower doses of TPM and low-dose OCs showed non-significant minor changes <12% in PK parameters, with TPM 50–200 mg/day [26]. Therefore, TPM is considered a weak inducer with induction impacting EE but not progestins (Table 7.2).

Lamotrigine: LTG is considered a weak inducer of contraceptive progestins. A cross-over study in 16 healthy women on a medium dose OC (30 mcg EE/150 mcg LNG) and moderate dose of LTG (300 mg/day) demonstrated that EE pharmacokinetics were unchanged. The Cmax, AUC, and trough levels of LNG, however, decreased about 20% with co-administration of LTG. FSH and LH concentrations were increased by 3.4- to 4.7-fold, and ovulation was not detected by single progesterone measurements. Intermenstrual bleeding was reported by 32% of subjects [27].

Rufinamide: Co-administration of rufinamide (800 mg BID for 14 days) and a COC (35 mcg EE/1 mg norethindrone) resulted in a mean decrease in the EE AUC_{0-24} of 22% and Cmax by 31% and norethindrone AUC_{0-24} by 14% and Cmax by 18% [28]. Rufinamide should be considered a weak inducer.

Clobazam: Clobazam and N-desmethylclobazam induce CYP3A4 activity in a concentration-dependent manner. There are no specific PK studies published with COCs, but the manufacturer recommends that additional non-hormonal forms of contraception should be used [29]. Data are lacking to clearly categorize clobazam as a strong or weak inducer, but it is more likely a weak inducer.

Eslicarbazepine acetate: Drug interaction studies suggest that eslicarbazepine may have some weak effects as a CYP 3A4 inducer. Two studies of COC interactions were performed, both in 20 healthy female subjects at doses of 800 mg and 1200 mg QD of eslicarbazepine [30]. Design for both studies was a two-way, crossover, two-period, randomized, open-label study, and an oral single dose of 30 mcg of EE and 150 mcg LNG was administered. Eslicarbazepine significantly decreased the exposure to EE and LNG with geometric mean ratios (90% CI) for AUC_{0-24} of EE of 68–75% and LNG of 76–89%, in a dose-dependent manner. Eslicarbazepine acetate should be considered a weak inducer as exposure led to minimal decreases in trough levels of progestins.

Perampanel: As reported in the package insert, studies in healthy controls revealed that daily doses of 4 and 8 mg/day of perampanel (PRM) did not have a significant effect on the Cmax or for AUC_{0-24} of EE or LNG [31]. However, at 12 mg/day of PRM, the LNG AUC_{0-24} and Cmax were decreased by 42% and 40%, respectively, and the EE Cmax was decreased by 18% and the EE AUC_{0-24} was not altered. Parampanel should be considered a weak inducer at lower doses but a strong inducer at higher daily doses.

Non-inducers

Non-inducers: Pharmacokinetic interaction studies have been performed with the other AEDs and various formulations of hormonal contraceptives and reported in journal articles and package inserts. Findings support lack of significant induction of metabolism of hormonal contraceptive agents with both older and newer AEDs: ethosuximide, valproate, gabapentin, clonazepam, tiagabine, levetiracetam, zonisamide, pregabalin, vigabatrin, lacosamide, and ezogabine (Table 7.2) [18].

Recommendations: Many authors have recommended "high-dose" OCs (≥50 mcg EE) with enzyme-inducing AEDs assuming enzyme induction will lower levels to what occurs with an effective lower dose OC [7]. A few OCs with higher doses of EE and progestin remain available but are infrequently used in practice for healthy women. While reasonable in the context of EIAEDs, no direct evidence supports efficacy in this situation. The CDC Medical Eligibility Criteria for contraception classified certain AEDs (PHT, CBZ, PB, PRM, TPM, and OXC) as a Category 3: the risks generally outweigh the benefits. In this category, the risk refers to birth control failure. The authors clarify that although the interaction of certain AEDs with COCs, POP, or the vaginal ring is not harmful to women, it is likely to reduce the effectiveness. The authors further state that if a COC is chosen, a preparation containing a minimum of 30 μg EE should be used [15].

Oral contraceptives, as well as patches, rings, and the implant, are not first-line contraceptive methods for women who use EIAEDs known to cause substantial changes in progestin levels (Table 7.2). For these women, the copper or LNG IUD are excellent choices. The LNG IUD prevents pregnancy by local hormonally mediated changes in cervical mucous which are not likely to be impacted by hepatic changes in cytochrome P450 enzyme induction. One reassuring prospective registry study in the United Kingdom demonstrated a pregnancy rate of 1.1 per 100 women-years for 56 women using the LNG-IUD with enzyme-inducing AEDs, a rate slightly higher than expected but still very low compared to other contraceptive methods available [32]. The DMPA is another choice with enzyme-inducing AEDs. No direct evidence examines how DMPA metabolism is impacted by enzyme-inducing AEDs; however, the dose of DMPA even at 12 weeks significantly exceeds the level needed for ovulation inhibition. Use of DMPA has to be considered in light of side effects discussed in this chapter.

Effects of hormonal contraceptives on AEDs

Earlier studies highlighted the finding that lamotrigine clearance is markedly enhanced during pregnancy. This observation prompted specific investigations of the effects of hormonal contraceptives. An early retrospective comparative study in WWE on LTG, ages 15–30 years

old enrolled 22 COC users and 30 non-users. The authors reported that LTG clearance [(LTG dose/body weight)/plasma concentration] was over twofold higher in the COC group compared to the non-user group [33]. A study investigating the mechanism of the enhanced clearance measured the main metabolite, lamotrigine-2-N-glucuronide, in WWE taking COC ($n = 31$), in WWE with the LNG IUD ($n = 12$), and in WWE on no contraceptive ($n = 20$) [34]. Compared to controls, the LTG dose/concentration ratio was 56% higher in the COC group and the N-2-glucuronide/LTG ratio was 82% higher ($P < 0.01$ in both). There were no differences between the control and the IUD group. Findings indicate that the enhanced metabolism of LTG is primarily by induction of the N-2-glucuronide pathway. Another study demonstrated increased LTG clearance in women on COC but a lack of difference in LTG clearance between non-hormonal users and those using POP, DMPA, progestin implant, or the LNG IUD, further supporting the theory that the enhanced glucuronidation is due to the estrogenic component [35]. A small study of seven women also reported lower plasma concentrations with COC use, but added information about the time course; baseline LTG levels were reached at an average of 8.0 (SD 3.69) days after the start of COCs. Two of the seven women experienced seizure worsening that correlated with reduced LTG concentrations [36].

The CDC Medical Eligibility Criteria specifically labels lamotrigine monotherapy as Category 3 (risks generally outweigh the benefits) for use with COC, given that PK studies have shown not only decreased LTG levels but also associated increased seizures [15].

Valproate and oxcarbazepine also undergo hepatic glucuronidation as a major elimination pathway. Similar PK interaction principles likely apply with estrogens decreasing AED concentrations, although surprisingly, this is not reported with OXC in the literature. However, enhanced clearance of OXC during pregnancy is reported. A later study investigated the effects of OCs on

Table 7.3 Antiepileptic drugs with increased clearance with concomitant use of a combined oral contraceptive

---

Antiepileptic drugs

Lamotrigine
Valproate
Oxcarbazepine[a]

---

[a]Reports in the literature are lacking, but increased clearance is probable given that hepatic glucuronidation is the major route of elimination.

VPA as well as LTG serum concentrations [37]. They enrolled four groups of WWE, with 12 women in each group: VPA, VPA plus OC, LTG, and LTG plus COC. The VPA concentrations were lower in the VPA plus COC group than the VPA alone group, with a median decrease of 23.4%. The LTG concentrations were 32.6% lower in the LTG plus COC group compared to LTG alone group (Table 7.3).

Preconception planning

Transitioning from contraception to preconception planning provides a valuable window of opportunity for the clinician. Not only does it allow the clinician to reassess the type of AED(s) prescribed and reinforce supplemental folic acid and prenatal vitamins, it also provides an opportunity to reassess the dose prescribed. This is especially important for the AEDs that undergo glucuronidation as a major metabolic pathway of elimination. Cessation of any hormonal contraceptives that contain an estrogen will result in a rise in the level of these AEDs (lamotrigine, valproic acid, and oxcarbazepine). If this is not considered, it can result in symptomatic toxicity and unnecessary overexposure of the fetus to the AED during the critical period of organogenesis. Findings from EURAP demonstrated that for each AED studied (LTG, VPA, PB, and CBZ), the odds ratio for an MCM increased with the higher dose ranges at the time of conception [5].

The clinician cannot wait until the diagnosis of pregnancy to determine the optimal lowest dose for the individual patient. Nor should he/she wait until the decision to become pregnant. As in healthy women, many pregnancies in women on AEDs will be unplanned. However, if a patient does decide to stop an estrogen-containing contraceptive, this provides a window of opportunity to lower fetal risk by adjusting the AED dose downward if she is on an AED with a metabolic route that is induced by estrogens (e.g., lamotrigine, valproic acid, and oxcarbazepine) and to perform a follow-up blood test to determine whether the AED concentration is still in the individual target range. The general principle that teratogens act in a dose-dependent manner for MCMs likely holds true for other effects of *in utero* AED exposure including fetal brain development.

Summary and conclusions

Effective contraception in women on AEDs is essential to allow for preconception planning and to implement the measures known to improve pregnancy outcomes. However, concomitant use of AEDs and hormonal contraceptives is complicated because of the bidirectional PK interactions, the pharmacodynamic consequences, and the potential effects on disease control. In summary, if a woman is on a weak inducer of metabolism of hormonal contraceptive agents, then avoid use of a very low-dose COC or POPs; other hormonal methods are likely to be effective. If she is on a strong inducer, either IUD is a first-line method for those who desire pregnancy in the future and sterilization for those who have completed childbearing or do not wish to have children (Tables 7.1 and 7.2). This chapter provides the groundwork necessary for practitioners from neurology, gynecology, and primary care to counsel this vulnerable patient population appropriately and to make informed prescribing choices.

References

1 Adedinsewo DA, Thurman DJ, Luo YH, Williamson RS, Odewole OA, Oakley GP. Valproate prescriptions for nonepilepsy disorders in reproductive-age women. *Birth Defects Res A Clin Mol Teratol.* 2013;97(6):403–408.

2 Bobo WV, Davis RL, Toh S, et al. Trends in the use of antiepileptic drugs among pregnant women in the US, 2001–2007: a medication exposure in pregnancy risk evaluation program study. *Paediatr Perinat Epidemiol.* 2012;26(6):578–588.

3 Harden CL, Meador KJ, Pennell PB, et al. American Academy of Neurology; American Epilepsy Society. Practice parameter update: management issues for women with epilepsy–focus on pregnancy (an evidence-based review): teratogenesis and perinatal outcomes: report of the Quality Standards Subcommittee and Therapeutics and Technology Assessment Subcommittee of the American Academy of Neurology and American Epilepsy Society. *Neurology.* 2009;73(2):133–141.

4 Meador KJ, Baker GA, Browning N, et al. NEAD study group. Fetal antiepileptic drug and folate exposure: cognition at age 6 years. *Lancet Neurol.* 2013;12(3):244–252.

5 Tomson T, Battino D, Bonizzoni E, et al. for the EURAP study group. Dose-dependent risk of malformations with antiepileptic drugs: an analysis of data from the EURAP epilepsy and pregnancy registry. *Lancet Neurol.* 2011;10(7):609–617.

6 Mosher WD, Jones J. Use of contraception in the United States: 1982–2008, Vital and Health Statistics, 2010, Series 23, No. 29.

7 Practice Parameter. Management issues for women with epilepsy (summary statement). Report of the Quality Standards Subcommittee of the American Academy of Neurology. *Neurology.* 1998;51(4):944–948.

8 Davis AR, Pack AM, Kritzer J, Yoon A, Camus A. Reproductive history, sexual behavior and use of contraception in women with epilepsy. *Contraception.* 2008;77(6):405–409.

9 Krauss GL, Brandt J, Campbell M, Plate C, Summerfield M. Antiepileptic medication and oral contraceptive interactions: a national survey of neurologists and obstetricians. *Neurology.* 1996;46(6):1534–1539.

10 Pack A, Davis AR, Kritzer J, Yoon A, Camus A. Anti-epileptic drugs: are women aware of interactions with oral contraceptives and potential teratogenicity? *Epilepsy Behav.* 2009;14(4):640–644.

11 Winner B, Peipert JF, Zhao Q, et al. Effectiveness of long-acting reversible contraception. *N Engl J Med.* 2012;366(21):1998–2007.

12 Ortiz ME, Croxatto HB. Copper-T intrauterine device and levonorgestrel intrauterine system: biological bases of their mechanism of action. *Contraception.* 2007;75(6 Suppl):S16–30.

13 Committee on Adolescent Health Care Long-Acting Reversible Contraception Working Group. The American College of Obstetricians and Gynecologists. Committee Opinion no. 539: adolescents and long-acting reversible contraception: implants and intrauterine devices. *Obstet Gynecol.* 2012;120(4):983–988.

14 Isley MM, Kaunitz AM. Update on hormonal contraception and bone density. *Rev Endocr Metab Disord.* 2011;12(2):93–106.

15 Centers for Disease Control and Prevention (CDC). U. S. Medical Eligibility Criteria for Contraceptive Use, 2010. *MMWR Recomm Rep.* 2010;59(RR-4): 1–86.

16 Dinger J, Minh TD, Buttmann N, Bardenheuer K. Effectiveness of oral contraceptive pills in a large U.S. cohort comparing progestogen and regimen. *Obstet Gynecol.* 2011;117(1):33–40.

17 Kenyon IE. Unplanned pregnancy in an epileptic. *Br Med J.* 1972;1:686–687.

18 Gaffield ME, Culwell Kelly R, Lee CR. The use of hormonal contraception among women taking anticonvulsant therapy. *Contraception.* 2011;83: 16–29.

19 Stoffel-Wagner B, Bauer J, Flügel D, Brennemann W, Klingmüller D, Elger CE. Serum sex hormones are altered in patients with chronic temporal lobe epilepsy receiving anticonvulsant medication. *Epilepsia.* 1998;39:1164–1173.

20 Davis AR, Westhoff CL, Stanczyk FZ. Carbamazepine coadministration with an oral contraceptive: Effects on steroid pharmacokinetics, ovulation, and bleeding. *Epilepsia.* 2011;52(2): 243–247.

21 Back D, Bates M, Bowden A, et al. The interaction of phenobarbital and other anticonvulsants with oral contraceptive steroid therapy. *Contraception.* 1980;22:495–503.

22 Crawford P, Chadwick DJ, Martin C, Tjia J, Back DJ, Orme M. The interaction of phenytoin and carbamazepine with combined oral contraceptive steroids. *Br J Clin Pharmacol.* 1990;30:892–896.

23 Fattore C, Cipolla G, Gatti G, et al. Induction of ethinyl estradiol and lovonorgestrel metabolism

by oxcarbazepine in healthy women. *Epilepsia*. 1999;40:783–787.

24 Saano V, Glue P, Banfield CR, et al. Effects of felbamate on the pharmacokinetics of a low-dose combination oral contraceptive. *Clin Pharmacol Ther*. 1995;58:523–531.

25 Rosenfeld WE, Doose DR, Walker SA, Nayak RK. Effect of topiramate on the pharmacokinetics of an oral contraceptive containing norethindrone and ethinyl estradiol in patients with epilepsy. *Epilepsia*. 1997;38(3):317–323.

26 Doose DR, Wang SS, Padmanabhan M, Schwabe S, Jacobs D, Bialer M. Effect of topiramate or carbamazepine on the pharmacokinetics of an oral contraceptive containing norethindrone and ethinyl estradiol in healthy obese and nonobese female subjects. *Epilepsia*. 2003;44(4):540–549.

27 Sidhu J, Job S, Singh S, Philipson R. The pharmacokinetic and pharmacodynamic consequences of the co-administration of lamotrigine and a combined oral contraceptive in healthy female subjects. *Br J Clin Pharmacol*. 2006;61(2):191–199.

28 Rufinamide (Banzel) Package Insert. Eisai Inc. http://dailymed.nlm.nih.gov/dailymed/lookup .cfm?setid=0a3fa925-1abd-458a-bd57-4ae780a1ef2d.

29 Clobazam (Onfi) Package Insert. Lundbeck Inc. http://dailymed.nlm.nih.gov/dailymed/lookup .cfm?setid=de03bd69-2dca-459c-93b4-541fd3e9571c.

30 Falcao A, Vaz-da-Silva M, Gama H, et al. Effect of eslicarbazepine acetate on the pharmacokinetics of a combined ethinylestradiol/levonorgestrel oral contraceptive in healthy women. *Epilepsy Res*. 2013;105:368–376.

31 Perampanel (Fycompa) Package Insert. Eisai Inc. http://dailymed.nlm.nih.gov/dailymed/drugInfo .cfm?setid=71cf3309-e182-473c-8b0b 280cabd0e122.

32 Bounds W, Guillebaud J. Observational series on women using the contraceptive Mirena concurrently with anti-epileptic and other enzyme-inducing drugs. *J Fam Plann Reprod Health Care*. 2002;28:78–80.

33 Sabers A, Ohman I, Christensen J, Tomson T. Oral contraceptives reduce lamotrigine plasma levels. *Neurology*. 2003;61(4):570–571.

34 Ohman I, Luef G, Tomson T. Effects of pregnancy and contraception on lamotrigine disposition: new insights through analysis of lamotrigine metabolites. *Seizure*. 2008;17:199–202.

35 Reimers A, Helde G, Brodtkorb E. Ethinyl estradiol, not progestogens, reduces lamotrigine serum concentrations. *Epilepsia*. 2005;46(9):1414–1417.

36 Wegner I, Edelbroek PM, Bulk S, Lindhout D. Lamotrigine kinetics within the menstrual cycle, after menopause, and with oral contraceptives. *Neurology*. 2009;73(17):1388–1393.

37 Herzog AG, Blum AS, Farina EL, et al. Valproate and lamotrigine level variation with menstrual cycle phase and oral contraceptive use. *Neurology*. 2009;72:911–914.

CHAPTER 8

Epilepsy

Mark S. Yerby

North Pacific Epilepsy Research, Oregon Health Sciences University, Portland, OR, USA

Introduction

In previous eras, issues of fertility, sexuality, and pregnancy were not considered important for neurologists. Women with chronic disease were not considered "eligible" for marriage and child rearing and were often counseled against doing so. Yet clearly women with epilepsy had been having children despite the discrimination and bias. Medical practice has gradually given way to an atmosphere in which marriage and child rearing are considered acceptable for women with epilepsy and physicians now see it as their responsibility to assist, not obstruct their patients.

The majority of women with epilepsy can and do have healthy children. The management of epilepsy in pregnant women, however, presents unique challenges. To be effective, neurologists need to understand several issues. Fluctuations in sex steroid hormones can have an impact on seizure control. Sexual dysfunction is seen more often in persons with epilepsy. Infertility is more common in women with epilepsy. It is unclear whether this is a function of anticonvulsant treatment or the underlying epilepsy. Enzyme-inducing antiepileptic drugs may reduce the effectiveness of hormonal contraceptives. Hormonal contraceptives may impact plasma concentrations of specific antiepileptic drugs. Women with epilepsy are at greater risk for complications of pregnancy and adverse pregnancy outcomes. The following is a practical discussion of the management of these problems.

Fertility

Epidemiological studies have demonstrated that women with epilepsy have only one-fourth to one-third as many children as women in the general population [1], [2]. Although social factors undoubtedly play some role, women with epilepsy do have higher rates of infertility and of reproductive and endocrine disorders than women without. In a large clinical center, 50% of women with epilepsy experienced menstrual abnormalities. In total, 20% of those with abnormalities were amenorrheic and 35% were anovulatory [3]. Lack of libido is driven by both hormonal and psychosocial elements and also contributes to lower birth rates. Libido is significantly reduced in one-third of men and women with epilepsy [4].

Menses can be considered a neurological event. A normal menstrual cycle requires normal central nervous system function. At puberty, the hypothalamic neurons in the basal aspect of the third ventricle begin to secrete gonadotropic-releasing hormone (GnRH). This hormone is released in pulses and is carried by the portal circulation to the anterior pituitary and regulates the secretion of prolactin,

Neurological Illness in Pregnancy: Principles and Practice, First Edition.
Edited by Autumn Klein, M. Angela O'Neal, Christina Scifres, Janet F. R. Waters and Jonathan H. Waters.

luteinizing hormone (LH), and follicle-stimulating hormone (FSH). Following menses increased FSH is released and stimulates the ovarian follicles to mature. Luteinizing hormone is then secreted and the combination results in the follicular cells of the ovary releasing estrogen. Luteinizing hormone is released from the pituitary in a pulsatile fashion reflecting the pulses of GnRH. In men, the LH pulses vary little. In women, LH pulses are of low amplitude 5–7 mIU/mL every 60–90 minutes during the follicular phase and accelerate just prior to ovulation. During the luteal phase, the amplitude is higher 8–12 mIU/mL and the frequency is lower, every 3–4 hours. As estrogen levels rise, there is a reciprocal braking effect on the secretion of FSH. Follicle-stimulating hormone levels fall, LH and estrogen levels peak, and an ovarian follicle moves to the ovarian surface and is released or "ovulates." Luteinizing hormone levels continue to rise and estrogen levels drop briefly. The remnant of the cells which surrounded the ova (the corpus luteum) is stimulated by LH to produce progesterone. Both estrogen and progesterone now rise to a peak and FSH and LH decline. Without continued stimulation by FSH, the corpus luteum will fail and estrogen and progesterone levels as well. The uterine endometrium can no longer be supported. There is necrosis and sloughing leading to menstrual flow. The hypothalamus drives anterior pituitary function and thus ovulation and menstruation.

The hypothalamus has connections from the amygdala and hippocampus. Localization-related epilepsies often have their origin in these regions. Epileptiform discharges may therefore have a direct effect on the hypothalamus and pituitary and disrupt ovulation. It appears as though the proportion of estrogens and progesterone rather than their absolute concentrations permits a normal menstrual cycle. The cyclic production of these sex steroid hormones responds to pituitary hormone secretion. Pituitary hormone secretion depends upon normal hypothalamic function. Considering this feedback system, it is not surprising that women with epilepsy whose cortices produce epileptiform discharges may experience reproductive dysfunction.

Various studies confirm the effects of seizure activity on hormone levels. Women with epilepsy experience more variation in LH pulse frequency and lower LH concentrations than controls. Frequency of seizure activity may have a differential effect on hormone levels. Increasing seizure frequency appears to decrease sexual desire, while there is no difference in libido between treated and untreated women with epilepsy.

The site of epileptiform discharge activity also has an effect on fertility and reproductive and endocrine disorders. In one study, women with left-sided ictal epileptiform foci had polycystic ovarian disease while those with right-sided foci had hypogonadotropic hypogonadism. Herzog and coworkers [5] were among the first to demonstrate increased reproductive and endocrine disorders in women with temporal lobe epilepsy. In total, 19 of 50 women experienced significant reproductive problems. Seven had polycystic ovarian disease, seven had hypergonadotropic hypogonadism, and six had hypogonadotrophic hypogonadism. Women with primary generalized epilepsies may also experience heightened rates of reproductive and endocrine disorders. Of 20 women studied by Bilo and colleagues [1], 3 had polycystic ovarian disease and 2 had hypogonadotrophic hypogonadism. Ascertainment bias may account for the high proportion of women with epilepsy with reproductive and endocrine disorders in these studies. Nonetheless, clinicians should be aware of these potential problems.

Different seizure types also cause varying effects. Electroconvulsive therapy increases prolactin concentrations over fivefold within 15–20 minutes and, in premenopausal women, also produces an acute increase in LH and FSH. Generalized seizures have been shown to triple prolactin serum concentrations within

15–20 minutes. This fact is used to assist physicians in differentiating epileptic from non-epileptic seizures [6]. Partial seizures do not increase serum prolactin, and they account for the majority (60%) of the epilepsies.

To add to the complexity, antiepileptic drugs may interfere with the hypothalamic–pituitary axis. Amenorrhea, oligomenorrhea, prolonged, or irregular cycles were seen in 20% of 238 women with epilepsy [7]. Though only 12% of the 238 women were treated with valproate, 45% of those on valproate monotherapy and 25% on valproate polytherapy had menstrual disturbances. Polycystic ovaries were found in 43% of valproate-treated women. Furthermore, 80% of women treated with valproate younger than 29 years had polycystic ovarian disease.

Libido is significantly reduced in one-third of men and women with epilepsy [4]. Increasing seizure frequency appears to decrease sexual desire. There appears to be no difference in libido between treated and untreated women with epilepsy making a drug effect less likely. Hyposexuality and orgasmic dysfunction have been reported in between 8% and 68% of women with epilepsy [8]. Persons with localization-related epilepsies appear to have higher rates of sexual dysfunction compared to those with primarily generalized epilepsies. Shukla and colleagues [9] have demonstrated 64% of women with partial, compared to 8% of generalized epilepsies reporting hyposexuality and sexual dysfunction.

The problem of infertility in women with epilepsy is complex. There are multiple factors: seizure type, frequency, and the site of ictal onset, as well as antiepileptic drugs, which may affect an individual patient. Infertility in a couple deserves a careful evaluation of both partners. For women with epilepsy, ultrasonography to rule out polycystic ovarian disease, serum LH and FSH concentrations, and an evaluation of antiepileptic drug use will help one narrow the focus of treatment. There is evidence that valproate may adversely impact the fertility of some women.

Contraception

A discussion of pregnancy needs to be preceded by reviewing the problems of contraception. Oral contraceptives have not been associated with exacerbation of epilepsy [10]. The effectiveness of hormonal contraceptives can, however, be reduced by enzyme-inducing antiepileptic drugs (carbamazepine, phenytoin, phenobarbital, felbamate, and topiramate). Hormonal contraceptives come in three formulations: oral (estrogen–progesterone combinations or progesterone only); subcutaneous (Implanon, Nexplanon) or intrauterine (NuvaRing, Paragaurd, and Mirena), implants; and injectable (depoprovera). All three forms can be adversely impacted by enzyme-inducing antiepileptic drugs.

Antiepileptic drugs may lower concentrations of estrogens by 40–50%. They also increase sex hormone-binding globulin (SHBG), which increases the binding of progesterone and reducing the unbound fraction. The result is that hormonal contraception is less reliable with enzyme-inducing antiepileptic drugs.

The low or mini dose oral contraceptives (<35 µg) are therefore to be used with caution. Because it is the progesterone not the estrogen that inhibits ovulation, using higher doses of estrogens alone may not be effective. The more rapid clearance of the oral contraceptive when used in conjunction with an enzyme-inducing antiepileptic drug will reduce the likelihood of unwanted side effects from higher dose tablets.

Failure of implantable hormonal contraceptives has also occurred [11]. Mid-cycle spotting or bleeding is a sign that ovulation is not suppressed. If this occurs, alternative or supplementary methods of contraception are required. Contraceptive failure may not always be predicable, even when mid-cycle spotting does not occur. Failure of basal body temperature to rise at mid-cycle can be used to document ovulatory suppression.

Medroxyprogesterone injections should be given every 10 weeks instead of 12 weeks to women on enzyme-inducing antiepileptic drugs. This shorter cycle is less likely to result in unintended pregnancy [12].

For many women with epilepsy, modern intrauterine devices (Mirena, Paragaurd) may be an excellent contraceptive choice. Paragaurd is a copper device and appears to have more adverse effects than the progesterone-imbedded Mirena. The Mirena's progesterone does not appear to be adversely effected by enzyme-inducing antiepileptic drugs. Alternatively, an intravaginal contraceptive the NuvaRing is well tolerated and effective.

Topiramate at doses higher than 200 mg may reduce ethinyl estradiol concentrations by 18% on 200 mg, 21% with 400 mg, and 30% with 800 mg of topiramate a day [13]. The importance of the potential impact on enzyme-inducing antiepileptic drugs cannot be underestimated. In a survey of 294 general practices in the General Practice Research Database, 16.7% of women with epilepsy aged 15–45 years were taking an oral contraceptive. Among them, 200 were on enzyme-inducing antiepileptic drugs and 56% on low estrogen (<50 μg) hormonal contraceptives [14].

There is at least one circumstance in which oral contraceptives affect antiepileptic drugs concentration. A marked reduction in lamotrigine concentrations may occur when oral contraceptives are taken concomitantly [15]. The average plasma concentration in 22 women on lamotrigine monotherapy with oral contraceptive use was 13 μmol/L. In a similar group of women on lamotrigine monotherapy with no oral contraceptive use, the plasma concentrations averaged 28 μmol/L, a significant reduction in antiepileptic drugs concentration of over 50%. Oral contraceptives may induce the metabolism of glucuronidated drugs such as lamotrigine. In addition, during the portion of the cycle in which women are taking the non-active form of oral contraceptives (days 21–28), lamotrigine concentrations may increase by 60%. These potentially relatively rapid fluctuations in plasma concentrations of lamotrigine

when oral contraceptives are used may either reduce the effectiveness of lamotrigine or result in adverse effects.

Pregnancy

The majority of women with epilepsy can conceive and bear normal healthy children. The pregnancies of women with epilepsy do present a greater risk for complications of pregnancy. They are more likely to have difficulties during labor, and there is a higher risk of adverse pregnancy outcomes.

Increased seizure frequency

Approximately one-quarter of women with epilepsy will have an increase in seizure frequency during pregnancy. This increase is unrelated to seizure type, duration of epilepsy, or seizure frequency in a previous pregnancy. While most studies have demonstrated that the increase tends to occur toward the end of pregnancy, a study by Cahill et al. [16] found that a substantial number (31%) had their increase in the first trimester. A recent report from India confirms that the period of greatest risk is peripartum but also found that localization-related epilepsies had bimodal peaks for gestational seizures, one at 2 to 3 months of gestational age (GA) and another at 6 months. Women with primarily generalized epilepsy tended to have exacerbations in the first trimester [17]. A large multicenter prospective study (EURAP) found that 17% of 1956 pregnancies had an increase in seizure frequency. Seizures occurred during delivery in 3.5%. Status epilepticus was fortunately uncommon occurring in 36 (1.8%) and only one-third of these were convulsive. There was one adverse outcome of a stillbirth as a result [18].

Seizures during pregnancy increase the risk of fetal loss. Generalized, tonic–clonic seizures increase the risk for hypoxia and acidosis [19] as well as injury from blunt trauma. Canadian researchers have found that maternal seizures during gestation increase the risk of developmental delay [20]. Although rare, stillbirths have occurred following a single generalized convulsion [21, 22] or series of [23, 18] convulsions.

Generalized convulsions occurring during labor can have a profound effect on fetal heart rate [24]. The increased rate of neonatal hypoxia and low Apgar scores may be related to such events [25]. Partial seizures may also have similar effects if less often [26].

Plasma concentrations of anticonvulsant drugs decline as pregnancy progresses, even in the face of constant and in some instances increasing doses [27–32]. Plasma concentrations tend to rise postpartum [33–36]. Although reduction in plasma drug concentration is not always accompanied by an increase in seizure frequency, virtually all women with increased seizures in pregnancy have subtherapeutic drug levels [37–40]. The decline of anticonvulsant levels during pregnancy is largely a consequence of decreased plasma protein binding [25, 41, 42], and increased drug clearance [38, 43–45]. The clearance rates are greatest during the third trimester.

Newer antiepileptic drugs tend to be more sensitive to increased clearance than their more protein-bound predecessors. The concentration–dose ratios (CD ratio) of topiramate are 34% lower in the third trimester than prior to conception. The CD ratio for levetiracetam is 50% lower in the third trimester and for lamotrigine 66% lower than prepregnancy [35, 46, 47]. The impact of pregnancy on lamotrigine is quite striking. Its clearance is increased by 167% in the first, 236% and 248% in the second and third trimesters, respectively, reaching 264% increase over baseline at delivery [36]. Postpartum, the clearance of lamotrigine rapidly returns to preconception values by the third week [36]. Unlike most antiepileptic drugs, lamotrigine is largely metabolized by glucuronidation. Estradiols increase glucuronidation and as

its concentrations raise in pregnancy, the clearance of lamotrigine follows. The rapid drop in estradiol postpartum reverses this process [48].

The dramatic changes in lamotrigine concentrations in pregnancy make managing women taking it a challenge. Sabers [49] has developed an algorithm for dose adjustment that can be helpful for clinicians. First, a reference plasma concentration should be established ideally prior to pregnancy. This is the concentration associated with seizure control in that individual patient. Lamotrigne concentration should be measured every 4 weeks. When the concentration falls below the reference, the dose should be increased by 20–25%. Postpartum the concentration should be measured every 1–2 weeks and if higher than the reference, the dose reduced by 20–25% until the patient's concentration returns to the reference level.

Complications in the offspring

The infants of epileptic mothers are at greater risk for a variety of adverse pregnancy outcomes. These include fetal death, congenital malformations, neonatal hemorrhage, low birth weight, developmental delay, feeding difficulties, and childhood epilepsy.

Infant mortality

Fetal death or stillbirths (defined as fetal loss after 20 weeks gestation) appear to be as common and perhaps as great a problem as congenital malformations and anomalies. Studies comparing stillbirth rates found higher rates in infants of mothers with epilepsy (IME) (1.3–14.0%) compared to infants of mothers without epilepsy (1.2–7.8%) [50].

Spontaneous abortions, defined as fetal loss prior to 20 weeks of gestation, do appear to occur more commonly in IME [51, 52]. Spontaneous abortions (miscarriages) are extremely difficult to quantify and rates are elusive, though the EURAP Registry reports 530/8476 pregnancies or 6.3% rate of spontaneous abortions and the Australian Registry a 4% rate [53], and the North American Registry a 4.4% rate [54].

Women with localization-related epilepsies appear to be at greater risk for spontaneous abortions than those with other seizure types [55]. Other studies have demonstrated the increased rates of neonatal and perinatal death. Perinatal death rates range from 1.3% to 7.8% compared to 1.0% to 3.9% for controls.

Malformations

Fetal malformations have been associated with *in utero* exposure to antiepileptic drugs. Congenital malformations are defined as a physical defect requiring medical or surgical intervention and resulting in a major functional disturbance.

Infants of mothers with epilepsy who are exposed to anticonvulsant drugs *in utero* are twice as likely to develop birth defects as infants not exposed to these drugs. Malformation rates in the general population range from 2% to 3%. Reports of malformation rates in various populations of exposed infants range from 1.25% to 12.5% [53, 54, 56–68]. These combined estimates yield a risk of malformations in a pregnancy of women with epilepsy of 4–6%. Cleft lip, cleft palate, or both and congenital heart disease account for many of the reported cases. Orofacial clefts are responsible for 30% of the increased risk of malformations in these infants [69–71].

A wide variety of congenital malformations have been reported, and every anticonvulsant drug has been implicated as a cause. No anticonvulsant drug can be considered absolutely safe in pregnancy, yet most of these drugs do not produce any specific pattern of major malformations. There are, however, two antiepileptic drugs which may be associated with specific malformations. Meningomyelocele has been found to be associated with intrauterine exposure to sodium valproate and carbamazepine. The prevalence of neural tube defects with valproate exposure is approximately 1–2% [72], and with carbamazepine it is 0.5% [73, 74].

Methodological problems have made frequency estimates imprecise. Most published data are case reports, case series, or small cohorts not designed to evaluate pregnancy outcomes. Prior to the development of pregnancy registries, data were lacking with regard to the relative risk of specific antiepileptic drugs in monotherapy or polytherapy. When one looked at specific drugs, there was tremendous diversity of findings. In addition, 11 new antiepileptic drugs have been introduced into the North American market since 1993. Gabapentin, felbamate, lamotrigine, levetiracetam, oxcarbazepine, tiagabine, topiramate, zonisamide, vigabatrin, lacosimide, and clobazam are all now available in the United States. The number of reported pregnancies with exposure to these drugs is, in many cases, very small and unfortunately not large enough for one to determine whether there is an increased risk for adverse outcome with fetal exposure. These drugs were all initially introduced for use as adjunctive therapy, and there has been little information about their safety in monotherapy or relative safety in pregnancy.

Pregnancy registries were developed as a solution to the lack of data on new-drug safety. These registries for prospective data collection can serve as an "early warning system" by looking for clusters of specific abnormalities or rates of malformation in excess of those expected. They have many limitations, however. They are hampered by not being truly population-based. They have no accurate data on the number of exposed women with epilepsy who give birth. Therefore, no population-based denominator exists to permit the estimation of rates. Registries in different regions use different definitions of malformations, thus data are not comparable across registries. There are difficulties in ascertaining the time of antiepileptic drugs exposure and verifying pregnancy outcomes [75]. It is difficult to maintain enrollees in a registry that has little personal connection with the participants; therefore, the rate of loss to follow-up is fairly high. The data are collected by telephone interview or written questionnaire, making it difficult to collect information about or to verify comorbidities. The period of follow-up is limited to a modest interval after delivery. Such systems can only accurately identify major malformations of the type diagnosable at birth. Despite these limitations, however, they remain the only method currently available for surveillance, and physicians and patients are encouraged to enroll.

Provided that these limitations are kept in mind, pregnancy registries have the best utility short of prospective, double-blind monitoring studies. There are some principles that if applied will strengthen a registry and minimize bias. When evaluating the data from a registry, one should know whether these principles have been followed and thus whether one can rely on the information in the report.

Patient recruitment should start as close to the beginning of pregnancy as possible to ensure that enrollment precedes knowledge of the pregnancy outcome. Outcomes, even the knowledge of a fetal ultrasound, can bias a study's findings. Some data should be collected that will permit one to determine whether the subjects enrolled are representative of the population and not simply persons at very high or very low risk.

Quality of data collection should be verifiable and systematic, so that the same queries are addressed to each person enrolled. Standardized forms are required to ensure consistency. The initial interview should be conducted as soon as possible after the pregnancy is identified to record any fetal losses, as well as to eliminate dropouts due to therapeutic abortion secondary to malformations discovered by ultrasound. Other risk factors for adverse outcome of pregnancy should also be identified.

Subjects should be followed up until the outcome of the pregnancy is known, whether or not it results in a live birth. It is therefore important to have means of contacting the subjects intermittently and to encourage them to contact the registry if there is any change in their health status. For example, the birth rate of anencephalic infants has fallen by 60–70% and the rates of spinal bifida by 20–30% since the inception of earlier and more effective ultrasonography [76]. Thus, early enrollment and careful follow-up are necessary to avoid missing these types of abnormalities.

While congenital malformations are the issue of greatest concern, other adverse pregnancy outcomes need to be evaluated. Spontaneous abortions (fetal loss before 20 weeks), therapeutic abortions, and fetal deaths or stillbirths (failure of the conceptus to survive after 20 weeks) also need to be recorded. The definitions of congenital malformations should also be clear, and conditions appropriate for the GA. Patent ductus arteriosus and inguinal hernias should be excluded. The distinction between malformations and minor congenital anomalies should be made before any data collection, and methods of identifying which of these types are being reported should be established.

After the number of adverse outcomes is established, statistical techniques are used to determine the upper and lower limits of that risk or the confidence interval. Any report of risk should include such a range, because by the nature of registries, the true denominator is unknown. The risk is only an estimate. The more narrow the confidence interval, the better the estimate. Risk can only be discussed in the aggregate. Registries by their nature are usually (but not always) unable to provide a control group. Therefore, the registry must state which control group or population its rates are being compared against. Internal comparisons, such as those comparing adverse outcomes between women using different antiepileptic drugs for the same condition, must be made with care. Epilepsy is a heterogeneous set of conditions, and one must be careful about the potential differences between various epilepsy types, some of which, such as juvenile myoclonic epilepsy, have strong genetic components. Newer antiepileptic drugs may be used preferentially in persons with more severe epilepsy who have failed to respond to older medications. The ideal control group would be women with the same syndrome, in a randomized treatment. Such a group does not exist in sufficient numbers for comparison, as few persons with genuine epilepsy can remain seizure-free for prolonged intervals with no treatment. A registry should also be able to report the power of its findings to determine a difference in rates.

Individual registries

There are now two major regional pregnancy registries for antiepileptic drugs: European (EURAP) and North American (NAREP). All are prospective and collect information for all antiepileptic drugs. They differ in the source of subjects. The NAREP requires patients themselves to report while the other relies on physicians.

There is also a toll-free number for the NA-AEDR: 1-888-233-2334. Established in 1996, this registry has prospectively enrolled over 6857 women, 5278 of whom were receiving antiepileptic drugs monotherapy in the first trimester. The risk of major malformations was 9.5% (30/317) for valproate, 5.6% (11/197) for phenobarbital, 3.4% (11/321) for topiramate, 3.0% (12/407) for phenytoin, 2.9% (29/1012) for carbamazepine, 2.1% (8/378) for levetiracetam, and 1.9% (28/1441) for lamotrigine exposed pregnancies [54].

This registry also looked at the malformation rates in mono- versus polytherapy antiepileptic drug exposure and found that polytherapy did not increase the risk of malformations unless valproate was one of the medications used.

The EURAP has been in operation since 1999. It has a central registry in Milan and 41 reporting countries including not only Europe but also Asia, India, Latin America, and Australia. Over 8476 women have been enrolled before the 16th week of GA. Among them, 80% (6774/8476) were receiving monotherapy. Eighty-nine percent of pregnancies were live births, 6.3% spontaneous abortions, and 1.4% fetal deaths. A total of 431 malformations (5.4%) have been identified, including 320 (5%) after monotherapy exposure and 108 (7.4%) after polytherapy exposure [52].

To date, the most productive pharmaceutical registry has been the Lamotrigine Pregnancy Registry, with 1558 prospectively registered first-trimester monotherapy pregnancies. Thirty-five infants with major congenital malformations (MCMs) were identified giving a rate of 2.2% (95% CI 1.5–5.0%). Lamotrigine polytherapy with valproate was 0.7% (95% CI 6.4–17.0%) and without valproate 2.8% (95% CI 1.5–5.0%) [77].

A Swedish birth registry study has reviewed 1398 antiepileptic drugs-exposed infants. The odds ratio for malformations in infants exposed to antiepileptic drugs was 1.86 (95% CI 1.4–2.4). Malformation rates for specific antiepileptic drugs in monotherapy were 4.0% for carbamazepine, 4.4% for lamotrigine, 6.8% for phenytoin, and 9.7% for valproic acid [66]. The maternal risk for preeclampsia was increased OR = 1.66 (95% CI 1.32–2.08) and IME had an increased risk of respiratory distress OR = 2.06 (95% CI 1.6–2.6) [78].

An Australian pregnancy registry has combined prospective and retrospective data in an unusual approach. They have reported on the malformation rates of infants of women with epilepsy in 1317 pregnancies. Malformation rates with levetiracetam 0% (0/22), phenytoin 2.9% (1/35), topiramate 3.2% (1/31), lamotrigine 5.2% (12/231), carbamazepine 6.3% (19/301), and valproate 16.3% (19/301) [79].

A registry from the United Kingdom reported on 3607 pregnancies. The overall malformation rate for all antiepileptic drugs-exposed infants was 4.2% (95% CI 3.6–5.0). The malformation rate was 3.7% for those exposed to monotherapy and 6.0% exposed to polytherapy. There were higher rates of malformations in polytherapy with valproate than without (OR 2.49). Carbamazepine monotherapy exposures resulted in the lowest malformation rates of 2.1% followed by gabapentin 3.7%, lamotrigine 3.5%, phenytoin 4.1%, and valproate 6.1% [67].

Exposure to antiepileptic drugs *in utero* increases the risk of MCMs by a factor of two compared to control populations. The risk associated with first trimester exposure varies with specific antiepileptic drugs ranging from 1.9% for lamotrigine to 9.5% for valproate. Oral facial clefts are overrepresented; 1/1000 live births in the general population, >10/1000 in infants exposed to phenobarbital, valproate, or topiramate. Valproate is also associated with an increased risk of hypospadias, neural tube, and cardiac defects.

Folic acid has been demonstrated to reduce the risk of malformations in general. The Center of Disease Control recommends that women of childbearing age should take folate supplementation of 400 µg/d.

Low birth weight

Low birth weight (less than 2500 gm or 5 lbs. 8 oz.) and prematurity have been described in IME. The average rates range from 7% to 10% for low birth weight and 4–11% for prematurity [80–84]. These studies do not analyze the effect of specific seizure types, frequency, or antiepileptic drugs on this aspect of fetal development.

A prospective study which pooled data from three countries (Canada, Japan, and Italy) on 870 IME found that 7.8% were below the 10th percentile in weight at birth [85]. The risk was greater with polytherapy.

Body dimensions of IME have been studied by Wide and colleagues [86]. Infants exposed to polytherapy, not surprisingly, were shorter and smaller than those exposed to monotherapy. Exposure to monotherapy with carbamazepine revealed a tendency toward small size for GA, birth weight, and head circumference but it was not statistically significant.

Topiramate has been associated with weight loss in patients taking it for epilepsy. It appears to have a similar effect on fetal growth. Infants exposed to topiramate averaged 300 g less at birth than controls in a prospective study of 289 monotherapy-exposed pregnancies. This increased risk of low birth weight persists even after controlling for maternal smoking (Hernandez-Diaz et al., In Press).

Developmental delay

With a prevalence of 0.6% to 1%, it is estimated that there are 24,000 deliveries to women with epilepsy in the United States each year. If 75–95% of these persons take antiepileptic drugs, we can expect 18,000 to 22,800 infants exposed to antiepileptic drugs *in utero* per year. It is estimated that half of all antiepileptic drug prescriptions are used for conditions other than epilepsy. Though these patient populations may have fewer women of childbearing years, the number of exposed children is substantial.

Most investigators have focused on congenital malformations as the primary adverse outcomes for children of mothers with epilepsy. The rates are approximately double those of the general population. The magnitude of developmental delay may be similar.

Infants of mothers with epilepsy have been reported to have higher rates of mental retardation than the general population. This risk is increased by a factor of two- to sevenfold according to various authors [87, 88].

Leavitt and colleagues found that IME display lower scores in measures of verbal acquisition at both 2 and 3 years of age. Though there was no difference in physical growth parameters between IME and controls, IME scored significantly lower in the Bayley Scale of Infant Development's mental developmental index (MDI) at 2 and 3 years. They also performed significantly less well on the Bates Bretherton early language inventory ($P \leq 0.02$) and in the Peabody Picture Vocabulary's scales of verbal reasoning ($P \leq 0.001$) and composite IQ ($P \leq 0.01$), and they displayed significantly shorter mean lengths of utterance ($P \leq 0.001$) [89].

Leonard et al. [90] addressed the question of whether maternal seizures or *in utero* exposure to antiepileptic drugs are responsible for the developmental delay seen. A group of children of mothers with epilepsy who were followed until they reached school age were found to have a rate of intellectual deficiency of 0.6%. The Wechler Intelligence Scale for Children revealed significantly lower scores for children exposed to seizures during gestation (100.3), than for children whose mother's seizures were controlled (104.1) or controls (112.9). All antiepileptic drugs are clearly not created equal and Koch and coworkers [91] have demonstrated that primidone particularly when used in polytherapy is associated with lower Wechler score of intelligence.

Both maternal epilepsy and antiepileptic drugs were associated with a delayed development of offspring in a study by Koch et al. [91]. Severity of outcomes increased from control group to maternal epilepsy/no-drug group to monotherapy group and was most marked in the polytherapy group. These differences may reflect neural vulnerability to social, genetic, and teratogenic factors.

An intensive retrospective analysis of 100 consecutive pregnancies seen at a tertiary epilepsy center found that 3.9% of the children were premature, 1.1% had congenital malformations, and 6.2% had developmental delay. This occurred despite the fact that 59% of the mothers were seizure-free and 98% took folic acid during their pregnancy [93].

A retrospective study from the United Kingdom demonstrated that 16% of 594 children of mothers with epilepsy exposed to antiepileptic drugs *in utero* required additional education assistance in school, compared to 11% of 176 of children with no antiepileptic drugs' exposure. The mothers in the study had no history of a fixed severe neurologic deficit or significant learning disabilities. Developmental delay occurred in 30% of children exposed to valproate monotherapy, 24% exposed to valproate polytherapy, and 3.2% of

carbamazepine monotherapy-exposed children [93]. Monotherapy with other antiepileptic drugs had rates of 6% and polytherapy without valproate 16%. Children with no antiepileptic drugs exposure had an 11% use of additional educational services.

The same cohorts of children were studied to determine IQ scores. Of 251 children tested, the mean IQ for valproate-exposed children was 82 compared to 95 for carbamazepine-exposed and 92 for antiepileptic drugs unexposed children [94].

The authors followed up their initial cohort eventually studying 249 children of mothers with epilepsy from ages 6 to 16. The numbers in monotherapy included 41 exposed to valproate, 52 to carbamazepine, 21 to phenytoin, 49 to polytherapy, and 80 unexposed children. They used regression analysis to demonstrate that both exposure to valproate and frequently generalized tonic–clonic seizures in pregnancy increased the risk of low verbal IQ scores [95].

A retrospective study of mothers with epilepsy delivering in Scotland between 1976 and 2000 used non-exposed siblings as controls. Developmental delay was demonstrated in 19% of 293 antiepileptic drugs-exposed children compared to just 3% of their non-exposed siblings. The rate of delay in valproate-exposed children was, particularly high, 37% [96].

In one of the best-designed prospective studies of outcomes of mothers with epilepsy, Gaily and colleagues [97] measured the intelligence of 182 children of mothers with epilepsy and 141 controls. The investigators performing the testing were blinded as to the child's exposure. Mean verbal, performance, and full-scale IQ scores were consistently lower in valproate-exposed children ranging from 6 to 13 points lower than children exposed to carbamazepine, other antiepileptic drugs in monotherapy or unexposed children.

In an attempt to determine whether certain antiepileptic drugs are more hazardous in terms of child development, the NEAD study was devised. It is a prospective multicenter

Table 8.1 Mean IQ scores of infants exposed to AED *in utero*

Medication	N	Mean IQ	95% CI
Carbamazepine	53	106	102–109
Lamotrigine	72	106	102–109
Phenytoin	40	105	102–109
Valproate	38	96	91–100

AED, antiepileptic drug.

study which has compared neurodevelopmental differences in children exposed to monotherapy with carbamazepine, lamotrigine, phenytoin, or valproate. In total, 203 mother–child pairs were studied at 2, 3, 4.5, and 6 years of age. The differential ability scale was used to determine differences at age of 4.5 years. Valproate-exposed infants had lower adjusted IQ scores than any other antiepileptic drugs exposed group. Table 8.1 demonstrates the findings [98].

The magnitude of developmental delay in infants of women with epilepsy is on a par with that of congenital malformations. Exposure to maternal gestational convulsions, valproate, and antiepileptic drug polytherapy are consistently associated with poor cognitive performance.

Specific effects of antiepileptic drugs and other interventional therapies

New antiepileptic drugs in pregnancy

Since 1993, a number of effective new antiepileptic drugs have been introduced in North America. Their diminished side effect profiles have made them increasingly popular. Gabapentin, felbamate, lamotrigine, levetiracetam, oxcarbazepine, pregabalin, tiagabine, topiramate, zonisamide, vigabatrin, lacosimide, and clobazam are all now available in the United States. There is some tendency to think that since we know that the older antiepileptic drugs

have hazards, the new ones might be acceptable substitutes. We have good data for lamotrigine, levetiracetam, and topiramate. Unfortunately, for the other drugs, there is little information to support their safety. The numbers of reported exposed pregnancies with these drugs, particularly, those approved for use in adjunctive therapy is very low, and unfortunately not large enough for one to determine whether there is an increased risk of adverse outcome with fetal exposure to these compounds. Below is the current information about other antiepileptic drugs.

Gabapentin: A registry for gabapentin and pregnancy combined retrospective and prospectively collected cases. It reported on 44 children born to 39 mothers with epilepsy taking gabapentin; 2 of 44 or 4.5% had major malformations. One child had hypospadias and was exposed to gabapentin and valproic acid. The other was exposed to gabapentin monotherapy until the 16th week of gestation and then switched to phenobarbital and had only one kidney [99].

A population-based study covering deliveries in Denmark from 1996 to 2008 described a very small population of gabapentin-exposed pregnancies, 59 of 1532 pregnancies. One or 1.7% of the gabapentin-exposed pregnancies developed malformations [100].

The North American Registry has demonstrated a malformation rate of 0.7% or 1% of 142 monotherapy pregnancies (95% CI 0.02–3.9%) [54].

Oxcarbazepine: A retrospective study from Finland of 133 women with epilepsy, 101 monotherapy exposures had no malformations and in 17 polytherapy exposures, there was one malformation, a ventriculoseptal defect [101]. A prospective series of 55 oxcarbazepine-exposed pregnancies from Argentina found no malformations in the 35 monotherapy-exposed cases. One child with a ventricular septal defect was exposed to oxcarbazepine and phenobarbital [102]. A 2.4% rate of malformations (6/248 pregnancies) were described in a review of the literature [103].

Oxcarbazepine's primary metabolite 10-monohydroxy derivative (MHD) falls significantly in pregnancy starting in the first trimester and continuing through the third trimester [104, 105]. This can result in an increase in maternal seizures in as many as 50% of pregnancies [105].

Topiramate has been best studied by the NAREP. Of 289 monotherapy first trimester exposures, there were 11 major malformations or 3.8%. Of 11 malformations, 4 were orofacial clefts. This compares unfavorably with the malformation rate in the control group of 1.3%. The relative risk of malformations with topiramate exposure is 2.8 (95% CI 1.0–8.1).

Topiramate is also associated with an increased risk of low birth weight. Infants exposed to topiramate weigh an average of 307 g less than those born to controls. This is significantly less than the effect of maternal smoking on birth weight in which such children average 200 g less than controls (Hernandez-Diez et al., In Press).

Despite the fact that zonisamide is the most commonly used antiepileptic drug in Japan, there has been little study of pregnancy outcomes. There is one case series of 26 reported pregnancies with zonisamide exposure. Of 26, 2 (7.7%) had congenital malformations. One child was also exposed to phenytoin and the other to both phenytoin and valproic acid [106]. A report from post-marketing surveillance has found a high 16.7% malformation rate, from a very small group only 1 of 6 polytherapy pregnancies [107].

There is a single case series describing visual field changes in four infants exposed to vigabatrin *in utero* [108]. Vigabatrin has been demonstrated to lower maternal folate and increase fetal loss and skeletal hypoplasia in mice [109].

The North American Registry of Antiepileptic Drugs and Pregnancy has the most thoroughly evaluated prospective cohort of monotherapy exposures. For many individual antiepileptic drugs, the sample sizes are too small to calculate accurate rates. The Registry does, however, have a concurrent comparator group and thus its data on malformations are the strongest to date. Table 8.2 demonstrates the rates and their confidence limits [54].

Complications of pregnancy

Most of the attention with regard to pregnancy in women with epilepsy has focused on fetal outcome and maternal seizures. These patients have, however, also been described as having more complications of pregnancy and labor than women in the general population. Older studies report that hyperemesis gravidarum, vaginal bleeding, eclampsia, premature labor, and cesarean section rates are all higher in women with epilepsy [110, 25].

Subsequent studies have found conflicting types and rates of complications. Some have demonstrated little or no such problems [111–113]. Others have found increased risks of preeclampsia, hypertension, and maternal bleeding [114–116]. It remains unclear whether these issues are a function of maternal epilepsy, maternal seizures in pregnancy, use of antiepileptic drugs or socioeconomic factors that may accompany women with epilepsy. The diagnosis of epilepsy in and of itself may effect some obstetrical practices. Knowing that a patient has epilepsy could lead some obstetricians to prefer cesarean section. A study done at the University of Washington found that although the cesarean section rate was twice that of controls, all cesarean sections had followed an appropriate period of failure to progress [89].

The disparity of results found in the literature may be secondary to the difficulty of finding a comparable control group or differences in the population of women with epilepsy in terms of treatment and epilepsy types. The ability to control for other risk factors makes a Norwegian hospital-based study (though retrospective) more helpful [117]. The authors compared a group of 104 women with treated epilepsy, a

Table 8.2 Risk of major malformations of specific AED in monotherapy

AED	Lamotrigine	Carbamazepine	Phenytoin	Levetiracetam	Topiramate	Valproate	Phenobarbital	Oxcarbazepine	Gabapentin	Zonisamide	Clonazepam
N	1441	1012	407	378	321	317	197	171	142	76	56
Malformations (%)	28 (1.9%)	24 (2.9%)	12 (3.0%)	8 (2.1%)	11 (3.4%)	30 (9.5%)	11 (5.6%)	3 (1.8%)	1 (0.7%)	0 (0%)	2 (3.6%)
95% CI	(1.3–2.8%)	(1.9–4.1%)	(1.5–5.1%)	(0.9–4.1%)	(1.7–6.1%)	(6.5–13.2%)	(2.8–9.8%)	(0.4–5.0%)	(0.02–3.9%)	(0.0–3.9%)	(0.0–8.4%)
RR	1.6	2.3	2.4	1.7	2.8	7.7	4.6	1.4	0.6	NA	2.9

AED, antiepileptic drug; RR, relative risk.

Table 8.3 Pregnancy complications of women with epilepsy compared to controls

Complication	Control N (%)	Women with epilepsy N (%)	OR (95% CI)
Preeclampsia	11 (5.4)	26 (12.7)	2.3 (1.1–5.0)
Vaginal bleeding	8 (3.9)	25 (12.2)	3.8 (1.7–8.8)
Induction	23 (11.2)	43 (21.0)	1.8 (1.0–3.2)
Cesarean section	26 (12.7)	51 (24.9)	1.8 (1.0–3.1)

Reproduced from Reference 117 with permission of John Wiley & Sons.

group of 101 untreated women who had been seizure-free for 5 years, and a control group of 205 women. They controlled for other medical conditions, education, smoking, folate use, and body mass index. Women with epilepsy were more likely to have preeclampsia, early pregnancy bleeding, induction of labor, and cesarean sections (Table 8.3). All of the increased risks seen in women with epilepsy were also found in those treated with antiepileptic drugs, opposed to untreated women.

Breastfeeding

Breastfeeding is generally safe in terms of infants as they have been exposed to the antiepileptic drugs for 9 months and have induced hepatic microsomal enzyme systems. Breastfeeding should be done cautiously by women receiving phenobarbital or primidone due to the risk of infant sedation.

Summary and conclusions

Women with epilepsy and their caregivers face a dilemma. Seizures need to be prevented because they increase the risk of maternal injury and fetal loss and to some extent developmental delay. Fetal exposure to anticonvulsant drugs needs to be minimized because they may increase the risk of major malformations, developmental delay, and pregnancy complications. Withdrawing the patient from anticonvulsants prior to conception is not a realistic option. Women are likely to be employed and the potential disruption of their lifestyle by seizures, and risk of loss of driver's license, makes elimination of anticonvulsants impractical, and to some extent dangerous.

The major organ systems have formed by late in the first trimester. The posterior neuropore closes by day 27 and the palate by the 47th day of gestation. By the time, most women realize they are pregnant, any malformations have likely already developed. Women with epilepsy of childbearing age need to be informed of the risks of pregnancy associated with anticonvulsant use prior to conception and also need to know that seizures can be harmful to both the mother and the fetus. Risks can be reduced with proper management.

Healthy parents without epilepsy or antiepileptic drug exposure have a 2–3% risk of having a child with a malformation. One cannot guarantee a successful pregnancy but risk of complications can be managed. In general, risks can be minimized by the preconceptual use of multivitamins with folate, using antiepileptic drugs in monotherapy with the lowest effective dose that prevents maternal seizures. Sufficient studies of many antiepileptic drugs are lacking, but the data to date support the relative safety of lamotrigine and levetiracetam whose rates of malformations in monotherapy are modest at 1.9% and 2.1%, respectively. Unfortunately, valproate, phenobarbital, and topiramate carry relative high risks of malformations 9.5%, 5.6%, and 3.4%, respectively. Topiramate also carries a significant risk for low birth weight. Polytherapy appears to be of greater risk, and even higher when valproate is used. Monitoring drug levels both prior to and during pregnancy will permit accurate assessment of concentrations in a situation where antiepileptic drug clearance is dynamic. Dose adjustment, however, should be made on both an empirical and clinical basis. Plasma anticonvulsant drug concentrations will fall in pregnant women, but only a quarter will have an increase in seizures. We tend to keep dosage as low as possible during conception and organogenesis, but may raise dosage during the third trimester to reduce the risk of seizures during labor and the perinatal period.

There is unfortunately no clear evidence to support either the safety or hazards of vagal nerve stimulation therapy in pregnancy.

There is no clear evidence of the most effective folate dose for pregnant women. Supplementation with at least 0.4 mg/day of folate is recommended by the Center for Disease Control for all women of childbearing age whether or not they have epilepsy. In the United States, supplementation of cereals and grains with folate has greatly reduced the chances of folate deficiency.

In those using older antiepileptic drugs, vitamin K, 10 mg/day, should be initiated late in the third trimester to prevent neonatal hemorrhage. Such hemorrhages appear to be rare with newer antiepileptic drugs.

Valproate may be the most effective antiepileptic drug for some women and such patients should avail themselves of prenatal diagnostic techniques such as ultrasound and alpha fetoprotein measurements. Ultrasonography has become much more accurate and in experienced hands can identify the vast majority of structural defects. Current prenatal testing recommendations are as follows.

1 Anatomic ultrasound at 11–13 weeks. This can identify the most severe defects such as anencephaly.
2 Maternal serum alpha fetoprotein
3 Repeat anatomic ultrasound at 16 weeks. This can identify abnormalities such as orofacial clefts, heart defects, and caudal neural tube defects

When a woman with epilepsy initially presents to her physician pregnant, her gestational age (GA) needs to be established with reasonable accuracy. One cannot rely on last menstrual period (LMP) alone but an early

ultrasound should be obtained to date the pregnancy. Once GA is established, a calendar can be established with the dates for monthly antiepileptic drugs level checks and prenatal testing. Anticonvulsant levels need to be monitored regularly through the eighth postpartum week, particularly for the medications levetiracetam and lamotrigine which may have rapid concentration elevations in these first few weeks. A treatment plan for managing acute seizures should be developed in conjunction with the patient's neurologist and obstetrician.

The management of women with epilepsy presents unique challenges and potential rewards. Confirmation of diagnosis and verification of the most appropriate antiepileptic drugs for the individual is the starting point. Effective patient education, careful and consistent management including a coordinated treatment plan with neurologists and obstetricians allow patients to have successful pregnancies. Neural tube defects are serious malformations lacking effective therapeutic interventions. Their risk can be reduced by careful management and theoretically eliminated by prenatal diagnosis and therapeutic abortion. In our role as advisors, we need to recognize that all patients may not share our value systems or even begin to perceive what it really means to care for a child with a neural tube defect. Physicians must be sensitive to their patient's anxieties and be prepared to manage not simply their seizures but their emotional concerns as well.

References

1 Bilo L, Meo R, Nappi C, et al. Reproductive endocrine disorders in women with primary generalized epilepsy. *Epilepsia*. 1988;29(5):612–619.
2 Isojarvi JI, Laatikainen TJ, Pakarinen AJ, Juntunen KT, Myllyla VV. Polycystic ovaries and hyperandrogenism in women taking valproate for epilepsy. *N Engl J Med*. 1993;329(19):1383–1388.
3 Herzog AG. Psychoneuroendocrine aspects of temporolimbic epilepsy, Part II: epilepsy and

reproductive steroids. *Psychosomatics*. 1999;40: 102–108.

4   Morrell MJ. Sexual dysfunction in epilepsy. *Epilepsia*. 1991;32(Suppl 6):S38–S45.

5   Herzog AG, Seibel MM, Schomer DL, Vaitukaitis JL, Geswind N. Reproductive and endocrine disorders in women with partial seizures of temporal lobe origin. *Arch Neurol*. 1986;43:341–346.

6   Trimble MR. Serum prolactin in epilepsy and hysteria. *Br Med J*. 1978;2(6153):1682.

7   Drislane FW, Coleman AE, Schomer DL, et al. Altered pulsatile secretion of luteinizing hormone in women with epilepsy. *Neurology*. 1994;44(2): 306–310.

8   Lambert MV. Seizures, hormones and sexuality. *Seizure*. 2001;10(5):319–340.

9   Shukla GD, Srivastava ON, Katiyar BC. Sexual disturbances in temporal lobe epilepsy: a controlled study. *Br J Psychiatry*. 1979;134:288–292.

10   Mattson RH, Cramer JA, Darney PD, Naftolin F. The use of oral contraceptives by women with epilepsy. *JAMA*. 1986;256(2):238–240.

11   Shane-McWhorter L, Cerveny JD, MacFarlane LL, Osborne C. Enhanced metabolism of levonrgestrel during phenobarbital treatment and resultant pregnancy. *Pharmacotherapy*. 1998; 18(6):1360–1364.

12   Crawford P. Interactions between antiepileptic drugs and hormonal contraception. *CNS Drugs*. 2002;16(4):263–272.

13   Doose DR, Jacobs D, Squires L, Wang SS, Bialer M. Oral contraceptive-AED interaction: no effect of topiramate as monotherapy at clinically effective doses of 200 mg or less. *Epilepsia*. 2002; 43(Suppl. 7):205.

14   Shorvon SD, Tallis RC, Wallace HK. Antiepileptic drugs: coprescription of proconvulsant drugs and oral contraceptives: a national study of antiepileptic drug prescribing practice. *J Neurol Neurosurg Psychiatry*. 2002;72(1):114–115.

15   Sabers A, Ohman I, Christensen J, Tomson T. Oral contraceptives reduce lamotrigine plasma levels. *Neurology*. 2003;61(4):570–571.

16   Cahill WT, Kovilam OP, Pastor D, et al. Neurologic and fetal outcomes of pregnancies of mothers with epilepsy. *Epilepsia*. 2002;43(Suppl. 7): 289

17   Thomas SV, Syam U, Devi JS. Predictors of seizures during pregnancy in women with epilepsy. *Epilepsia*. 2012;53(5):385–388. doi: 10.1111/j.1528-1167

18   EURAP Study Group. Seizure control and treatment in pregnancy. *Neurology*. 2006;66(3): 354–360.

19   Stumpf DA, Frost M. Seizures, anticonvulsants, and pregnancy. *Am J Dis Child*. 1978;132:746–748.

20   Leonard G, Andermann E, Pitno A, Schopflocher C, Cognitive effects of antiepileptic drug therapy during pregnancy on school age offspring. *Epilepsia*. 1997;38(S3):170.

21   Burnett CWF. A survey of the relation between epilepsy and pregnancy. *J Obstet Gynecol*. 1946;53: 539–556.

22   Higgins TA, Commerford JB. Epilepsy in pregnancy. *J Ir Med Assoc*. 1974;67:317–329.

23   Suter C, Klingman WO. Seizure states and pregnancy. *Neurology*.1957;7:105–118.

24   Teramo K, Hiilesmaa VK, Bardy A, et al. Fetal heart rate during a maternal grand mal epileptic seizure. *J Perinat Med*. 1979;7:3–5.

25   Yerby MS, Koepsell T, Daling J. Pregnancy complications and outcomes in a cohort of women with epilepsy. *Epilepsia*. 1985;26:631–635.

26   Sahoo S, Klein P. Maternal complex partial seizures associated with fetal distress. *Arch Neurol*. 2005 Aug;62(8):1304–1305.

27   Nau H, Rating D, Koch S, Hauser I, Helge H. Valproic acid and its metabolites: placental transfer, neonatal pharmacokinetics, transfer via mother's milk and clinical status in neonates of epileptic mothers. *J Pharmacol Exp Ther*. 1981;219(3):768–777.

28   Tomson T, Lindbom U, Ekqvist B, Sundqvist A. Epilepsy and pregnancy: a prospective study of seizure control in relation to free and total plasma concentrations of carbamazepine and phenytoin. *Epilepsia*. 1994;35(1):122–130.

29   Rodriguez-Palomares C, Belmont-Gomez A, Amancio-Chassin O, Estrad-Altamirano A, Herrerias-Cunedo T, Hernandez-Sserrano M. Phenytoin serum concentration monitoring during pregnancy and puerperium in Mexican epileptic women. *Arch Med Res*. 1995;26(4):371–377.

30   Tomson T, Ohman I, Vitols S. Lamotrigine in pregnancy and lactation: a case report. *Epilepsia*. 1997;38(9):1039–1041.

31   Pennell PB, Hovinga CA. Antiepileptic drug therapy in pregnancy1: gestation-induced effects on AED pharmacokinetics. *Int Rev Neurobiol*. 2008;83:227–240.

32 Burakgazi E, Pollard J, Harden C. The effect of pregnancy on seizure control and antiepileptic drugs in women with epilepsy. *Rev Neurol Dis.* 2011;8(1–2):16–22.

33 Yerby MS, Friel PN, McCormick K. Antiepileptic drug disposition during pregnancy. *Neurology.* 1992 Apr;42(4 Suppl. 5):12–16.

34 Ohman I, Vitols S, Tomson T. Lamotrigine in pregnancy: pharmacokinetics during delivery, in the neonate, and during lactation. *Epilepsia.* 2000;41(6):709–713.

35 Westin AA, Reimers A, Helde G, Nakken KO, Brodtkorb E. Serum concentration/dose ratio of levetiracetam before, during and after pregnancy. *Seizure.* 2008 Mar;17(2):192–198.

36 Fotopoulou C, Kretz R, Bauer S, et al. Prospectively assessed changes in lamotrigine-concentration in women with epilepsy during pregnancy, lactation and the neonatal period. *Epilepsy Res.* 2009 Jul;85(1):60–64.

37 Dansky LV, Andermann E, Andermann F, Sherwin AL, Kinch RA. Maternal epilepsy and congenital malformations: correlation with maternal plasma anticonvulsants levels during pregnancy. In: Janz D, Dam M, Richens A, Bossi L, Helge H, Schmidt D, eds., *Epilepsy, Pregnancy and the Child.* New York: Raven Press, 1982; pp. 251–258.

38 Janz D. Antiepileptic drugs and pregnancy: altered utilization patterns and teratogenesis. *Epilepsia.* 1982;23(Suppl. 1):853–863.

39 Schmidt D, Canger R, Avanzini G, et al. Change of seizure frequency in pregnant epileptic women. *J Neurol Neurosurg Psychiatry.* 1983;46:751–755.

40 Otani K. Risk factors for the increased seizure frequency during pregnancy and the puerperium. *Folia Psychiar Neurol Jpn.* 1985;39:33–44.

41 Perruca E, Crema A. Plasma protein binding of drugs in pregnancy. *Clin Pharmacokinet.* 1982;7:336–352.

42 Tomson T, Lindbom U, Ekqvist B, Sundqvist A. Epilepsy and pregnancy: a prospective study of seizure control in relation to free and total plasma concentrations of carbamazepine and phenytoin. *Epilepsia.* 1994;35(1):122–130.

43 Nau H, Rating D, Koch S, Hauser I, Helge H. Valproic acid and its metabolites: placental transfer, neonatal pharmacokinetics, transfer via mother's milk and clinical status in neonates of epileptic mothers. *J Pharmacol Exp Ther.* 1981;219(3):768–777.

44 Dam M, Christiansen J, Munck O, Mygind KJ. Antiepileptic drugs: metabolism in pregnancy. *Clin Pharmacokinet.* 1979;4:53–62.

45 Philbert A, Dam M. The epileptic mother and her child. *Epilepsia.* 1982;23:85–99.

46 Westin AA, Nakken KO, Johannessen SI, Reimers A, Lillestolen KM, Brodtkorb E. Serum concentration/dose ratio of topiramte during pregnancy. *Epilepsia.* 2009;50(3):480–485.

47 Ohman I, Luef G, Tomson T. Effects of pregnancy and concentration on lamotrigine disposition: new insights through analysis of lamotrigine metabolites. *Seizure.* 2008;17(2):199–202.

48 Reimers A, Helde G, Brathen G, Brodtkorb E. Lamotrigine and its N2-glucuronide during pregnancy: the significance of renal clearance and estradiol. *Epilepsy Res.* 2011 [Epub ahead of print].

49 Sabers A. Algorithm for lamotrigine dose adjustment before, during and after pregnancy. *Acta Neurol Scand.* 2012;126(1): e1-4.

50 Yerby MS. Pregnancy and the mother with epilepsy. In: Jerome Engel, Timothy A. Pedley, eds., *A Comprehensive Textbook.* Philadelphia: Lippincott Williams & Wilkins Publishers, 2008; pp. 2067–2074.

51 Yerby MS. Contraception, pregnancy and lactation in women with epilepsy. *Baillieres Clin Neurol.* 1996;5(4):887–908.

52 Battino D, Tomson T. EURAP. *Interim Report.* November 2011.

53 Vajda FJ, O'Brien TJ, Hitchcock A, Graham J, Lander C. Australian registry of anti-epileptic drugs in pregnancy: experience after 30 months. *J Clin Neurosci.* 2003;10(5):543–549.

54 Hernández-Díaz S, Smith CR, Shen A, et al. North American AED Pregnancy Registry; North American AED Pregnancy Registry. Comparative safety of antiepileptic drugs during pregnancy. *Neurology.* 2012;78(21):1692–1699.

55 Schupf N, Ottman R. Reproduction among individuals with idiopathic/cryptogenic epilepsy: risk factors for spontaneous abortion. *Epilepsia.* 1997;38(7):824–829.

56 Fedrick J. Epilepsy and pregnancy: a report from the Oxford record linkage study. *Br Med J.* 1973;2:442–448.

57 Kelly TE. Teratogenicity of anticonvulsant drugs 1: review of literature. *Am J Med Genet.* 1984;19:413–434.

58 Nakane Y, Okuma T, Takahashi R, et al. Multi-institutional study on the teratogenicity and fetal

toxicity of antiepileptic drugs: report of a collaborative study group in Japan. *Epilepsia*. 1980;21:663–680.

59 Philbert A, Dam M. The epileptic mother and her child. *Epilepsia*. 1982;23:85–99.

60 Steegers-Theunissen RP, Reiner WO, Borm GF, et al. Factors influencing the risk of abnormal pregnancy outcomes in epileptic women: a multi-center prospective study. *Epilepsy Res*. 1994;18(3):261–269.

61 Jick SS, Terris BZ. Anticonvulsants and congenital malformations. *Pharmacotherapy*. 1997;17(3):561–564.

62 Kaneko S, Battino D, Andermann E, et al. Congenital malformations due to antiepileptic drugs. *Epilepsy Res*. 1999;33(2–3):145–158.

63 Canger R, Battino D, Canevini MP, et al. Malformations in offspring of women with epilepsy: a prospective study. *Epilepsia*. 1999;40(9):1231–1236.

64 Thomas SV, Indrani L, Devi GC, et al. Pregnancy in women with epilepsy: preliminary results of Kerala registry of epilepsy and pregnancy. *Neurol India*. 2001;49:60–66.

65 Kaaja E, Kaaja R, Hiilesmaa V. Major malformations in offspring of women with epilepsy. *Neurology*. 2003;60(4):575–579.

66 Wide K, Winbladh B, Kallen B. Major malformations in infants exposed to antiepileptic drugs in utero, with emphasis on carbamazepine and valproic acid: a nation-wide, population-based register study. *Acta Paediatr*. 2004;93(2):174–176.

67 Morrow JI, Russell A, Gutherie E, et al. Malformation risks of anti-epileptic drugs in pregnancy: a prospective study from the UK Epilepsy and Pregnancy Register. *J Neurol Neurosurg Psychiatry*. 2006;77(2):193–198.

68 Tomson T, Battino D, Bonizzoni E, et al. EURAP study group. Dose-dependent risk of malformations with antiepileptic drugs: an analysis of data from the EURAP epilepsy and pregnancy registry. *Lancet Neurol*. 2011;10(7):609–617.

69 Kelly TE, Rein M, Edwards P. Teratogenicity of anticonvulsant drugs. IV: the association of clefting and epilepsy. *Am J Med Genet*. 1984;19(3):451–458.

70 Friis ML, Holm NV, Sindrup EH, et al. Facial clefts in sibs and children of epileptic patients. *Neurology*. 1986;36(3):346–350.

71 Abrishamchian AR, Khoury MJ, Calle EE. The contribution of maternal epilepsy and its treatment to the etiology of oral clefts: a population based case-control study. *Genet Epidemiol*. 1994;11(4):343–351.

72 Lindhout D, Schmidt D. In-utero exposure to valproate and neural tube defects. *Lancet*. 1986;1(8494):1392–1393.

73 Rosa FW. Spina bifida in infants of women treated with carbamazepine during pregnancy. *N Engl J Med*. 1991;324(10):674–677.

74 Hiilesmaa VK. Pregnancy and birth in WWE. *Neurology*. 1992;42(Suppl. 5):8–11.

75 Weiss SR, Cooke CE, Bradley LR, Manson JM. Pharmacist's guide to pregnancy registry studies. *J Am Pharm Assoc* (Wash). 1999;39(6):830–834.

76 Cragen JD, Roberts HE, Edmonds LD. Surveillance for anencephaly and spina bifida and the impact of prenatal diagnosis – United States, 1985–1994. *MMWR*. 1995;44:1–13.

77 Cunnington MC, Weil JG, Messenheimer JA, Ferber S, Yerby MS, Tennis P. Final results from 18 years of the International Lamotrigine Registry. *Neurology*. 2011;76(21):1817–1823.

78 Pilo C, Wide K, Winbladh B. Pregnancy, delivery, and neonatal complications after treatment with antiepileptic drugs. *Acta Obstet Gynecol Scand*. 2006;85(6):643–646.

79 Vajda FJ, Graham J, Roten A, Lander CM, O'Brien TJ, Eadie M. Teratogenicity of the newer antiepileptic drugs—the Australian experience. *J Clin Neurosci*. 2012 Jan;19(1):57–59.

80 Svigos JM. Epilepsy and pregnancy. *Aust NZ J Obstet Gynaecol*. 1984;24:182–185.

81 Teramo K, Hiilesmaa VK. Pregnancy and fetal complications in epileptic pregnancies: review of the literature. In: Janz D, Bossi L, Dam M, et al., eds. *Epilepsy, Pregnancy and the Child*. New York: Raven Press, 1982; pp. 53–59.

82 Nakane Y, Oltuma T, Takahashi R, et al. Multi-institutional study on the teratogenicity and fetal toxicity of anticonvulsants: a report of a collaborative study group in Japan. *Epilepsia*. 1980;21:663–680.

83 Annegers JF, Elveback LR, Hauser WA, et al. Do anticonvulsants have a teratogenic effect? *Arch Neurol*. 1974;31:364–373.

84 Hvas CL, Henriksen TB, Ostergaard JR, Dam M. Epilepsy and pregnancy: effect of antiepileptic drugs and lifestyle on birthweight. *BJOG*. 2000;107(7):896–902.

85 Battino D, Kaneko S, Andermann E, et al. Interuterine growth in the offspring of epileptic

women: a prospective multicenter study. *Epilepsy Res.* 1999;36(1):53–60.

86 Wide K, Winbladh B, Tomson T, Kallen B. Body dimensions of infants exposed to antiepileptic drugs in utero: observations spanning 25 years. *Epilepsia.* 2000;41(7):854–861.

87 Speidel BD, Meadow SR. Anticonvulsant drugs and congenital anomalies. *Lancet.* 1968;2: 1296.

88 Hill RM, Verniaud WM, Horning MG, McCulley LB, Morgan NF. Infants exposed in utero to antiepileptic drugs. A prospective study. *Am J Dis Child.* 1974 May;127(5):645–653.

89 Leavitt AM, Yerby MS, Robinson N, Sells CJ, Erickson DM. Epilepsy and pregnancy: developmental outcomes at 12 months. *Neurology.* 1992;42(Suppl. 5):141–143.

90 Leonard G, Andermann E, Pitno A, Schopflocher C. Cognitive effects of antiepileptic drug therapy during pregnancy on school age offspring. *Epilepsia.* 1997;38(S3):170.

91 Koch S, Titze K, Zimmermann RB, Schroder M, Lehmkuhl U, Rauh H. Long-term neuropsychological consequences of maternal epilepsy and anticonvulsant treatment during pregnancy for school age children and adolescents. *Epilepsia.* 1999;40(9):1237–1243.

92 Katz JM, Pacia SV, Devinsky O. Current management of epilepsy and pregnancy: fetal outcome, congenital malformations, and developmental delay. *Epilepsy Behav.* 2001;2(2):119–123.

93 Adab N, Jacoby A, Smith D, Chadwick D. Additional educational needs in children born to mothers with epilepsy. *J Neurol Neurosurg Psychiatry.* 2001;70:15–21.

94 Vinten J, Gorry J, Baker GA. The long term neuropsychological development of children exposed to antiepileptic drugs in utero (the Liverpool and Manchester Neurodevelopmental Study Group). *Epilepsia.* 2001;42(Suppl. 2):36.

95 Adab N, Kini U, Vinten J, et al. The longer term outcome of children born to mothers with epilepsy. *J Neurol Neurosurg Psychiatry.* 2004;75(11):1517–1518.

96 Dean JC, Hailey H, Moore SJ, Lloyd DJ, Turnpenny PD, Littler J. Long term health and neurodevelopment in children exposed to antiepileptic drugs before birth. *J Med Genet.* 2002;39(4): 251–259.

97 Gailey E, Kantola-Sorsa E, Hiilesmaa V, et al. Normal intelligence in children with prenatal exposure to carbamazepine. *Neurology.* 2004; 62(1):28–32.

98 Meador KJ, Baker GA, Browning N, et al.NEAD Study Group. Effects of fetal antiepileptic drug exposure: outcomes at 4.5 years. *Neurology.* 2012; 78(16):1207–1214.

99 Montouris G. Gabapentin exposure in human pregnancy: results from the Gabapentin Pregnancy Registry. *Epilepsy Behav.* 2003;4(3):310–317.

100 Molgaard-Nielsen D, Hvid A. Newer-generation antiepileptic drugs and the risk of major birth defects. *JAMA.* 2011;305(19):1996–2002.

101 Isojarvi JI. Reproductive dysfunction in women with epilepsy. *Neurology.* 2003;61(6 Suppl. 2): S27–S34.

102 Meischenguiser R, D'Giono CH, Ferraro SM. Oxcarbazepine in pregnancy: clinical experience in Argentina. *Epilepsy Behav.* 2004;5:163–167.

103 Montouris G. Safety of newer antiepileptic drug oxcarbazepine during pregnancy. *Curr Med Res Opin.* 2005;21(5):693–701.

104 Christensen J, Sabers A, Sidenius P. Oxcarbazepine concentrations during pregnancy: a retrospective study in patients with epilepsy. *Neurology.* 2006;67(8):1497–1499.

105 Petrenaite V, Sabers A, Hansen-Schwartz J. Seizure deterioration in women treated with oxcarbazepine during pregnancy. *Epilepsy Res.* 2009;84(2–3):245–249.

106 Kondo T, Kaneko S, Amano Y, Egawa I. Preliminary report on teratogenic effects of zonisamide in the offspring of treated women with epilepsy. *Epilepsia.* 1996;37(12):1242–1244.

107 Ohtahara S, Yamatogi Y. Safety of zonisamide therapy: prospective follow up survey. *Seizure.* 2004;13(Suppl. 1):S50–S55.

108 Lawthon C, Smith PE, Wild JM. In utero exposure to vigabatirn: no indication of visual field loss. *Epilepsia.* 2009;50(2):318–321.

109 Pdmanabhan R, Abdulrazzaq YM, Bastaki SM, Nurulain M, Shafiullah M. Vigabatrin (VGB) administered during late gestation lowers maternal folate concentration and causes pregnancy loss, fetal growth restriction and skeletal hypoplasia in the mouse. *Reprod Toxicol.* 2010;29(3):366–377.

110 Bjerkdal T. Bahna SL. The course and outcome of pregnancy in women with epilepsy. *Acta Obstet Gynecol Scand.* 1973;52:245–248.

111 Endo SS, Hagimoto HH, Yamazawa HH, Kajihara SS, Kubota SS, Kamijo AA. Statistics on

deliveries of mothers with epilepsy at Yokohama City University Hospital. *Epilepsia*. 2004;45 (Suppl. 8):42–47.

112 Viinikainen K, Heinonen S, Eriksson K, Kalviainen R. Community based prospective, controlled study of obstetric and neonatal outcome of 179 pregnancies in women with epilepsy. *Epilepsia*. 2006;47:186–192.

113 Katz O, Levy A, Wiznitzer A, Sheiner E. Pregnancy and perinatal outcome in epileptic women: a population based study. *J Matern Fetal Neonatal Med*. 2006;19:21–25.

114 Richmond JR, Krishnomoorthy P, Andermann EQ, Benjamin A. Epilepsy and pregnancy: an obstetric perspective. *Am J Obstet Gynecol*. 2004; 190:371–379.

115 Pilo C, Wide K, Winbladh B. Pregnancy, delivery and neonatal complications after treatment with antiepileptic drugs. *Acta Obstet Gynecol Scand*. 2006;85:643–646.

116 Borthern I, Eide MG, Veiby G, Daltveit AK, Gilhus NE. Complications during pregnancy in women with epilepsy: population based cohort study. *BJOG*. 2009;116:1736–1742.

117 Borthern I, Eide MG, Daltveit AK, Gilhus NE. Obstetric outcome in women with epilepsy: a hospital-based, retrospective study. *BJOG*. 2011; 118(8):956–965.

CHAPTER 9

Multiple sclerosis

Aiden Haghikia[1] & Kerstin Hellwig[2]

[1] Department of Neuroanatomy and Molecular Brain Research, Ruhr University, Bochum, German
[2] Department of Neurology, St Josef Hospital, Ruhr University, Bochum, Germany

Epidemiology

Multiple sclerosis (MS) is one of the most common diseases of the central nervous system, with an increasing incidence in young women [1, 2]. There is no single causative event that leads to MS, MS is likely driven by an auto-inflammatory process involving various components of cellular of humoral immunity and to a certain extent by neurodegeneration [3]. The disease is thought to develop in genetically susceptible individuals with certain HLA haplotyopes, (e.g., HLA-DRB1*15) it may be triggered by environmental factors, including smoking, vitamin D deficiency, and eventually by gut microbiota [4, 5]. Furthermore, both susceptibility and disease course appear to be influenced by hormonal factors including female sex, ovulatory age, pregnancy, and possibly lactation. Observations supporting this notion are (a) MS predominantly affects women in their childbearing years [2]; (b) onset of MS is rarely prior to menarche or after menopause; and (c) the disease is significantly ameliorated during pregnancy [6] and possibly during exclusive breastfeeding [7].

Hormonal influences

There are three main observations that support the assumption that hormonal factors have an influence on risk and prognosis of MS: (1) the female preponderance of MS; (2) decrease of relapse frequency and severity seen during pregnancy; and (3) the observation that onset of MS is rarely prior to menarche or after menopause. Despite these apparently plausible observations in favor of female hormones correlating with autoimmune activity, the actual hormonal influence on disease seems more complex. Early evidence for the hormonal influence on MS disease course and other auto-inflammatory diseases like arthritis accumulated from experimental results in the animal model of MS, the experimental autoimmune encephalomyelitis (EAE) [8]. The initial study showed that estrogen exerts a rather protective or therapeutic effect on EAE disease course, whereas progesterone—a gestagen derivate mainly secreted by the corpus luteum—had a contrary effect. Later studies attributed a similar anti-inflammatory and neuroprotective effect for both estrogen and progesterone by skewing the inflammatory response toward anti-inflammatory cytokines and chemokines, for example, interleukin-10 [9]. These data, however conclusive and reproducible, appear to be contradicted by findings on androgen. Androgen-affected T-lymphocytes reactive to myelin proteolipid protein caused less damage and disease activity if taken from male animals than from females before being transferred to naïve mice [10]. Translating these data into

Neurological Illness in Pregnancy: Principles and Practice, First Edition.
Edited by Autumn Klein, M. Angela O'Neal, Christina Scifres, Janet F. R. Waters and Jonathan H. Waters.
© 2016 John Wiley & Sons, Ltd. Published 2016 by John Wiley & Sons, Ltd.

the human system, testosterone treatment of male MS patients led to the improvement of clinical and paraclinical submeasures, including improved cognitive performance and reduction in brain atrophy [11]. There are still gaps to be filled in our understanding of the hormonal influence on MS and it is more likely that the complex interplay involving a whole array of sex hormones rather than single hormones have an impact on disease activity.

The suggested mechanisms by which hormones exert their effect on immune response are incomplete and contain uncertainties. Evidence from experimental works suggest that the beneficial estrogen effect observed in the EAE is achieved by a dual mechanism utilizing two different estrogen receptors (ERs). While the anti-inflammatory effect is mediated by ERalpha via suppression of Th1/Th17-mediated pro-inflammatory immune responses, the protective effect within the central nervous system is ERbeta dependent [12, 13]. Vitamin D, another proposed environmental factor for the pathogenesis of MS, has also been implicated in estrogen's mode of action in the EAE [14].

Susceptibility to develop MS

A few studies have investigated the role of oral contraceptives (OCs) on risk for developing MS [15] and their effect on disease course [16, 17]. These studies found conflicting results, with either a slight increase [15, 18], decrease [19], or no effect of OCs on MS [20]. These studies are limited by factors including small sample size [19, 20] and no consideration of OC subclasses in the analyses [15, 18]. Other studies have attempted to address the role of parity as a protective factor in MS. One study suggested that MS risk might be lower in women with 3 or more children [19]. In another recently published study, parity was associated with a reduced risk of developing a first demyelinating event [22]. Another study evaluating the combined effect of pregnancy and OC use revealed a

significant later age of onset in MS patients with longer OC use and childbirth [21].

Prognosis of MS and hormonal factors

A study done in 2011 suggested that OC use was associated with higher scores (6 or greater), in the expanded disability status scale in patients with progressive onset MS. The study did not find this association in patients with relapsing remitting MS [23]. Earlier studies [16, 17] found no increase or decrease in demyelinative disease activity in patients who used OCs.

Pregnancy has been associated with reduction in MS relapses and will be discussed further later in this chapter. Relapses during the postpartum period, however, are more common. The long-term effects of pregnancy on disability are less clear. At one point in time, there was concern that childbirth raised the likelihood of higher levels of disability. Recent studies do not support this postulation [24–27].

Menstrual cycle

Patients have self-reported increased MS symptoms in the menstrual and premenstrual periods [28–30]. One author proposed that increased symptomatology may be due to pseudo exacerbations related to fluctuations in body temperature [30]. Use of aspirin was found to be helpful in reducing premenstrual symptoms.

Preconception planning

Historically women with MS were discouraged from becoming pregnant, but today there is no reason to advise against pregnancy, as reliable data about the course of the disease during and after pregnancy is available [6, 31–34]. Management of MS medication before, during, and after pregnancy is an important issue and will be discussed in more detail later in the chapter. Some patients feel pressured by family members or health professionals either to abstain from pregnancy or to bear children as soon as possible while they are in an early stage of disease. Women themselves might be concerned about their own and their child's well being and dealing with parenthood [36].

MS experts advise patients to become pregnant when the disease is controlled. Fortunately, the overall disease course with a decreased number of relapses during pregnancy makes medical intervention unnecessary in most cases. It is important for women with a chronic disease to take care of themselves and accept help from their environment.

Genetics/inheritance

Despite the identification of disease-associated genetic variants [37], MS is not inherited in Mendelian fashion. Young MS patients planning to have children often worry about transmitting the disease to their offspring. The associated genetic variants in large cohorts are well described, and the risk of transmitting MS to offspring remains relatively low. Considering the overall prevalence of MS in the general population is 50–150 per 100,000 in Europe, a 10-fold increase in risk for children of parents with MS means that roughly 2% of affected individuals will have children with MS [38, 39]. Monozygotic twin studies have demonstrated only a 15–20% concordance for MS between twin pairs, highlighting the complexity of factors contributing to the development of this disease. Interestingly, a recent study that compared monozygotic twins, discordant for MS at the genomic, epigenetic, and transcriptional level did not find any differences that would explain the occurrence of disease in only one twin. Taken together, these data support the notion that MS patients planning a family should not be discouraged from procreating due to a genetic risk for their children.

Fertility

A study conducted in Finland in 2010 suggests that women with MS tend to have fewer children than those without MS. They also more commonly underwent assisted reproductive techniques (ARTs) than healthy aged matched controls [41]. It is unclear whether this study reflects a biological fertility issue or psychosocial considerations. Other studies have found no significant impairment in fertility in the MS population [40].

Some drugs used to treat MS have been shown to have an impact on contraception. Immunosuppressant therapy with mitoxanrone has been shown to cause permanent amenorrhea in 30% of women older than 35 years [43]. Similar findings occur in women using cyclophosphamide. These medications are generally reserved for late stages of MS and are less likely to be used in women of childbearing age. Interferons are known to cause menstrual cycle disturbances [42], but do not appear to have a significant impact on contraception. There are, however, no controlled studies on the impact of MS treatment and fertility.

Assisted reproductive techniques

Although the disease process of MS does not appear to lead to infertility, MS patients do share the same rate of impaired fertility as the general population at 6%. Some of these couples pursue ARTs. Several small studies suggest that hormonal stimulation increases the risk of relapses, most often in those couples who fail to conceive. Two French studies attributed the increased relapse rate to the use of luteinizing hormone-releasing hormone (LHRH) agonists [44, 45]. This was not supported by other studies [46, 47]. While the reason for increased relapses in women using ART has yet to be elucidated, rapid changes in hormonal levels, stress, and discontinuation of MS medication may all

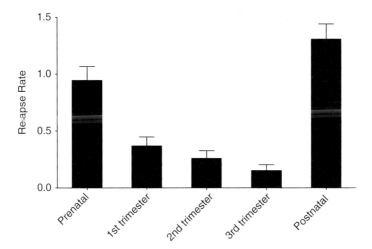

Figure 9.1 Relapse during pregnancy and postpartum.

be contributing. While use of ART in women with MS is not absolutely contraindicated, these women should be counseled on the increased relapse risk following the procedure.

Pregnancy

Disease changes during pregnancy and postpartum

Pregnancy (a period with tremendous increases in estrogen levels, particularly estriol a form of estrogen exclusively produced during pregnancy) significantly reduces the risk of MS relapses (Figure 9.1). There is no other known natural event or innovative MS therapy, able to reduce the relapse risk for up to 80% as seen in the last trimester of pregnancy. This short-term decrease of disease activity is generally followed by an increase of disease activity during the first 3 months postpartum with about 30% of women suffering from an exacerbation in this time period[6, 48]. As such, the postpartum period is the only clear-cut significant risk factor for MS relapses. Reasons for this pattern of pregnancy-amelioration and postpartum worsening of MS are not fully understood. Some experimental evidence suggests that estrogens play the key role in inducing a protective immune response through a Th1/Th17 to Th 2[49, 50] shift combined with higher immune tolerance during pregnancy.

Disease-modifying therapies and pregnancy

Several immunomodulatory drugs (DMD) are licensed worldwide for the treatment of relapsing remitting MS. None of the current MS treatment including interferon-beta, Glatiramer acetate (GLAT), natalizumab, fingolimod, or teriflunomide is categorized as FDA pregnancy category A. Table 9.1 lists the FDA categories for various MS medication recently reviewed [35, 51, 52]. In general, women with MS are advised to discontinue these medications during pregnancy. There is less agreement on whether it is advisable to discontinue the medication prior to conception. While in North America, the discontinuation of DMDs (especially interferon-beta) prior to pregnancy is still recommended [52, 53], in Europe, (particularly in Germany), women conceive more frequently while taking DMDs. Fortunately, there is thus far no evidence for an increased teratogenic risk, attributable to GLAT or natalizumab, in animal studies or in observational studies in humans [51, 54–61].

Table 9.1 FDA ranking pregnancy categories

Pregnancy category		MS medication
A	Adequate and well-controlled human studies have failed to demonstrate a risk to the fetus in the first trimester of pregnancy (and there is no evidence of risk in later trimesters).	None
B	Animal reproduction studies have failed to demonstrate a risk to the fetus and there are no adequate and well-controlled studies in pregnant women OR animal studies have shown an adverse effect, but adequate and well-controlled studies in pregnant women have failed to demonstrate a risk to the fetus in any trimester.	Glatiramer acetate
C	Animal reproduction studies have shown an adverse effect on the fetus and there are no adequate and well-controlled studies in humans, but potential benefits may warrant use of the drug in pregnant women despite potential risks.	Interferon-beta, natalizumab, fingolimod
D	There is positive evidence of human fetal risk based on adverse reaction data from investigational or marketing experience or studies in humans, but potential benefits may warrant use of the drug in pregnant women despite potential risks.	Mitoxantron
X	Studies in animals or humans have demonstrated fetal abnormalities and/or there is positive evidence of human fetal risk based on adverse reaction data from investigational or marketing experience, and the risks involved in use of the drug in pregnant women clearly outweigh potential benefits.	Teriflunomide

Fingolimod and teriflunomide have been shown in animal studies to pose teratogenic risk. A prospective world wide data collection of exposed pregnancies is ongoing to determine the risk in humans.

Interferon-beta

Results from clinical trials, post-marketing observation, and smaller observations are available. A recent systematic review identified 761 published pregnancies with interferon (IFN)-beta exposure during pregnancy [53]. Best evidence studies suggested that IFN-beta exposure might be associated with a lower mean birth weight, shorter mean birth length, and preterm birth. The IFN-beta exposure was not associated with increased rate of cesarean section, spontaneous abortion, teratogenicity, or low birth weight. The authors conclude that women with MS should discontinue IFN-beta before a planned pregnancy [53].

Women with MS who become pregnant while undergoing treatment with interferon can be reassured that IFN-beta is not teratogenic and an elective termination of the pregnancy due to

IFN-beta exposure is not necessary. In general, women are advised to stop IFN-beta when they become aware of the pregnancy.

Glatiramer actetate

Ninety-seven GLAT-exposed pregnancies [62, 66–68] were identified by Lu et al. [53]. Together with older post-marketing company data (>200 pregnancies), these data, although limited by the quality and quantity, did not demonstrate teratogenicity, lower birth weight or length, earlier gestational age nor an elevated risk for spontaneous abortion. Some advocate interuption of treatment with GA during pregnancy.

Natalizumab

Preliminary data in a study done by the author did not reveal a teratogenic risk attributable to natalizumab in 35 pregnancies [57]. Neither was the birth weight reduced, nor the risk of spontaneous abortion increased. Limited by the small sample, more data to better estimate the risk of natalizumab exposure is needed. Treatment with natalizumab is mainly indicated in patients with high disease activity. This raises some concern about the safety of interruption of the drug prior to conception. The disease activity is likely to return after 4–6 months after treatment interruption. Pregnancy protects to a certain extent from relapses, but about 40% of women whose natalizumab was discontinued experienced relapses during pregnancy (AH and KH unpublished data). After careful risk–benefit consideration (return of relapses vs. limited experience in humans with natalizumab exposure), this author supports women with an aggressive form of the disease controlled with natalizumab to become pregnant under natalizumab and stop further treatment in the course of the pregnancy. If severe disease activity returns despite pregnancy, natalizumab could be readministered during pregnancy. However, a thorough hematological monitoring of the newborns is necessary after birth.

Fingolimod

Because of the potential risk for the fetus, mainly based on animal studies, and its long half-life (approximately 9 days), fingolimod should be stopped 2 months prior to a planned pregnancy. So far, the experience with human pregnancies especially with its potential effect on the fetus is limited. In clinical trials, 81 fingolimod-exposed pregnancies resulted in 3 congenital abnormalities. A worldwide registry with prospective follow-up of fingolimod-exposed pregnancies is under way.

Teriflunomide

Teriflunomide selectively and reversibly inhibits the mitochondrial enzyme dihydroorotate dehydrogenase, important for the pyrimidine *de novo* synthesis. Teratogenic effects have been observed in animal studies and with the prodrug of teriflunomide, leflunomide, which is approved in the treatment of rheumatoid arthritis. Clinical experience again is limited. But as presented at the AAN meeting in 2012, 33 pregnancies occurred during clinical trials under teriflunomide: 8 healthy newborns were born, 13 pregnancies were terminated electively, 9 spontaneous abortions occurred, and 3 pregnancies were still ongoing. In this very limited sample, pregnancies were full term and birth weight in the normal range [69].

It is recommended to employ effective contraception while under treatment with teriflunomide. Teriflunomide has a very long biological half-life, but can be washed out rapidly and effectively with activated charcoal or cholestyramine if a pregnancy is planned or has occurred while on this medication.

Mitoxantron

Only 2 case reports of MS patients with accidental mitoxantron exposure are published [70, 71]. In one case of periconceptional exposure, a child with Pierre Robin sequence was born. In another case report, mitoxantron exposure during midst of pregnancy resulted in a healthy, small for gestational age baby. Because of its potential genotoxicity, both men and women should be advised not to procreate for at least 6 months after infusion.

In conclusion, available data are very limited for disease-modifying drugs during pregnancy. Particularly lacking is data for the newer treatments including teriflunomide, fingolimod, and natalizumab but even GA, which has been available for more than 10 years, has limited data with regard to outcomes of pregnancy. Further research is warranted.

Obstetrical issue and pregnancy outcome

In general, obstetrical complications are not more common in women with MS. Birth weight might be reduced compared to newborns of healthy mothers, although this was not confirmed in all studies [33, 64, 65, 72]. Spontaneous abortion, malformations, or other pregnancy complications were not found to be increased in women with MS [63, 65, 73, 74]. In general, women with MS can be reassured that neither obstetrical nor adverse events in the newborns are increased because of the underlying disease.

Mode of delivery/anesthetics

The diagnosis of MS might increase the likelihood of assisted vaginal delivery or cesarean section [64, 73], although not all investigators could not confirm these results [72].

In women with MS with a higher degree of disability, assisted forms of delivery may be needed. It is important to note that the relapse rate postpartum is not influenced by the mode of delivery [75]. Therefore, the mode of delivery should be dependent upon obstetrical considerations.

Although, delivery is rarely impaired by MS symptoms, spasticity of the pelvic floor or extreme fatigue can effect delivery options. In the Prims study, the largest prospective study investigating the risk of postpartum relapses, epidural anesthesia was not associated with an increased risk of postpartum relapses. Therefore, epidural anesthesia should not be denied to women with MS [75].

Breastfeeding

In the scientific world, there is considerable controversy regarding the effect of breastfeeding on the postpartum relapse rate. In a recently published meta-analysis, breastfeeding was associated with a 50% risk reduction of postpartum relapses [76]. Two retrospective studies [58, 77] and a prospective pilot study by Langer-Gould et al. [7] also showed that exclusive breastfeeding was associated with a reduction in postpartum relapses. Other scientists could not confirm these results [16, 78, 79].

Exclusive breastfeeding may induce a hormonal state with anovulation that partial breastfeeding is not able to establish and may be particularly helpful in reducing the MS relapse rate in postpartum women. In non-placebo controlled studies, intravenous immunoglobulin (IVIG) was also shown to reduce the postpartum

relapse rate [80, 81]. Breastfeeding is feasible during treatment with IVIG. Safety of breastfeeding while undergoing DMT is unknown and merits further study. Exclusive breastfeeding may be encouraged for postpartum patients with MS and DMT may be offered after delivery in those patients who do not wish to breastfeed.

Menopause

The impact of menopause on MS symptoms is unknown. Multiple sclerosis is rarely diagnosed during menopause. In some women, MS symptoms might worsen during menopause. Hormone replacement therapy does not seem to have a major impact on MS symptoms. As our knowledge about the effect of menopause and MS course and symptoms is very limited, more research should focus on the relationship between menopause and MS.

KEY POINTS

1 Multiple sclerosis is a common neurological disease in young women.

2 Women with MS should not be discouraged from becoming pregnant.

3 Relapse rate decreases during pregnancy and increases after birth.

4 Mode of delivery is independent of MS in most cases.

5 Epidural anesthesia is not correlated with postpartum relapse risk.

6 Most women with MS can breastfeed if they wish to do so.

7 Individualized counseling with regard to disease modifying therapies is important.

Certainly, pregnancy is not contraindicated in women with MS. Women with MS can be reassured that neither the course of the disease nor the course of pregnancy will be negatively impacted. Future investigations should focus on the interactions of hormones on the immune system, provide safety data for old and new DMTs, and elucidate the role of (exclusive) breastfeeding or DMT reintroduction after birth.

References

1 Orton SM, Herrera BM, Yee IM, et al. Sex ratio of multiple sclerosis in Canada: a longitudinal study. *Lancet Neurol.* 2006;5(11):932–936.

2 Koch-Henriksen N, Sorensen PS. The changing demographic pattern of multiple sclerosis epidemiology. *Lancet Neurol.* 2010;9(5):520–532.

3 Weiner HL. The challenge of multiple sclerosis: how do we cure a chronic heterogeneous disease? *Ann Neurol.* 2009;65(3):239–248.

4 Handel AE, Giovannoni G, Ebers GC, Ramagopalan SV. Environmental factors and their timing in adult-onset multiple sclerosis. *Nat Rev Neurol.* 2010;6(3):156–166.

5 Berer K, Mues M, Koutrolos M, et al. Commensal microbiota and myelin autoantigen cooperate to trigger autoimmune demyelination. *Nature.* 2011;479(7374):538–541.

6 Confavreux C, Hutchinson M, Hours MM, Cortinovis-Tourniaire P, Moreau T. Rate of pregnancy-related relapse in multiple sclerosis. Pregnancy in Multiple Sclerosis Group. *N Engl J Med.* 1998;339(5):285–291.

7 Langer-Gould A, Huang SM, Gupta R, et al. Exclusive breastfeeding and the risk of postpartum relapses in women with multiple sclerosis. *Arch Neurol.* 2009;66(8):958–963.

8 Arnason BG, Richman DP. Effect of oral contraceptives on experimental demyelinating disease. *Arch Neurol.* 1969;21(1):103–108.

9 Yates MA, Li Y, Chlebeck P, Proctor T, Vandenbark AA, Offner H. Progesterone treatment reduces disease severity and increases IL-10 in experimental autoimmune encephalomyelitis. *J Neuroimmunol.* 2010;220(1–2):136–139.

10 Bebo BF Jr, Schuster JC, Vandenbark AA, Offner H. Androgens alter the cytokine profile and reduce encephalitogenicity of myelin-reactive T cells. *J Immunol.* 1999;162(1):35–40.

11 Sicotte NL, Giesser BS, Tandon V, et al. Testosterone treatment in multiple sclerosis: a pilot study. *Arch Neurol.* 2007;64(5):683–688.

12 Lelu K, Laffont S, Delpy L, et al. Estrogen receptor alpha signaling in T lymphocytes is required for estradiol-mediated inhibition of Th1 and Th17 cell differentiation and protection against experimental autoimmune encephalomyelitis. *J Immunol.* 2011;187(5):2386–2393.

13 Tiwari-Woodruff S, Morales LB, Lee R, Voskuhl RR. Differential neuroprotective and antiinflammatory effects of estrogen receptor (ER)alpha and ERbeta ligand treatment. *Proc Natl Acad Sci U S A* 2007;104(37):14813–14818.

14 Nashold FE, Spach KM, Spanier JA, Hayes CE. Estrogen controls vitamin D3-mediated resistance to experimental autoimmune encephalomyelitis by controlling vitamin D3 metabolism and receptor expression. *J Immunol.* 2009;183(6):3672–3681.

15 Alonso A, Jick SS, Olek MJ, Ascherio A, Jick H, Hernan MA. Recent use of oral contraceptives and the risk of multiple sclerosis. *Arch Neurol.* 2005;62(9):1362–1365.

16 Holmqvist P, Wallberg M, Hammar M, Landtblom AM, Brynhildsen J. Symptoms of multiple sclerosis in women in relation to sex steroid exposure. *Maturitas.* 2006;54(2):149–153.

17 Poser S, Raun NE, Wikstrom J, Poser W. Pregnancy, oral contraceptives and multiple sclerosis. *Acta Neurol Scand.* 1979;59(2–3):108–118.

18 Thorogood M, Hannaford PC. The influence of oral contraceptives on the risk of multiple sclerosis. *Br J Obstet Gynaecol.* 1998;105(12):1296–1299.

19 Villard-Mackintosh L, Vessey MP. Oral contraceptives and reproductive factors in multiple sclerosis incidence. *Contraception.* 1993;47(2):161–168.

20 Hernan MA, Hohol MJ, Olek MJ, Spiegelman D, Ascherio A. Oral contraceptives and the incidence of multiple sclerosis. *Neurology.* 2000;55(6):848–854.

21 Holmqvist P, Hammar M, Landtblom AM, Brynhildsen J. Age at onset of multiple sclerosis is correlated to use of combined oral contraceptives and childbirth before diagnosis. *Fertil Steril.* 2010;94(7):2835–2837.

22 Ponsonby AL, Lucas RM, van der Mei IA, et al. Offspring number, pregnancy, and risk of a first clinical demyelinating event: The AusImmune Study. *Neurology.* 2012;78(12):867–874.

23 D'Hooghe MB, Haentjens P, Nagels G, D'Hooghe T, De Keyser J. Menarche, oral contraceptives, pregnancy and progression of disability in relapsing onset and progressive onset multiple sclerosis. *J Neurol.* 2012; 259(5):855–861.

24 D'Hooghe MB, Nagels G, Uitdehaag BM. Long-term effects of childbirth in MS. *J Neurol Neurosurg Psychiatry.* 2010;81(1):38–41.

25 Thompson DS, Nelson LM, Burns A, Burks JS, Franklin GM. The effects of pregnancy in multiple sclerosis: a retrospective study. *Neurology*. 1986;36(8):1097–1099.

26 Weinshenker BG, Hader W, Carriere W, Baskerville J, Ebers GC. The influence of pregnancy on disability from multiple sclerosis: a population-based study in Middlesex County, Ontario. *Neurology*. 1989;39(11):1438–1440.

27 Ramagopalan S, Yee I, Byrnes J, Guimond C, Ebers G, Sadovnick D. Term pregnancies and the clinical characteristics of multiple sclerosis: a population based study. *J Neurol Neurosurg Psychiatry*. 2012;83(8):793–795.

28 Zorgdrager A, De Keyser J. Premenstrual exacerbations of multiple sclerosis. *J Neurol Neurosurg Psychiatry*. 1998;65(2):279–280.

29 Zorgdrager A, De Keyser J. Menstrually related worsening of symptoms in multiple sclerosis. *J Neurol Sci*. 1997;149(1):95–97.

30 Wingerchuk DM, Rodriguez M. Premenstrual multiple sclerosis pseudoexacerbations: role of body temperature and prevention with aspirin. *Arch Neurol*. 2006;63(7):1005–1008.

31 Dwosh E, Guimond C, Duquette P, Sadovnick AD. The interaction of MS and pregnancy: a critical review. *Int MS J / MS Forum*. 2003;10(2):38–42.

32 Dwosh E, Guimond C, Sadovnick AD. Reproductive counselling for MS: a rationale. *Int MS J/MS Forum*. 2003;10(2):52–59.

33 Hellwig K, Brune N, Haghikia A, et al. Reproductive counselling, treatment and course of pregnancy in 73 German MS patients. *Acta Neurol Scand*. 2008;118(1):24–28.

34 Hellwig K HA, Gold R. Multiple sclerosis and pregnancy: experience from a nationwide database. *Neurology*. 2011;76(4):A272.

35 Borisow N, Doring A, Pfueller CF, Paul F, Dorr J, Hellwig K. Expert recommendations to personalization of medical approaches in treatment of multiple sclerosis: an overview of family planning and pregnancy. *EPMA J*. 2012;3(1):9.

36 Prunty M, Sharpe L, Butow P, Fulcher G. The motherhood choice: themes arising in the decision-making process for women with multiple sclerosis. *Mult Scler*. 2008;14(5):701–704.

37 Sawcer S, Hellenthal G, Pirinen M, et al. Genetic risk and a primary role for cell-mediated immune mechanisms in multiple sclerosis. *Nature*. 2011;476(7359):214–219.

38 Compston A, Coles A. Multiple sclerosis. *Lancet*. 2008;372(9648):1502–1517.

39 Carton H, Vlietinck R, Debruyne J, et al. Risks of multiple sclerosis in relatives of patients in Flanders, Belgium. *J Neurol Neurosurg Psychiatry*. 1997;62(4):329–333.

40 Cavalla P, Rovei V, Masera S, et al. Fertility in patients with multiple sclerosis: current knowledge and future perspectives. *Neurol Sci*. 2006;27(4):231–239.

41 Jalkanen A, Alanen A, Airas L. Pregnancy outcome in women with multiple sclerosis: results from a prospective nationwide study in Finland. *Mult Scler*. 2010;16(8):950–955.

42 Fachinformation. Betaferon® 250 Mikrogramm/ml. http://www.deutschesapothekenportal.de/fileadmin/bestellungen/fi_betaferon.pdf. 2012.

43 Cocco E, Sardu C, Gallo P, et al. Frequency and risk factors of mitoxantrone-induced amenorrhea in multiple sclerosis: the FEMIMS study. *Mult Scler*. 2008;14(9):1225–1233.

44 Laplaud DA, Leray E, Barriere P, Wiertlewski S, Moreau T. Increase in multiple sclerosis relapse rate following in vitro fertilization. *Neurology*. 2006;66(8):1280–1281.

45 Michel L, Foucher Y, Vukusic S, et al. Increased risk of multiple sclerosis relapse after in vitro fertilisation. *J Neurol Neurosurg Psychiatry*. 2012;83(8):796–802.

46 Hellwig K, Beste C, Brune N, et al. Increased MS relapse rate during assisted reproduction technique. *J Neurol*. 2008;255(4):592–593.

47 Hellwig K, Schimrigk S, Beste C, Muller T, Gold R. Increase in relapse rate during assisted reproduction technique in patients with multiple sclerosis. *Eur Neurol*. 2009;61(2):65–68.

48 Trooster WJ TA, Kampinga J, Loof JG, Nieuwenhuis P, Minderhoud JM. Suppression of acute experimental allergic encephalomyelitis by the synthetic sex hormone 17-alpha-ethinylestradiol: an immunological study in the Lewis rat. *Int Arch Allergy Immunol*. 1993;102(2):133–140.

49 Devonshire V, Duquette P, Dwosh E, Guimond C. The immune system and hormones: review and relevance to pregnancy and contraception in women with MS. *Int MS J Forum*. 2003;10(2):44–50.

50 Airas L, Saraste M, Rinta S, Elovaara I, Huang YH, Wiendl H. Immunoregulatory factors in multiple sclerosis patients during and after pregnancy: relevance of natural killer cells. *Clin Exp Immunol*. 2008;151(2):235–243.

51 Houtchens MK, Kolb CM. Multiple sclerosis and pregnancy: therapeutic considerations. *J Neurol*. 2012; 260(5):1202–1214.

52 Alwan S, Sadovnick AD. Multiple sclerosis and pregnancy: maternal considerations. *Women's health*. 2012;8(4):399–414.

53 Lu E, Wang BW, Guimond C, Synnes A, Sadovnick D, Tremlett H. Disease modifying drugs for multiple sclerosis in pregnancy: a systematic review. *Neurology*. 2012; 79(11):1130–1135.

54 Hellwig K, Agne H, Gold R. Interferon beta, birth weight and pregnancy in multiple sclerosis. *J Neurol*. 2009;256(5):830–831.

55 Hellwig K, Beste C, Schimrigk S, Chan A. Immunomodulation and postpartum relapses in patients with multiple sclerosis. *Ther Adv Neurol Disord*. 2009;2(1):7–11.

56 Hellwig K, Gold R. Glatiramer acetate and interferon-beta throughout gestation and postpartum in women with multiple sclerosis. *J Neurol*. 2011;258(3):502–503.

57 Hellwig K, Haghikia A, Gold R. Pregnancy and natalizumab: results of an observational study in 35 accidental pregnancies during natalizumab treatment. *Mult Scler*. 2011;17(8):958–963.

58 Hellwig K, Haghikia A, Rockhoff M, Gold R. Multiple sclerosis and pregnancy: experience from a nationwide database in Germany. *Ther Adv Neurol Disord*. 2012;5(5):247–253.

59 Amato MP, Portaccio E, Ghezzi A, et al. Pregnancy and fetal outcomes after interferon-beta exposure in multiple sclerosis. *Neurology*. 2010;75(20):1794–1802.

60 Sandberg-Wollheim M, Alteri E, Moraga MS, Kornmann G. Pregnancy outcomes in multiple sclerosis following subcutaneous interferon beta-1a therapy. *Mult Scler*. 2011;17(4):423–430.

61 Sandberg-Wollheim M, Frank D, et al. Pregnancy outcomes during treatment with interferon beta-1a in patients with multiple sclerosis. *Neurology*. 2005;65(6):802–806.

62 Weber-Schoendorfer C, Schaefer C. Multiple sclerosis, immunomodulators, and pregnancy outcome: a prospective observational study. *Mult Scler*. 2009;15(9):1037-1042.

63 De Las Heras V, De Andres C, Tellez N, Tintore M. Pregnancy in multiple sclerosis patients treated with immunomodulators prior to or during part of the pregnancy: a descriptive study in the Spanish population. *Mult Scler*. 2007;13(8):981–984.

64 Dahl J, Myhr KM, Daltveit AK, Hoff JM, Gilhus NE. Pregnancy, delivery, and birth outcome in women with multiple sclerosis. *Neurology*. 2005;65(12):1961–1963.

65 Dahl J, Myhr KM, Daltveit AK, Gilhus NE. Pregnancy, delivery and birth outcome in different stages of maternal multiple sclerosis. *J Neurol*. 2008;255(5):623–627.

66 Fragoso YD, Finkelsztejn A, Kaimen-Maciel DR, et al. Long-term use of glatiramer acetate by 11 pregnant women with multiple sclerosis: a retrospective, multicentre case series. *CNS Drugs*. 2010;24(11):969–976.

67 Finkelsztejn A, Fragoso YD, Ferreira ML, et al. The Brazilian database on pregnancy in multiple sclerosis. *Clin Neurol Neurosurg*. 2011;113(4):277–280.

68 Salminen HJ, Leggett H, Boggild M. Glatiramer acetate exposure in pregnancy: preliminary safety and birth outcomes. *J Neurol*. 2010;257(12):2020–2023.

69 Stuve O BM, Benzerdjeb H, Kieseier B. Pregnancy outcomes from the teriflunomide clinical development program: retrospective analysis of a global pharmacovigilance database. *Neurology*. 2012;78(April 22):P06.190.

70 Hellwig K, Schimrigk S, Chan A, Epplen J, Gold R. A newborn with Pierre Robin sequence after preconceptional mitoxantrone exposure of a female with multiple sclerosis. *J Neurol Sci*. 2011;307(1–2):164–165.

71 De Santis M, Straface G, Cavaliere AF, Rosati P, Batocchi AP, Caruso A. The first case of mitoxantrone exposure in early pregnancy. *Neurotoxicology*. 2007;28(3):696–697.

72 van der Kop ML, Pearce MS, Dahlgren L, et al. Neonatal and delivery outcomes in women with multiple sclerosis. *Ann Neurol*. 2011; 70(1):41–50.

73 Kelly VM, Nelson LM, Chakravarty EF. Obstetric outcomes in women with multiple sclerosis and epilepsy. *Neurology*. 2009;73(22):1831–1836.

74 Finkelsztejn A, Brooks JB, Paschoal FM Jr, Fragoso YD. What can we really tell women with multiple sclerosis regarding pregnancy? A systematic review and meta-analysis of the literature. *BJOG*. 2011;118(7):790–797.

75 Vukusic S, Hutchinson M, Hours M, et al. Pregnancy and multiple sclerosis (the PRIMS study): clinical predictors of post-partum relapse. *Brain: J Neurol*. 2004;127(Pt 6):1353–1360.

76 Pakpoor J, Disanto G, Lacey MV, Hellwig K, Giovannoni G, Ramagopalan SV. Breastfeeding and multiple sclerosis relapses: a meta-analysis. *J Neurol*. 2012.

77 Hellwig K KM, Gold R, Langer-Gould A. Exclusive breastfeeding reduces the risk of postpartum relapses-a prospective study from the German MS and pregnancy registry: Experience from a nationwide database. *Neurology.* 2011;76(4): A272.

78 Airas L, Jalkanen A, Alanen A, Pirttila T, Marttila RJ. Breast-feeding, postpartum and prepregnancy disease activity in multiple sclerosis. *Neurology.* 2010;75(5):474–476.

79 Portaccio E, Ghezzi A, Hakiki B, et al. Breastfeeding is not related to postpartum relapses in multiple sclerosis. *Neurology.* 2011; 77(2):145–150.

80 Haas J, Hommes OR. A dose comparison study of IVIG in postpartum relapsing-remitting multiple sclerosis. *Mult Scler.* 2007;13(7):900–908.

81 Achiron A, Kishner I, Dolev M, et al. Effect of intravenous immunoglobulin treatment on pregnancy and postpartum-related relapses in multiple sclerosis. *J Neurol.* 2004;251(9):1133–1137.

CHAPTER 10

Neuromuscular disorders

Mohammad Kian Salajegheh & Kathy Chuang

Department of Neurology, Brigham and Women's Hospital, Harvard Medical School, Boston, MA, USA

Pregnancy, with the subsequent stages of labor and delivery, is associated with many well-studied physiologic changes. It is not surprising that neuromuscular conditions may fluctuate with the multisystemic adaptations during these periods. During pregnancy, these conditions may have their initial presentation; the course or treatment may be altered; or a preexisting condition may lead to adverse fetal or obstetric outcomes. Therefore, it is important for neurologists to have a level of understanding of these diseases during pregnancy. This chapter will review the effect of pregnancy on the acquired and hereditary neuromuscular disorders listed in Table 10.1.

Of note, the discussion of the genetics of hereditary conditions (including the probability of transmission, prenatal testing, and diagnosis) requires extensive multidisciplinary counseling, but is beyond the scope of this chapter.

Acquired generalized neuromuscular disorders

Acquired inflammatory myopathies

Knowledge of the pathogenesis and different subtypes of inflammatory myopathies has grown significantly in the past few decades. This topic encompasses such diverse entities as dermatomyositis (DM), polymyositis (PM), connective tissue disease-associated myopathies,

immune-mediated necrotizing myopathy (including that associated with HMGCR antibody), and inclusion body myositis, amongst others [1].

With the exception of inclusion body myositis, which is more prevalent in males older than age 50, the majority of inflammatory myopathies are more prevalent in females [2]. PM and DM are the most common forms, with prevalence cited to be approximately 2.4–10.7 cases per 100,000 [3]. Only 14% of patients with PM and DM present during their childbearing years [4]. A small prospective study also demonstrated that the majority of patients with inflammatory myopathies present after their childbearing years, and that only 11.5% became pregnant before or at onset of their disease [5]. Thus, despite the female predominance and multiple subtypes, inflammatory myopathies are fairly rare during pregnancy.

Several case reports and prospective studies have demonstrated that outcome in pregnancy is linked to the overall disease course. While mothers with active myositis are at higher risk for prematurity and fetal loss, mothers whose symptoms are in remission are more likely to have healthy babies [6, 7]. For example, in one prospective study, two patients with active disease had fetal loss, whereas the other two had healthy newborns [8]. A subsequent literature review of 37 cases found that 43% of pregnancies with active inflammatory myopathy

Neurological Illness in Pregnancy: Principles and Practice, First Edition.
Edited by Autumn Klein, M. Angela O'Neal, Christina Scifres, Janet F. R. Waters and Jonathan H. Waters.
© 2016 John Wiley & Sons, Ltd. Published 2016 by John Wiley & Sons, Ltd.

Table 10.1 Neuromuscular disorders in pregnancy

Acquired disorders

1 Acquired general disorders of muscle
   a Inflammatory myopathies: dermatomyositis (DM) and polymyositis (PM)
2 Acquired disorders of neuromuscular junction
   a Myasthenia gravis
3 Motor neuron disease
   a Amyotrophic lateral sclerosis (ALS)
4 Acquired disorders of nerve
   a Acute inflammatory demyelinating polyradiculoneuropathy (AIDP)
   b Chronic inflammatory demyelinating polyradiculoneuropathy (CIDP)
   c Multifocal motor neuropathy (MMN)
5 Focal disorders of root, plexus or peripheral nerve
   a Median neuropathy at the wrist (carpal tunnel syndrome)
   b Bell's palsy
   c Lateral femoral cutaneous neuropathy (meralgia paresthetica)
   d Femoral and obturator neuropathies
   e Lumbar radiculopathy and plexopathy
   f Postpartum foot drop

Hereditary disorders

1 Hereditary disorders of muscle
   a Myotonic dystrophies: type 1 and type 2
   b Muscular dystrophies/congenital myopathies: limb-girdle muscular dystrophy (LGMD) and facioscapulohumeral muscular dystrophy (FSHD)
2 Hereditary disorders of peripheral nerve/motor neuron
   a Charcot–Marie–Tooth (CMT) or hereditary sensorimotor neuropathy (HSMN)
   b Spinal muscular atrophy (SMA)

were complicated by fetal death, and 33% had intrauterine growth restriction, compared to 13.6% and 13.6% in patients with controlled disease, respectively. Worse outcomes were seen in patients with new diagnosis during pregnancy or flare during the first trimester of pregnancy [8]. Of note, DM and PM are not transmitted to the fetus, though asymptomatic newborns may have transiently increased creatine kinase for 2–4 months [9].

During pregnancy, symptoms of inflammatory myositis may improve, worsen, or

remain stable [10], and those with inflammatory myopathies should be considered high-risk pregnancies. Experts have recommended monitoring respiratory function and strength for worsening disease [11]. Treatment options are limited, with several immunosuppressive medications contraindicated during pregnancy. Table 10.2 lists several immunosuppressants used in neuromuscular disorders and their possible side effects during pregnancy and lactation. It is preferable for the patients to have their disease brought under control with the lowest dose of prednisone possible prior to becoming pregnant. Overall, flares during pregnancy can be treated with increasing doses of prednisone, and for steroid-resistant cases, intravenous immunoglobulin (IVIG) [12]. There have been case reports of symptoms of myositis improving after pregnancy termination [13] and delivery [10]. Though there have not been any studies done on the mode of delivery in inflammatory myopathies, some physicians have recommended Caesarian section for mothers with active myositis, to avoid maternal exertion and decrease the risk of rhabdomyolysis [14]. Fortunately, occurrence of PM during one pregnancy does not predict recurrence of symptoms in a subsequent pregnancy [13].

Disorders of the neuromuscular junction—myasthenia gravis

Myasthenia gravis (MG) is an autoimmune disorder of neuromuscular transmission, in which antibodies against the postsynaptic neuromuscular junction inhibit transmission, leading to fatigable weakness of skeletal muscle. It is seen in an estimated one in 20,000 pregnancies [15]. Myasthenia gravis may be exacerbated by certain medications (including some anesthetic agents), surgery, infection, and emotional stress. Like other autoimmune disorders, symptoms may worsen, improve, or remain unchanged during pregnancy and the postpartum period [16]. Unfortunately, the degree of remission does not predict the probability of exacerbation [17]. Exacerbations occur most frequently in the

Table 10.2 Common medications used for neuromuscular diseases and risk category during pregnancy

Medication	Potential adverse advents during pregnancy and lactation	FDA Class
Corticosteroids *Oral prednisone* *IV methylprednisolone*	Less than 10% of active form of prednisone and methylprednisolone reach the fetus. Risk of elevated blood pressure, hyperglycemia, and osteopenia. Studies on animals have shown corticosteroids cause birth defects. A meta-analysis demonstrated a 3.3-fold increase (from 1/1000 to 3/1000) in cleft/lip or palate after first trimester exposure, though not consistent in other studies. May correlate with premature rupture of amniotic membranes and low birth weight. Prednisolone levels measured in breast milk are less than 0.1% of ingested dose and less than 10% of infants' endogenous corticosteroid production. Peak levels occur 2 hours after a dose and decline rapidly. With long-term therapy, adrenal suppression may occur, and stress dose steroids may be needed during labor and delivery.	C
Azathioprine	Known to cross placenta. Lack of specific pattern of congenital abnormalities, though anecdotal evidence of malformations. Associated with intrauterine growth restriction and preterm delivery. Felt to have fewer adverse effects than MTX, MMF, or cyclophosphamide. Undetectable to very low levels in breast milk, and no adverse events reported in breast-fed infants.	D
Methotrexate (MTX)	Known risk of fetal abnormalities and miscarriage. Pregnancy should be avoided for either partner—men should wait 3 months after cessation of therapy, women should wait at least one ovulatory cycle. Medication can persist in the liver up to 4 months after exposure. Unknown whether safe in lactation—should be avoided.	X
Mycophenolate mofetil (MMF)	Shown to be teratogenic in animal studies. National Transplantation Pregnancy Registry (NTPR) data showed 45% of pregnancies ended in spontaneous abortions. 22% of live-born babies had birth defects. EMFO tetrad: ear (microtia/auditory canal atresia), mouth (cleft lip/palate), fingers (brachydactyly and hypoplastic toenails), and organs (cardiac, renal, CNS, diaphragmatic, and ocular). Use of reliable contraception is mandatory on this medication. Women should discontinue mediation at least 6 weeks before conception. No data on secretion in breast milk—use during breastfeeding is contraindicated.	D
Cyclophosphamide	May affect fertility in men and women. Use by father prior to conception can be associated with birth defects. Associated with craniosynostosis, facial anomalies, distal limb malformations and developmental delays. Absolutely contraindicated in early pregnancy. Used with extreme caution in severely ill patients in second half of pregnancy. Contraindicated in breastfeeding.	D
Cyclosporine	Known to cross placenta. Associated with premature birth and low birth weight. Analysis of data from 15 studies did not show evidence of increase in birth defects. Low to moderate secretion into breast milk—use during breastfeeding is not recommended.	C

(continued)

Table 10.2 (*Continued*)

Medication	Potential adverse advents during pregnancy and lactation	FDA Class
IVIG	Known to cross placenta after 32 weeks gestation. Successful outcomes in pregnancy have been observed. Hemolytic disease of the newborn and transmission of hepatitis C have been reported. No reports published for breastfeeding. However, the World Health Organization (WHO) reports IVIG is compatible with breastfeeding.	C
Rituximab	No adequate human studies have been conducted. B-cell lymphopenia seen in infants exposed *in utero*—lasts less than 6 months. One successful pregnancy in a patient on R-CHOP for lymphoma. Excreted into human milk—breastfeeding contraindicated.	C
Plasma exchange	May alter blood volume and cause hypotension in mother and fetus. Left lateral decubitus position and close monitoring of fluid status protect against hypotension. In third trimester, fetal monitoring is recommended.	N/A
Pyridostigmine	No adequate studies in humans. Unknown whether it crosses placenta. Limited data indicate use near-term and/or during labor may result in neonatal myasthenia, which improves with neostigmine. Normal births have also been reported. Infants receive about 0.1% of maternal dose. Weight of an adequate body of evidence and/or expert consensus suggests this drug poses minimal risk to the infant when used during breastfeeding. WHO states compatible with breastfeeding.	C
Riluzole	No adequate studies in humans. The use of riluzole during human pregnancy has been described in two case reports. One infant was light for age, but was otherwise healthy, and the other had intrauterine growth retardation and an asymptomatic small atrial communication and a small ductus arteriosus. The pregnancies for both children were otherwise uneventful. It is unknown whether riluzole is excreted into human breast milk.	C
Mexiletine	One human case report and few animal studies did not find teratogenic effects associated with use of mexiletine during pregnancy. Excreted into human breast milk, but small amounts excreted are unlikely to be harmful. American Academy of Pediatrics: compatible with breastfeeding.	C

Source: U.S. Food and Drug Administration, http://www.accessdata.fda.gov/scripts/cdrh/cfdocs/cfcfr/cfrsearch.cfm?fr=201.57
Pregnancy category A: Adequate and well-controlled studies in pregnant women have failed to demonstrate a risk to the fetus in the first trimester of pregnancy and there is no evidence of a risk in later trimesters.
Pregnancy category B: Animal reproduction studies have failed to demonstrate a risk to the fetus and there are no adequate and well-controlled studies in pregnant women.
Pregnancy category C: Animal reproduction studies have shown an adverse effect on the fetus, if there are no adequate and well-controlled studies in humans, and if the benefits from the use of the drug in pregnant women may be acceptable despite its potential risks.
Pregnancy category D: There is positive evidence of human fetal risk based on adverse reaction data from investigational or marketing experience or studies in humans, but the potential benefits from the use of the drug in pregnant women may be acceptable despite its potential risks.
Pregnancy category X: Studies in animals or humans have demonstrated fetal abnormalities or if there is positive evidence of fetal risk based on adverse reaction reports from investigational or marketing experience, or both, and the risk of the use of the drug in a pregnant woman clearly outweighs any possible benefit.

first trimester, the last 4 weeks of gestation, during delivery, and the postpartum period [12, 18].

Myasthenic symptoms are often controlled with cholinesterase inhibitors such as pyridostigmine and/or immunosuppressants. Although there are no clinical trials on the safety of pyridostigmine in pregnancy, clinical experience and reports in the literature suggest that it is reasonably safe to use if indicated [19]. The use of immunosuppressants in MG during pregnancy is similar to the approach used in inflammatory myopathies. It is preferable for the patients to have their disease brought under control with a combination of pyridostigmine and the lowest dose of prednisone possible prior to becoming pregnant. Worsening symptoms are managed with increasing doses of these medications, and myasthenic crises or flares unresponsive to steroids are treated with IVIG or plasmapheresis [19].

Other possible complications with pregnancy include transient neonatal myasthenia gravis (TNMG) and arthrogryposis multiplex congenita. TNMG occurs with placental transfer of maternal antibodies against the acetylcholine receptor. It occurs in approximately 4–12% of infants born to mothers with MG [19] and presents with hypotonia, generalized weakness, difficulty with suck, and rarely with respiratory difficulties. All infants born to myasthenic mothers should be monitored after birth for these symptoms. TNMG resolves with clearance of maternal antibodies (usually within a few weeks to months), and treatment is supportive. Severe cases can be treated with cholinesterase inhibitors and plasmapheresis, though some may require short term ventilatory support.

Arthrogryposis multiplex congenita occurs when the transfer of placental antibodies causes intrauterine fetal paralysis, leading to dysmorphic features, arthrogryposis, and possibly even central nervous system (CNS) abnormalities and death. It may occur in up to 2.2% of pregnancies [16]. The risk of developing TNMG or arthrogryposis multiplex congenita is increased if a prior pregnancy was complicated by either condition

[20, 21]. Of note, a large population study did not demonstrate a significantly increased prevalence of severe birth defects in infants born to mothers with MG than in the general population [15].

Labor and delivery may be complicated by MG as well, though there is some conflicting data about the degree of risk. One large population study in Norway suggested that there could be an increased risk of premature rupture of membranes (5.5% vs. 1.7%), and an increased number of obstetric interventions (such as Caesarian sections or forceps/vacuum use) in mothers with MG [15]. A more recent population study done in Taiwan did not show a statistically significant difference in preterm birth, low birth weight or prevalence of Caesarian section [22]. Like many other neuromuscular conditions, the unpredictable course and possible complications of MG and treatments should be managed with a multidisciplinary group with a neurologist [23].

Thymectomy is indicated in all myasthenic patients with thymoma. For patients without thymoma, thymectomy can be considered, though indications are not as strong. Although one retrospective study in 69 pregnant women suggested that mothers who had undergone thymectomies had a lower risk of having babies with TNMG (2/25 in post-thymectomy vs. 19/45), larger, more recent population-based studies have not supported this finding [15, 22, 24]. Experts currently recommend that thymectomies be performed prior to pregnancy or after the postpartum period due to the delayed therapeutic effect [12].

Lastly, medications and anesthesia given during labor and delivery may not be without risk. Magnesium is known to cause neuromuscular transmission blockade, and there has been a case report of bulbar and limb weakness precipitated by magnesium sulfate infusion for preeclampsia in a patient who was later diagnosed with MG [25]. A recent review published on anesthesia and MG suggested that pyridostigmine be continued pre-procedurally, given the risk of developing respiratory difficulties if it is withdrawn, that neuromuscular monitoring with train-of-four be used in patients with MG (as they are more sensitive to neuromuscular blockade), and that regional anesthesia be preferred to generalized anesthesia [26].

Motor neuron disease—amyotrophic lateral sclerosis

Amyotrophic lateral sclerosis (ALS) is a degenerative disease of the upper and lower motor neurons, which can be sporadic or inherited. Its incidence is approximately 1.8/100,000, and average age of onset is approximately 60 years [2]. It is rarely seen in pregnant women, in fact, since 1997, only 19 pregnancies have been reported in the English literature [27]. Overall, ALS does not seem to cause obstetric complications and does not inhibit uterine contractions; however, some patients can demonstrate rapid worsening, possibly with respiratory failure requiring tracheostomy and gastrostomy, and/or death postpartum [27, 28]. One case report suggests that the impact of pregnancy on ALS may be more severe in later stages—while the patient's first delivery was reported to be without complications, her second pregnancy (after she became bedridden) required tracheostomy, gastrostomy, and early Caesarian section at 34 weeks for rupture of the amniotic sac in the presence of severe abdominal weakness [29]. It has been recommended that women of childbearing age with ALS have anticipatory counseling about the possible requirement of invasive ventilation during pregnancy [12]. Both vaginal delivery and Caesarian sections have been reported in ALS patients with successful outcomes.

The use of riluzole during human pregnancy has been described in two case reports. One infant was light for age, but was otherwise healthy, and the other had intrauterine growth retardation, an asymptomatic small atrial communication, and a small ductus arteriosus. The pregnancies for both children were otherwise uneventful [27, 28]. Riluzole is classified as Food Drug Administration (FDA) pregnancy class C (Table 10.2).

Acquired generalized neuropathies
Acute inflammatory demyelinating polyneuropathy or Guillain–Barré syndrome

Acute inflammatory demyelinating polyneuropathy (AIDP) has an annual incidence of approximately 1–4 per 100,000 [2]. Population studies have suggested that the risk of acquiring AIDP during pregnancy is similar to the general population, though there appears to be an increased risk in the first 30 days postpartum (OR 2.93, CI 1.20–7.11) [30, 31]. In one literature review, approximately one-third of patients had respiratory failure, and approximately one-third of patients had preterm delivery—of these, 3 of 8 were spontaneous labor, and the other 5 were induced for neurological or obstetrical reasons. There were no cases of neonatal death, and termination of pregnancy did not affect duration of illness in the mother [32].

Compared to the general population, fewer pregnant women have evidence of *Campylobacter jejuni* infection. However, cases of AIDP have been associated with presence of infection by CMV (cytomegalovirus), EBV (Epstein–Barr virus), Rubella, hepatitis A, and VZV (varicella zoster virus) [32, 33] and infectious causes should be sought as they can have teratogenic effects on the fetus. Also, unlike the general population, the inactivated influenza vaccine has not been shown to be associated with an increased risk of AIDP in pregnant women [34, 35].

Treatment of AIDP, as in the general population, is IVIG or plasma exchange, which is well tolerated [32, 36]. Subcutaneous prophylaxis against deep vein thrombosis is recommended, as patients are hypercoagulable due to pregnancy, immobility, and possibly treatment with IVIG.

Vaginal delivery is possible, as normal uterine contractions are not inhibited by AIDP. In fact, AIDP is not a clear indication for Caesarian section [37]. If anesthesia is required, succinylcholine should be avoided due to risk of life-threatening hyperkalemia [38], and non-depolarizing neuromuscular blocking agents should be used with caution as they can be associated with prolonged blockade in patients with AIDP [39]. Overall, epidural anesthesia seems to be safe in patients with AIDP [39], although there is one case report of worsening of AIDP symptoms after epidural anesthesia [40].

The AIDP does not seem to affect the fetus; in fact, normal fetal activity has been seen even in mothers that are completely paralyzed [41]. There has been a case report of hypotonia and respiratory distress in a neonate in a mother with AIDP, which improved with IVIG [42].

Chronic inflammatory demyelinating polyneuropathy

Chronic inflammatory demyelinating polyneuropathy (CIDP) is an autoimmune demyelinating neuropathy that is characterized by a relapsing/remitting or progressive course. It is rare, estimated to occur in 1–7.7 out of 100,000 patients [43]. There is a significant increase in the number of relapses during pregnancy, especially during the third trimester or immediate postpartum period [44]. Treatment, similar to other autoimmune conditions, consists of escalation of steroid dose, IVIG, or plasmapheresis. Prolonged weakness has been described after epidural anesthesia, though there have also been other reports of uncomplicated administration [45]. Currently, there are no specific recommendations for anesthesia in patients with CIDP, and inferences are drawn from the AIDP literature. Of note, CIDP does not appear to alter the course of pregnancy or significantly affect the fetus [46].

Multifocal motor neuropathy

Multifocal motor neuropathy (MMN) is an immune-mediated demyelinating neuropathy characterized by asymmetric motor involvement in the distribution of individual peripheral nerves, often associated with anti-ganglioside antibodies. It is treated with IVIG and is not as responsive as other forms of CIDP to steroids or plasma exchange. Because it predominantly occurs in men and mostly in the fifth decade of life [2], it is not commonly seen in pregnant women. One case series of three women with MMN reported worsening during pregnancy. These women were treated with IVIG without reported treatment side effects; however, they were not able to regain normal strength during pregnancy. After delivery, all patients returned to their prepregnancy state [47]. Relapses in subsequent pregnancies have been reported [48]. There has been one case report of neonatal transmission, presenting with decreased fetal movement, neonatal weakness, and hyporeflexia that improved after 1 month without IVIG, though there was report of weakness and atrophy of distal limbs with foot drop at age four. The infant also had anti-GM1 IgG and IgG lambda monoclonal gammopathy, which normalized after several months [49].

Acquired focal neuropathies
Carpal tunnel syndrome/median neuropathy at the wrist

Carpal tunnel syndrome (CTS) is a common disorder, affecting 3–6% of the general population [50] and is the most frequent compression neuropathy that complicates pregnancy [11]. Risk factors for CTS include pregnancy, endocrine disorders (such as diabetes, hypothyroidism), rheumatoid arthritis, space occupying lesions, amyloidosis, and repetitive stress, among others [51].

The incidence of CTS in pregnancy reported in the literature varies widely and has been quoted to be between 0.34% and 62% [19]. Only a portion of these patients have electrodiagnostically confirmed median neuropathy at the wrist; for example, in a study done by the Italian CTS Study Group, though 62% of patients had clinical symptoms, only 43% had positive electrophysiological studies [52]. In another prospective study, incidence of electrodiagnostically confirmed median neuropathy at the wrist in pregnancy was approximately 17% [53]. Generally, patients develop CTS in the third trimester

[54]. Nulliparous patients and those with generalized edema seem to be at higher risk [55]. Gestational diabetes does not seem to increase the risk of developing CTS during pregnancy [56]. It has been proposed that the increased incidence of CTS in pregnancy may be due to increased fluid retention causing edema and compression on the median nerve [56].

Carpal tunnel syndrome does not always resolve after pregnancy. There is considerable variation in the natural history of pregnancy-related CTS, with approximately only half of cases resolving after 1 year and two-thirds after 3 years [53]. Though the American Academy of Orthopedic Surgeons does not provide specific recommendations for treatment for pregnancy-related CTS, consensus is to provide conservative care through pregnancy and to use surgical decompression for patients that are not responding to conservative care or those with significant compression on electrodiagnostic studies [57]. Conservative treatment is preferred, as up to 82% of pregnant patients have good relief with nighttime splints [55]. Local corticosteroid injections have been tried in the pregnant population, with overall good improvement in symptoms and electrophysiological studies [58, 59] though, there are no studies on the effect of steroid injections on fetal development. Similarly, there are no randomized trials comparing non-operative treatment for CTS in pregnant women.

Bell's palsy (idiopathic facial neuropathy)

Bell's palsy presents as unilateral lower motor neuron facial weakness. The incidence of Bell's palsy increases up to 3.3 times the expected incidence during pregnancy, up to 45 per 100,000 births, and occurs most often in the third trimester or early postpartum period [60]. It has been associated with preeclampsia during pregnancy [61] as well as chronic or gestational hypertension and obesity [62]. There are conflicting data as to whether Bell's palsy is associated with low Apgar scores, perinatal mortality, or fetal malformation [12, 62].

Though some reviews do suggest good outcomes [11, 60], one retrospective study has suggested that a higher percentage of pregnant women with Bell's palsy may progress to completion (65% vs. ~50% in nonpregnant) and that those patients may have less chance of recovery than nonpregnant patients with complete lesions (52% vs. ~80%). In this study, all patients with incomplete palsies recovered fully, and only 2 out of 48 patients had recurrence with subsequent pregnancies, with overall recurrence rate of 12% [63].

Treatment recommendations from the American Academy of Neurology (AAN) in nonpregnant patients include corticosteroids to help increase the probability of facial nerve recovery. Antiviral medications are thought to increase the probability of recovery of facial function, but benefit is modest at best and has not been definitively established (Level C) [64]. No specific recommendations are made in pregnancy, though corticosteroids are generally considered safe and antivirals are FDA pregnancy class B [12].

Lower extremity compression neuropathies/plexopathies

Lower extremity neuropathies are seen commonly in the postpartum period—in one large observational study done in a single hospital, 0.92% of women developed a lower extremity neuropathy after giving birth. The most common neuropathies were (listed in descending order): lateral femoral cutaneous, femoral, peroneal, lumbosacral plexus, sciatic, and obturator. The development of a lower extremity neuropathy was associated with nulliparity and a prolonged second stage of labor [65].

Meralgia paresthetica (lateral femoral cutaneous neuropathy) is associated with excessive weight gain or in combination with diabetes or a large fetus [66]. Meralgia paresthetica is treated by relieving pressure on the nerve, eliminating tight clothing, using abdominal binders to lift the weight off the nerve, or weight loss. Overall, treatment is supportive, as spontaneous recovery often occurs after delivery [50].

Femoral neuropathies are associated with prolonged periods of time in the lithotomy position, excessive weight gain, and tight clothing [50]. It is thought that the femoral nerve is compressed at the inguinal ligament during delivery by thigh flexion, abduction, and external rotation, or perhaps compression by the fetal head [11, 67]. Lesions are usually demyelinating and typically recover in 6 months or less [68].

Obturator neuropathies are thought to be caused by compression of the fetal head against the pelvic wall, the lithotomy position, or forceps delivery (which can compress the nerve as it passes over the pelvic brim) [12]. Rarely, pudendal nerve blocks can cause a local hematoma in the obturator foramen and subsequent compression neuropathy as well [65].

Postpartum foot drop

There are many possible etiologies for postpartum foot drop, including common peroneal and sciatic neuropathies, lumbosacral plexopathy, or lumbar radiculopathy. Common peroneal neuropathies are presumed to be caused by compression from prolonged knee flexion from squatting, the lithotomy position, or by pressure over the fibular head during delivery [19]. Patients may be more at risk with epidural anesthesia, due to the lack of sensory input that would normally signal the need for a position change [65].

Injury to the lumbosacral plexus is thought to occur from compression from the fetal head or possibly forceps delivery. Injury to the sciatic nerve is infrequent, and the etiology is not clearly understood, but is also presumed to be due to mechanical factors [12, 19].

Lumbar radiculopathies from disc herniation with objective findings during pregnancy are rare, and presents in only 1 in 10,000 pregnancies [69]. Low back pain is much more prevalent, occurring in 50% of women at some time during pregnancy [70]. Overall, the incidence of lumbar radiculopathy does not increase during pregnancy, and management should not be different than from nonpregnant patients [71]. Of

note, cauda equina syndrome from disc herniation during pregnancy is extremely uncommon (estimated at about 2% of lumbosacral disk herniations) but should be treated with emergent surgery [71, 72].

Hereditary disorders

Myotonic dystrophy type 1

Myotonic dystrophy type 1 (DM1) is the most common muscular dystrophy affecting pregnant women, affecting 1 in 8000 adults [11]. It is an autosomal dominant genetic condition with anticipation, caused by expansion of CAG trinucleotide repeats in the myotonic dystrophy protein kinase (*DMPK*) gene on chromosome 19q13.3 [2]. It is a multisystemic disease, which is known to cause gonadal atrophy and infertility in men. In women, its effects on fertility have been more controversial—both infertility and normal fertility have been reported [73, 74]. It is not uncommon for women to be diagnosed with DM1 during pregnancy or after delivery of an affected child. In one review of 31 women, 84% did not know of their diagnosis before their first pregnancy [75]. Only a small percentage of women, if any, have mild worsening of weakness during pregnancy, which often resolves after delivery [75, 76].

Despite the overall good maternal prognosis with DM1, these patients may have a higher obstetric complication rate than the general population. This is attributed to the risk of delivering a child with congenital myotonic dystrophy, a severe form of the disease with onset at birth, with weakness, hypotonia, respiratory difficulties, cognitive deficits, and higher risk of early mortality [19]. The congenital phenotype is an effect of anticipation, which for an unknown reason is more severe when the infant receives its affected gene from the mother. Mothers are also at higher risk of delivering a child with this disorder if they are symptomatic in multiple organ systems before the age of 30, inherited DM1 from their fathers, have a gene expansion greater than 1 kB or have previously had a child with congenital myotonic dystrophy [11]. Congenital myotonic dystrophy is associated with polyhydramnios, usually seen in the 7th month of pregnancy, and severe intrauterine movement restriction [77]. It also carries an increased risk of fetal death—in one recent study with 65 newborns born to mothers with DM1, 14 were affected, of which 5 died a few hours after birth or were stillborn [77].

Premature birth and labor are also significantly increased in patients with DM1, as well as ectopic pregnancy, placenta previa, and urinary tract infections [75, 77]. There may be an increased incidence of breech presentation and oblique fetal lie [77]. Mothers with DM1 are at risk for anesthetic complications. Depolarizing agents should be avoided due to risk of life-threatening muscle spasms, and opiates and barbiturates should be used cautiously due to the risk of respiratory depression [11].

Myotonic dystrophy type 2 or proximal myotonic myopathy

Myotonic dystrophy type 2 (DM2) is an autosomal dominant genetic condition caused by CCTG repeat expansion in first intron of the zinc finger protein 9 (*ZNF 9*) gene on chromosome 3 [2]. There is some retrospective data suggesting that pregnancy may hasten the onset or progression of DM2—women with prior pregnancies have an earlier onset of symptoms [78]. In small retrospective studies, symptoms of DM2 were first observed during pregnancy in 14–21% of patients. If onset of symptoms occurred before or during pregnancy, there was a higher rate of preterm labor and prematurity. Fortunately, patients did seem to improve after delivery [77,78]. Unlike DM1, there is no congenital form [74]. There is conflicting data about fetal loss, with one study suggesting an increased risk with pregnancy-related worsening, but another study without increased risk [77,78].

Muscular dystrophies and congenital myopathies

There are many forms of muscular dystrophies and congenital myopathies, which are very rare in the general population. Overall, fetal outcomes in disorders like facioscapulohumeral muscular dystrophy (FSHD), limb-girdle muscular dystrophy (LGMD), and congenital myopathies are generally good, with incidence of miscarriage, preterm birth, and neonatal/perinatal death comparable to the general population [77–80]. There may be a higher incidence of low birth weight in FSHD [79], and perhaps a slight increase in breech presentation in LGMD [77], though these studies are small and have not been reproduced. There is an increased rate of obstetric interventions such as Caesarian section or instrumental deliveries in FSHD, but the increased rate of obstetric interventions seen in LGMD and congenital myopathies did not reach statistical significance due to small patient populations. [74] Overall, significant proportions of women seem to worsen during pregnancy and have lasting weakness (FSHD 12–25%, LGMD 56%, congenital myopathy 16%), though it is unclear whether this is due to pregnancy or progression of disease [12, 77].

Charcot–Marie–Tooth disease or hereditary sensory motor neuropathy

Charcot–Marie–Tooth disease (CMT) is a heterogenous group of hereditary neuropathies with multiple genetic causes. Similar to other neuromuscular disorders, data on this topic are from small retrospective studies. Overall, one review found a higher occurrence of postpartum bleeding and breech presentation [81], though two reviews with 33 and 21 patients did not find any increase in obstetric complications [77, 82]. Worsening of symptoms did occur in 32–50% of patients and was persistent in 22–65%, and patients who experienced deterioration in one pregnancy were more likely to experience deterioration in subsequent pregnancies [77, 82].

Spinal muscular atrophy

Spinal muscular atrophies (SMAs) are a heterogeneous group of diseases with multiple genetic causes that are characterized by degeneration of anterior horn cells and motor cranial nerve nuclei [2]. Small retrospective studies of patients with SMA suggest a higher incidence of premature labor and Caesarian section, and possibly prolonged labor and delayed postpartum recovery. There was no evidence of increased incidence of adverse fetal events; however, there may be persistent worsening of symptoms during or after pregnancy [77, 83]. Respiratory failure leading to intrauterine death has been known to occur, especially for patients with poor lung function and severe scoliosis, though successful pregnancies have been reported [77]. Of note, fetal ultrasound has not been shown to predict severe neonatal spinal muscular atrophy [84].

General recommendations for pregnancy in neuromuscular disease

The 179th European Neuromuscular Centre (ENMC) workshop in 2010 reviewed existing literature on pregnancy in neuromuscular disorders and provided specific recommendations to improve maternal and fetal outcomes. Foremost amongst these recommendations were to define patients with diaphragm or cardiac involvement as high risk. In these patients, they recommended forced vital capacity (FVC), maximum inspiratory pressure (MIP), and peak cough flow (PCF) at baseline and in each trimester. An echocardiogram is recommended in each trimester if ejection fraction is 45–60%, and monthly if ejection fraction is <45%. Mothers with FVC < 50% predicted or less than 1 L, MIP < 60 cm H_2O or PCF < 160 L/min should receive an arterial blood gas and a respiratory sleep study. Holter or electrocardiogram should be considered in those with prior history of arrhythmias or palpitations. Further details can be found in the reference article cited [85].

References

1 Ernste FC, Reed AM. Idiopathic inflammatory myopathies: current trends in pathogenesis, clinical features and up-to-date treatment recommendations. *Mayo Clin Proc.* 2013;88:83–105.

2 Amato AA, Russell JA (eds.). *Neuromuscular Disorders*, New York: McGraw-Hill Medical, 2008.

3 Targoff IN. Polymyositis and dermatomyositis in adults. In: Maddison PJ, Isenberg DA, Woo P, Glass DN, eds., *Oxford Textbook of Rheumatology*. Oxford: Oxford University Press 1998; pp. 1240–1207.

4 Pinheiro GRC, Goldenberg J, Atra E, et al. Juvenile dermatomyositis and pregnancy: report and literature review. *J Rheumatol.* 1992;19:1798–1801.

5 Vancsa A, Ponyi A, Constantin T, et al. Pregnancy outcome in idiopathic inflammatory myopathy. *Rheumatol Int.* 2007;27:435–439.

6 Clowse ME. Managing contraception and pregnancy in the rheumatologic diseases. *Best Pract Res Clin Rheumatol.* 2010;24:373–385.

7 Chopra S, Suri V, Bagga R, et al. Autoimmune inflammatory myopathy in pregnancy. *Medscape J Med.* 2008;10:17–22.

8 Silva CA, Sultan SM, Isenberg DA. Pregnancy outcome in adult-onset idiopathic inflammatory myopathy. *Rheumatology (Oxford).* 2003;42:1168–1172.

9 Messina S, Fagiolari G, Lamperti C, et al. Women with pregnancy-related polymyositis and high serum CK levels in the newborn. *Neurology.* 2002;58:482–484.

10 Bauer KA, Siegler M, Lindheimer MA. Polymyositis complicating pregnancy. *Arch Int Med.* 1979;139:449.

11 Sax TW, Rosenbaum RB. Neuromuscular disorders in pregnancy. *Muscle Nerve.* 2006;34:559–571.

12 Guidon AC, Massey EW. Neuromuscular disorders in pregnancy. *Neurol Clin.* 2012;30:889–911.

13 Papapetropoulos T, Kanellakopoulou N, Tsibri E, et al. Polymyositis and pregnancy: report of a case with 3 pregnancies. *J Neurol Neurosurg Psychiatry.* 1998;64:406.

14 Mosca M, Strigini F, Carmignani A, et al. Pregnant patient with dermatomyositis successfully treated with intravenous immunoglobulin therapy. *Arthritis Rheum.* 2003;53:119–121.

15 Hoff JM, Daltveit AK, Gilhus NE. Myasthenia gravis: consequences for pregnancy, delivery and the newborn. *Neurology.* 2003;61:1362–1366.

16 Batocchi AP, Majolini L, Evoli A, et al. Course and treatment of myasthenia gravis during pregnancy. *Neurology.* 1999;52:447–452.

17 Ciafaloni E, Massey J. Myasthenia gravis and pregnancy. *Neurol Clin.* 2004;22:771–782.

18 Chaudhry SA, Vignarajah B, Koren G. Myasthenia gravis during pregnancy. *Can Fam Physician.* 2012;58:1346–1349.

19 Briemberg HR. Neuromuscular diseases in pregnancy. *Semin Neurol.* 2007;27:460–466.

20 Hoff JM, Dalveit AK, Gilhus NE. Arthrogryposis multiplex congenita – a rare fetal condition caused by maternal myasthenia gravis. *Acta Neurol Scand Suppl.* 2006;183:26–27.

21 Polizzi A, Huson SM, Vincent A. Teratogen update: maternal myasthenia gravis as a cause of congenital arthrogryposis. *Teratology.* 2000;62:332–341.

22 Wen JC, Llu TC, Chen YII, et al. No increased risk of adverse pregnancy outcomes for women with myasthenia gravis: a nationwide population-based study. *Eur J Neurol.* 2009;16:889–894.

23 Hoff JM, Daltveit AK, Gilhus NE. Myasthenia gravis in pregnancy and birth: identifying risk factors, optimizing care. *Eur J Neurol.* 2007;14:38–43.

24 Djelmis J, Sostarko M, Mayer D, et al. Myasthenia gravis in pregnancy: report on 69 cases. *Eur J Obstet Gynecol Reprod Biol.* 2002;104:21–25.

25 Barshuk RG, Krendel DA. Myasthenia gravis presenting as weakness after magnesium administration. *Muscle Nerve.* 1990;13:708–712.

26 Blichfeldt-Lauridsen L, Hansen BD. Anesthesia and myasthenia gravis. *Acta Anaesthesiol Scand.* 2012;56:17–22.

27 Scalco RS, Vieira MC, da Cunha Filho EV, et al. Amyotrophic lateral sclerosis and riluzole use during pregnancy: a case report. *Amyotroph Lateral Scler.* 2012;13:471–472.

28 Kawamichi Y, Makino Y, Matsuda Y, et al. Riluzole use during pregnancy in a patient with amyotrophic lateral sclerosis: a case report. *J Int Med Res.* 2010;38:720–726.

29 Sarafov S, Doitchinova M, Karagiozova Z, et al. Two consecutive pregnancies in early and late stage of amyotrophic lateral sclerosis. *Amyotroph Lateral Scler.* 2009;10:483–486.

30 Cheng Q, Jiang GX, Fredrikson S, et al. Increased incidence of Guillain-Barre syndrome postpartum. *Epidemiology.* 1998;9:601–604.

31 Jiang GX, de Pedro-Cuesta J, Strigard K, et al. Pregnancy and Guillain-Barre syndrome: a nationwide register cohort study. *Neuroepidemiology.* 1996;15:192–200.

32 Chan LYS, Tsui MH, Leung TN. Guillain-Barre syndrome in pregnancy. *Acta Obstet Gynecol Scand.* 2004;83:319–325.

33 Modi M, Singla M, Aggarwal N, et al. Guillain-Barre syndrome in pregnancy: a rare complication of varicella. *Taiwan J Obstet Gynecol.* 2010;49:364–365.

34 Nordin JD, Kharbanda EO, Benitez GV, et al. Maternal safety of trivalent inactivated influenza vaccine in pregnant women. *Obstet Gynecol.* 2013;121:519–525.

35 Steinhoff MC, MacDonald NE. Influenza pandemics – pregnancy, pathogenesis and perinatal outcomes. *JAMA.* 2012;308:184–185.

36 Fait G, Gull I, Kupferminc M, et al. Intravenous immune globulins in Guillain-Barre syndrome in pregnancy. *J Obstet Gynecol.* 1998;18:78–79.

37 Rockel A, Wissel J, Rolfs A. Guillain-Barre syndrome in pregnancy – an indication for caesarian section? *J Perinat Med.* 1994;22:393–398.

38 Feldman JM. Cardiac arrest after succinylcholine administration in a pregnant patient recovered from Guillain-Barre syndrome. *Anesthesiology.* 1990;72:942–944.

39 Kocabas S, Karaman S, Firat V, et al. Anesthetic management of Guillain-Barre syndrome in pregnancy. *J Clin Anesth.* 2007;19:299–302.

40 Wiertlewski S, Magot A, Drapier S, et al. Worsening of neurologic symptoms after epidural anesthesia for labor in a Guillain-Barre patient. *Anesth Analg.* 2004;98:825–827.

41 Nelson LH, McLean WT Jr. Management of Landry-Guillain-Barre syndrome in pregnancy. *Obstet Gynecol.* 1985;65(suppl):25S–29S.

42 Luijckx GI, Vles J, de Baets M, et al. Guillain-Barre syndrome in mother and newborn child. *Lancet.* 1997;349:27.

43 Latov N. Diagnosis of CIDP. *Neurology.* 2002;59(suppl 6):2–6.

44 McCombe PA, McManis PG, Frith JA, et al. Chronic inflammatory demyelinating polyradiculoneuropathy associated with pregnancy. *Ann Neurol.* 1987;21:102–104.

45 Richter T, Langer KA, Koch T. Spinal anesthesia for cesarean section in a patient with chronic inflammatory demyelinating polyradiculoneuropathy. *J Anesth.* 2012;26:280–282.

46 Nwosu EC, Tandon S, Breeze C, et al. Chronic demyelinating polyneuropathy in pregnancy treated with intravenous immunoglobulin. *Br J Obstet Gynecol.* 1999;106:174–176.

47 Chaudhry V, Escolar DM, Cornblath DR. Worsening of multifocal motor neuropathy during pregnancy. *Neurology.* 2002;59:139–141.

48 Ioannides XA, Airey C, Fagermo N, et al. Susac syndrome and multifocal motor neuropathy first manifesting in pregnancy. *Aust N Z J Obstet Gynaecol.* 2013;53:314–317.

49 Attarian S, Azulay JP, Chabrol B, et al. Neonatal lower motor neuron syndrome associated with maternal neuropathy with anti-GM1 IgG. *Neurology*. 2004;63:379–381.

50 Klein A. Peripheral nerve disease in pregnancy. *Clin Obstet Gynecol*. 2013;56:382–388.

51 Preston DC, Shapiro BE. *Electromyography and Neuromuscular Disorders*. Philadelphia: Elsevier, 2005.

52 Padua L, Aprile I, Caliandro P, et al. Symptoms and neurophysiological picture of carpal syndrome in pregnancy. *Clin Neurophysiol*. 2001;112:1946–1951.

53 Padua L, Di Pasquale A, Pazzaglia C, et al. Systematic review of pregnancy-related carpal tunnel syndrome. *Muscle Nerve*. 2010;42:697–702.

54 Mondelli M, Rossi S, Monti E. Prospective study of positive factors for improvement of carpal tunnel syndrome in pregnancy women. *Muscle Nerve*. 2007;36:778–783.

55 Ekman-Ordeberg G, Salgeback S, Orderberg G. Carpal tunnel syndrome in pregnancy: a prospective study. *Acta Obstet Gynecol Scand*. 1987;66:233–235.

56 Turgut F, Cetinsahinahin M, Turgut M, et al. The management of carpal tunnel syndrome in pregnancy. *J Clin Neurosci*. 2001;8:332–334.

57 Osterman M, Ilyas AM, Matzon JL. Carpal tunnel syndrome in pregnancy. *Orthop Clin North AM*. 2012;43:515–520.

58 Visser LH, Ngo Q, Groeneweg SJ, et al. Long term effect of local corticosteroid injection for carpal tunnel syndrome: a relation with electrodiagnostic severity. *Clin Neurophysiol*. 2012;123:838–841.

59 Moghtaderi AR, Moghtaderi N, Logmani A. Evaluating the effectiveness of local dexamethasone injection in pregnant women with carpal tunnel syndrome. *J Res Med Sci*. 2011;16:687–690.

60 Cohen Y, Lavie O, Granovsky-Grisaru S, et al. Bell's palsy complicating pregnancy: a review. *Obstet Gynecol Surv*. 2000;55:184–188.

61 Ragupathy K, Emovon E. Bell's palsy in pregnancy. *Arch Gynecol Obstet*. 2013;287:177–178.

62 Katz A, Sergienko R, Dior U, et al. Bell's palsy during pregnancy: is it associated with adverse perinatal outcome? *Laryngoscope*. 2011;121:1395–1398.

63 Gillman GS, Schaitkin BM, May M, et al. Bell's palsy in pregnancy: a study of recovery outcomes. *Otolaryngol Head Neck Surg*. 2002;126:26–30.

64 Gronseth GS, Paduga R. Evidence-based guideline update: steroids and antivirals for Bell's palsy: report of the Guideline Development Subcommittee of the American Academy of Neurology. *Neurology*. 2012;79:2209–2213.

65 Wong CA, Scavone BM, Dugan S, et al. Incidence of postpartum lumbosacral spine and lower extremity nerve injuries. *Obstet Gynecol*. 2003;101:279–288.

66 Van Diver T, Camann W. Meralgia paresthetica in the parturient. *Int J Obstet Anesth*. 1995;4:109–112.

67 al Hakim M, Katirji B. Femoral mononeuropathy induced by the lithotomy position – a report of 5 cases with a review of the literature. *Muscle Nerve*. 1993;16:891–895.

68 Tsen LC. Neurologic complications of labor analgesia and anesthesia. *Int Anesthesiol Clin*. 2002;40:67–88.

69 LaBan MM, Perrin JC, Latimer FR. Pregnancy and the herniated lumbar disc. *Arch Phys Med Rehabil*. 1983;64:319–321.

70 Fast A, Shapiro D, Ducommun EJ, et al. Low-back pain in pregnancy. *Spine*. 1987;12:368–371.

71 Han IH. Pregnancy and spinal problems. *Curr Opin Obstet Gynecol*. 2010;22:477–481.

72 Hakan T. Lumbar disk herniation presented with cauda equine syndrome in a pregnant woman. *J Neurosci Rural Pract*. 2012;3:197–199.

73 Jaffe R, Mock N, Abramowicz J, et al. Myotonic dystrophy and pregnancy: a review. *Obstet Gynecol Surv*. 1986;41:272–278.

74 Argov Z, de Visser. What we do not know about pregnancy in hereditary neuromuscular disorders. *Neuromusc Dis*. 2009;19:675–679.

75 Rudnik-Schoneborn S, Zerres K. Outcome in pregnancies complicated by myotonic dystrophy: a study of 31 patients and review of the literature. *Eur J Obstet Gynecol Reprod Biol*. 2004;114:44–53.

76 Rudnik-Schoneborn S, Nicholson GA, Morgan G, et al. Different patterns of obstetric complications in myotonic dystrophy in relation to the disease status of the fetus. *Am J Med Genet*. 1998;80:314–321.

77 Awater C, Zerres K, Rudnik-Schoneborn S. Pregnancy course and outcome in women with hereditary neuromuscular disorders: comparison of obstetric risks in 178 patients. *Eur J Obstet Gynecol Reprod Biol*. 2012;162:153–159.

78 Rudnik-Schoneborn S, Schneider-Gold C, Raabe U, et al. Outcome and effect of pregnancy in myotonic dystrophy type 2. *Neurology*. 2006;66:579–580.

79 Ciafaloni E, Pressman EK, Loi AM, et al. Pregnancy and birth outcomes in women with

facioscapulohumeral muscular dystrophy. *Neurology*. 2006;67:1887–1889.

80 Rudnik-Schoneborn S, Glauner B, Rohrig D, et al. Obstetric aspects in women with facioscapulohumeral muscular dystrophy, limb-girdle muscular dystrophy, and congenital myopathies. *Arch Neurol*. 1997;54:888.

81 Hoff JM, Gilhus NE, Daltveit AK. Pregnancies and deliveries in patients with Charcot-Marie-Tooth disease. *Neurology*. 2005;64:459–462.

82 Rudnik-Schoneborn S, Rohrig D, Nicholson G, et al. Pregnancy and delivery in Charcot-Marie-Tooth disease type 1. *Neurology*. 1993;43:2011–2016.

83 Rudnik-Schoenborn S, Zerres K, Ignatius J, et al. Pregnancy and spinal muscular atrophy. *J Neurol*. 1992;239:26–30.

84 Parra J, Martinez-Hernandez R, Also-Rallo E, et al. Ultrasound evaluation of fetal movements in pregnancies at risk for severe spinal muscular atrophy. *Neuromusc Dis*. 2011;21:97–101.

85 Norwood F, Rudnik-Schoneborn S. 179th ENMC international workshop: pregnancy in women with neuromuscular disorders 5–7 November 2010, Naarden, The Netherlands. *Neuromusc Dis*. 2012;22:183–190.

CHAPTER 11

Anterior and posterior pituitary disease and pregnancy

Mark E. Molitch

Northwestern University Feinberg School of Medicine, Chicago, IL, USA

Anterior pituitary

Anterior pituitary hormone changes in pregnancy

Pregnancy induces a number of changes in cardiovascular and renal function as well as causing changes in hormone levels via placental hormone and enzyme activity (Table 11.1). The normal pituitary gland enlarges considerably during pregnancy, due to placental estrogen-stimulated lactotroph hyperplasia [1, 2]. Concomitantly, prolactin (PRL) levels rise through gestation, preparing the breast for lactation [3]. This lactotroph hyperplasia results in an increase in overall pituitary size as seen on magnetic resonance imaging (MRI) scans, with the peak size occurring in the first few days postpartum when gland heights up to 12 mm may be seen [4, 5]. Following delivery, there is a rapid involution of the gland, so that normal pituitary size is found by 6 months postpartum [4, 5]. This stimulatory effect of pregnancy on the pituitary has important implications for the woman with a prolactinoma who desires pregnancy.

Circulating levels of a *growth hormone* (GH) variant made by the syncytiotrophoblastic epithelium of the placenta increase during the second half of pregnancy [6, 7]. The GH variant is biologically active, stimulating the production of insulin-like growth factor 1 (IGF-1) which causes a reduction in pituitary GH secretion

via negative feedback [6, 7]. In patients with *acromegaly* who have autonomous GH secretion and become pregnant, both forms of GH persist in the blood [8].

Over the course of gestation, *cortisol* levels rise progressively, due to an estrogen-induced increase in cortisol-binding globulin levels and an increase in cortisol production, so that the bioactive-"free" fraction, urinary-free cortisol levels, and salivary cortisol levels are also increased [9, 10]. Although there is placental production of adrenocorticotropic hormone (ACTH) and corticotropin-releasing hormone (CRH) with both reaching the circulation, they do not appear to be involved in the physiologic regulation of adrenal cortisol secretion during pregnancy [10]. The elevated cortisol and ACTH levels may also be due to an antiglucocorticoid action of the elevated progesterone levels of pregnancy, with a resultant increase in the set point for the negative feedback effects of cortisol [10].

Thyrotropin (TSH) levels fall in the first trimester, in response to the rise in thyroid hormone levels that are stimulated by placental chorionic gonadotropin (hCG), but return to the normal range by the third trimester [11]. In response to placental sex steroid production, hypothalamic gonadotropin-releasing hormone (GnRH), pituitary follicle-stimulating hormone (FSH), and luteinizing hormone (LH)

Neurological Illness in Pregnancy: Principles and Practice, First Edition.
Edited by Autumn Klein, M. Angela O'Neal, Christina Scifres, Janet F. R. Waters and Jonathan H. Waters.

Table 11.1 Changes in normal physiology that may affect endocrine tests

Cardiovascular
Increased plasma and RBC volume
Increased cardiac output
Lowered "osmostat" for vasopressin release and thirst

Renal
Increased GFR and renal plasma flow
Increased hormone and substrate clearance
Altered renal tubular function
Decreased T_m for glucose

Placental hormone production
Increased estrogen and progesterone production
    Stimulation of pituitary lactotrophs
Increased hormone-binding globulin production
Production of peptide hormones
    ACTH, CRH, GnRH, hCG, GH variant, hPL, cTSH, PRL

Placental enzyme production
Vasopressinase

ACTH adrenocorticotropic hormone; CRH, corticotropin-releasing hormone; GnRH, gonadotropin-releasing hormone; hCG, human chorionic gonadotropin; GH, growth hormone; hPL, human placental lactogen; cTSH, chorionic thyroid-stimulating hormone; PRL, prolactin.

levels decline in the first trimester of pregnancy, with a blunted gonadotropin response to GnRH [12].

Pituitary tumors

Pituitary adenomas cause problems because of hormone hypersecretion as well as by causing *hypopituitarism* because of mass effects. The pregnancy-induced alterations in hormone secretion complicate the evaluation of patients with pituitary adenomas. The influence on various types of therapy on the developing fetus also affects therapeutic decision-making.

Prolactinoma

Hyperprolactinemia commonly causes symptoms of galactorrhea, amenorrhea, and infertility [9]. The differential diagnosis of hyperprolactinemia is extensive [13], but this discussion will focus on the patient with a *prolactinoma*. The choice of treatment modality

has important consequences for decisions regarding pregnancy. Transsphenoidal surgery is curative in 50–60% of cases and rarely causes hypopituitarism when performed on patients with microadenomas (tumors <10 mm in diameter) [14]. However, for women with macroadenomas (tumors ≥10 mm in diameter), surgical cure rates are much lower and there is a considerably greater risk of causing hypopituitarism [14].

Medical therapy with the dopamine agonists, *bromocriptine* and *cabergoline*, is generally considered to be the preferred mode of therapy, restoring ovulatory menses in about 80% and 90%, respectively [14]. Macroadenoma size can be reduced by more than 50% in 50–75% of patients with bromocriptine and in more than 90% of patients with cabergoline [14].

Usually the dopamine agonist is stopped once a woman has missed her menstrual period and pregnancy is diagnosed, in order to limit fetal exposure. When used in this fashion, no increase in spontaneous abortions, ectopic pregnancies, trophoblastic disease, multiple pregnancies, or malformations were found in 6239 pregnancies in which bromocriptine was used and 789 pregnancies in which cabergoline was used [15].

The stimulatory effect of the hormonal milieu of pregnancy and the withdrawal of the dopamine agonist may result in significant prolactinoma enlargement (Table 11.2). Tumor enlargement requiring intervention during pregnancy has been reported in 2.7% women with microadenomas, 23% with macroadenomas that had not undergone prior surgery or radiotherapy, and 4.8% with macroadenomas that had undergone prior surgery or radiotherapy [15]. In almost all cases, such enlargement was successfully treated with reinstitution with a dopamine agonist. If the pregnancy is sufficiently advanced, another approach is to deliver the baby. Surgical decompression is only resorted to if these other approaches fail. In rare patients with very large prolactinomas, continued dopamine agonist therapy during

Table 11.2 Effect of pregnancy on prolactinomas

Tumor type	Prior therapy	Number of patients	Symptomatic enlargement
Microadenomas	None	658	18 (2.7%)
Macroadenomas	None	214	49 (22.9%)
Macroadenomas	Yes	148	7 (4.8%)

Data abstracted from Reference 15.

pregnancy may be considered, as the risk for fetal harm is likely very small and the risk from tumor enlargement may be much greater [15].

Patients with large macroadenomas should be assessed monthly for symptoms of tumor enlargement and visual fields should be tested each trimester. The PRL levels should not be measured during the pregnancy, as the levels may rise without tumor enlargement and also not rise with tumor enlargement and therefore are often misleading [16].

Case Vignette

This 31-year-old woman initially presented with galactorrhea and amenorrhea and was found to have hyperprolactinemia and a 12 mm macroadenoma. With bromocriptine, her PRL levels normalized, her menses returned, and she quickly became pregnant. Bromocriptine was then stopped and she did well until 7 months gestation, when she developed progressively severe headaches. An MRI showed substantial enlargement of the tumor (Figure 11.1); bromocriptine was then reinstituted and the headaches resolved. Following delivery, her tumor continued to shrink but she required continued bromocriptine treatment to maintain normal PRL levels and reduced tumor size.

Acromegaly

Conventional assays usually cannot distinguish between pituitary GH and the placental GH variant [6]. If it is critical to make a diagnosis during pregnancy, this may be possible by demonstrating GH pulsatility with frequent sampling, as GH secretion in acromegaly is highly pulsatile but that of the variant is not [6, 18]. Acromegaly

is associated with hypogonadism and infertility [19] (Table 11.3).

The primary therapy for most patients with acromegaly is surgery; those not cured by surgery are usually then treated with the somatostatin analogs *octreotide* and *lanreotide* [20]. Cabergoline may also be helpful in some cases [20]. More than half of patients who become pregnant are taking somatostatin analogs [21, 22].

Only one patient with a tumor secreting GH has been reported to have enlargement of her tumor without any hemorrhage into the tumor with a resultant visual field defect during pregnancy [23]. Two other patients have had demonstrated tumor enlargement without hemorrhage but did not develop visual field defects [24, 25] and in one of these cases, tumor enlargement likely was more due to octreotide withdrawal than the pregnancy itself [25]. Hemorrhage into the tumor causing headache and visual symptoms during pregnancy, however, has been reported several times [21]. Therefore, as with prolactinomas, patients with acromegaly with macroadenomas should be monitored clinically for headaches and visual symptoms. Because of the GH-induced insulin resistance, the risk of gestational diabetes is increased in acromegalic patients [26]. The risk of gestational hypertension is also increased [26]. Cardiac disease has not proved to be an issue in pregnant women with acromegaly [25, 26].

The considerations regarding the safety use of cabergoline in women with prolactinomas discussed earlier also apply to those with acromegaly being treated in this fashion. Fewer than 50 pregnant patients treated with

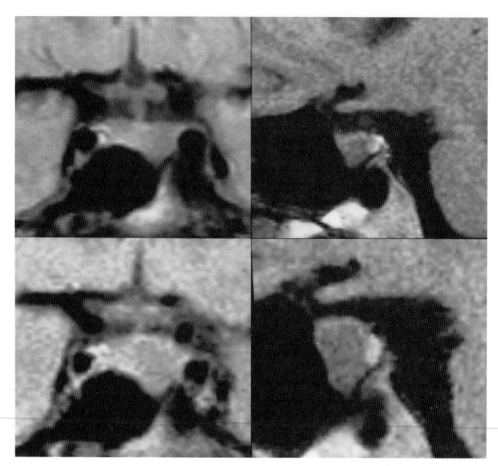

Figure 11.1 Coronal and sagittal MRI scans of an intrasellar prolactin-secreting macroadenoma in a woman prior to conception (above) and at 7 months of gestation (below). Note the marked tumor enlargement at the latter point, at which time the patient was complaining of headaches. Reproduced from Reference 17 with permission of Elsevier.

Table 11.3 Gonadal status in 55 women with acromegaly

Gonadal status	Percentage
Eugonadal with regular menses	31
Hyperprolactinemia and anovulatory	20
Hypopituitary	11
Anovulatory because of increased GH/IGF-1	13
Two or more reasons	25

Data from Grynberg et al.
GH, growth hormone; IGF, insulin-like growth factor 1.

somatostatin analogs have been reported; no malformations have been found in their children [21, 22, 26, 27]. However, a decrease in uterine artery blood flow has been reported with short-acting octreotide [27] and one fetus appeared to have intrauterine growth retardation that responded to a lowering of the dose of octreotide LAR [26]. Octreotide binds to somatostatin receptors in the placenta [27] and crosses the placenta [27] and therefore can affect developing fetal tissues where somatostatin receptors are widespread, especially in the brain. Because of the limited data documenting safety, I recommend that octreotide and other somatostatin analogs be discontinued if pregnancy is considered and that contraception be used when these drugs are administered and most [21, 22, 26] but not all [27] others concur. Considering the prolonged nature of the course of most patients with acromegaly, interruption of medical therapy for 9–12 months should not have a particularly adverse effect on the long-term outcome. On the other hand, these drugs can control tumor growth and for enlarging tumors, their reintroduction during pregnancy may be warranted versus operating. Pegvisomant, a GH receptor antagonist, has been given to two patients with acromegaly during pregnancy without harm [22, 28] but the safety of this is certainly not established.

Cushing's disease

Fewer than 150 cases of *Cushing's syndrome* in pregnancy have been reported [29–35]. Unlike the nonpregnant state, in which over 85% of patients have pituitary adenomas (Cushing's disease), less than 50% of the pregnant patients described had pituitary adenomas, a similar number had adrenal adenomas, and more than 10% had adrenal carcinomas [29–35]. In many cases, the hypercortisolism first became apparent during pregnancy, with improvement and even remission after parturition [31, 33, 35].

Diagnosing Cushing's syndrome during pregnancy may be difficult (Table 11.4). Both con-

Table 11.4 Clinical features of Cushing's syndrome versus normal pregnancy

Clinical feature	Cushing's	Pregnancy
Centripetal weight gain	+	+
Fatigue	+	+
Edema	+	+
Emotional lability	±	+
Glucose intolerance	+	+
Hypertension	+	+
Striae	Pigmented	Pale
Hirsutism	+	−

ditions may be associated with weight gain in a central distribution, fatigue, edema, emotional upset, glucose intolerance, and hypertension. The striae associated with normal pregnancy are usually pale and red or purple in Cushing's syndrome. Hirsutism and acne may point to excessive androgen production. Proximal myopathy and bone fractures point to Cushing's syndrome.

The laboratory evaluation is also difficult. Elevated total and free serum cortisol and ACTH levels, and urinary-free cortisol excretion may also be seen in normal pregnancy [10]. The overnight dexamethasone test usually demonstrates inadequate suppression during normal pregnancy as well as in patients with Cushing's syndrome [10, 34]. The ACTH levels are normal to elevated even with adrenal adenomas [10, 29–31, 34], perhaps due to the production of ACTH by the placenta or from the nonsuppressible stimulation of pituitary ACTH by placental corticotropin-releasing hormone. A persistent circadian variation in the elevated levels of total and free serum cortisol during normal pregnancy may be most helpful in distinguishing Cushing's syndrome from the hypercortisolism of pregnancy, because this finding is characteristically absent in all forms of Cushing's syndrome [9, 10]. Midnight levels of salivary cortisol during pregnancy have not yet been standardized [33]. In some cases, MRI scanning of the pituitary (without contrast) or ultrasound of the adrenal may be helpful. However, neuroradiologists are reluctant to perform MRIs with contrast during pregnancy despite no evidence of toxicity to the fetus [36] and the finding of a microadenoma on MRI is nonspecific, given the high rate of in finding pituitary incidentalomas [37]. Little experience has been reported with CRH stimulation testing or petrosal venous sinus sampling during pregnancy [31, 34, 35].

Cushing's syndrome is associated with a pregnancy loss rate of 25% due to spontaneous abortion, stillbirth, and early neonatal death because of extreme prematurity (Table 11.5) [29, 33–35]. The passage of cortisol across the placenta may rarely result in suppression of the

Table 11.5 Complications from Cushing's syndrome during pregnancy

Maternal complications		Fetal complications	
Hypertension	68%	Prematurity	43%
Glucose intolerance	25%	Stillbirths	6%
Preeclampsia	14%	Spontaneous abortion/IUD	5%
Osteoporosis/fracture	5%	IUGR	21%
Psychiatric disorders	4%	Hypoadrenalism	2%
Heart failure	3%		
Wound dehiscence	2%		
Maternal death	2%		

Data from Reference 34.
IUGR, intrauterine growth restriction; IUD, intrauterine death.

fetal adrenals [38]. Hypertension develops in most mothers with Cushing's and diabetes and myopathy are frequent [34, 35]. Postoperative wound infection and dehiscence are common after cesarean section [34, 35].

In a review of 136 pregnancies collected from the literature, Lindsay et al. found that the frequency of live births increased from 76% to 89% when active treatment was instituted by a gestational age of 20 weeks [34]. Therefore, treatment during pregnancy has been advocated [24, 34, 35]. Medical therapy for Cushing's syndrome during pregnancy with metyrapone and ketoconazole is not very effective [33, 34, 35]. Intrauterine growth retardation has been reported with ketoconoazole [32]. However, a recent case was described in whom ketoconazole was used during the first trimester and metyrapone in the second and third trimesters with a good fetal outcome [39]. Recently, the FDA has issued a black box warning for ketoconazole with respect to severe liver toxicity and so its use cannot be recommended. Aminoglutethimide and mitotane should be avoided because of potential fetal toxicity [34]. Two new medications have been approved for the treatment of Cushing's disease recently. Mifepristone, a cortisol receptor blocker, is highly effective but because it is also a progesterone receptor blocker and an abortifacient; it cannot be used during pregnancy [40]. Pasireotide is a new somatostatin analog with modest efficacy

in patients with Cushing's disease [40]; it has the adverse effect of hyperglycemia and there is no experience with its use during pregnancy. However, the same cautions discussed earlier for somatostatin analogs should also hold true for when they might be used in a patient with Cushing's disease.

Transsphenoidal resection of a pituitary ACTH-secreting adenoma has been carried out successfully in several patients during the second trimester [33, 34, 35]. Although any surgery poses risks for the mother and fetus [41], it appears that with Cushing's syndrome, the risks of not operating are considerably higher than those of proceeding with surgery.

Thyrotropin-secreting tumors

Only three cases have been reported of pregnancy occurring in women with TSH-secreting tumors [42–44]. In one, octreotide had to be reinstituted to control tumor size [42] and in a second, octreotide was continued during pregnancy for tumor size control [43]. Clinically, the most important issue with such tumors is the need to control hyperthyroidism during pregnancy and that can usually be done with standard antithyroid drugs [43]. However, with growing macroadenomas, octreotide may be necessary for tumor size control [42, 43] and it is possible that it may be necessary to control the hyperthyroidism if thionamides are ineffective.

Clinically nonfunctioning adenomas

Pregnancy would not expected to influence tumor size in patients with clinically nonfunctioning adenomas (CNFAs) and only two cases have been reported in which tumor enlargement during pregnancy resulted in a visual field defect [23, 45]. In the second case, the patient responded rapidly to bromocriptine treatment, probably due to shrinkage of the lactotroph hyperplasia with decompression of the chiasm and probably with little or no direct effect on the tumor itself [45].

Most CNFAs are actually gonadotroph adenomas. Two patients have been reported who had gonadotroph adenomas secreting intact FSH with a resultant ovarian hyperstimulation syndrome [46, 47]. Both of these became pregnant, one after having the FSH hypersecretion controlled by bromocriptine [45] and the second following surgical removal of the tumor [47].

Hypopituitarism

Hypopituitarism may be partial or complete and loss of gonadotropin secretion is common. Induction of ovulation may be difficult and a variety of techniques have been used, including administration of hCG and FSH [48,49], pulsatile gonadotropin-releasing hormone [48,49], and *in vitro* fertilization [50, 51]. Although the malformation rate is normal in such pregnancies, there seems to be an increased frequency of cesarean sections, miscarriages, and small for gestational age babies [48–51].

Because of increased thyroxine turnover and volume of distribution in pregnancy, thyroxine (T4) levels usually fall and TSH levels rise with a fixed *thyroxine* dose over the course of gestation [52]. The average increase in thyroxine need in these patients is about 0.05 mg/day (Table 11.6). Because patients with hypothalamic/pituitary dysfunction may not elevate their TSH levels normally in the face of increased need for thyroxine, it is reasonable to increase the thyroxine supplementation by 0.025 mg after the first trimester and by additional 0.025 mg

Table 11.6 Treatment of hypopituitarism during pregnancy

- Thyroxine
  - Can only follow Free T4 levels and not TSH
  - Average increase over pregnancy is 0.05 mg/d
  - So, increase by 0.025 mg at end of first trimester and then 0.025 mg at end of second trimester
- Cortisol
  - Hydrocortisone metabolized by placental 11β-hydroxysteroid dehydrogenase 2, so fetus protected from excess
  - No need to increase during pregnancy but need to give stress doses for infections and labor
- GH
  - No data to support its use in pregnancy

TSH, thyroid stimulating hormone; GH, growth hormone.

after the second trimester, also following free T4 levels.

In most patients, the dose of chronic glucocorticoid replacement does not usually need to be increased during pregnancy (Table 11.6) [10]. *Hydrocortisone* is metabolized by the placental enzyme 11β-hydroxysteroid dehydrogenase 2, so the fetus is generally protected from any overdose of hydrocortisone; the usual dose of hydrocortisone is in the range of 12–15 mg/m^2 given in two or three divided doses, for example, 10 mg in the morning and 5 mg in the afternoon [10]. Additional glucocorticoids are for the stress of labor and delivery, such as 75 mg of hydrocortisone intravenous (IV) every 8 hours with rapid tapering postpartum [10]. Prednisolone does not cross the placenta and prednisone crosses only minimally [53]. Suppression of neonatal adrenal function in offspring of women taking prednisone during pregnancy is very uncommon [54] and the amounts passed in breast milk are negligible [55].

There are few data on the use of GH during pregnancy in hypopituitary individuals and in most series GH therapy has been stopped at conception [56, 57]. Whether GH replacement in GH-deficient women facilitates fertility is controversial [57]. As the GH variant, which is biologically active, is produced by the placenta in substantial amounts beginning in the second half of pregnancy and can access the maternal circulation (see Anterior pituitary hormone changes in pregnancy), then at most the mother would be GH deficient only in the first half of pregnancy. When Curran et al. analyzed 25 pregnancies that occurred in 16 patients with GH deficiency during which GH therapy was not continued, they found that there was no adverse outcome of omitting GH therapy on either the fetus or mother and concluded that GH replacement therapy during pregnancy is not essential for GH-deficient women [56].

Sheehan's syndrome

Sheehan's syndrome consists of pituitary necrosis secondary to ischemia occurring within hours of delivery [58, 59]. It is usually secondary to hypotension and shock from an obstetric hemorrhage. The degree of ischemia and necrosis dictates the subsequent patient course (Table 11.7). It rarely occurs with current obstetric practice in the United States [60] and occurs more frequently in less developed areas [59].

Acute necrosis is suspected in the setting of an obstetric hemorrhage where hypotension and tachycardia persist following adequate replacement of blood products. Failure to lactate and hypoglycemia may also occur [58]. Investigation should include obtaining blood samples for ACTH, cortisol, prolactin, and free thyroxine.

Table 11.7 Symptoms and signs in patients with Sheehan's syndrome

Acute form	Chronic form
Hypotension	Light-headedness
Tachycardia	Fatigue
Failure to lactate	Failure to lactate
Hypoglycemia	Persistent amenorrhea
Extreme fatigue	Decreased body hair
Nausea and vomiting	Dry skin
Hyponatremia	Loss of libido
	Nausea and vomiting
	Cold intolerance

The ACTH stimulation test would be normal, as the adrenal cortex would not be atrophied. Free thyroxine levels may prove normal initially, as the hormone has a half-life of 7 days, and an additional sample should be sent after 1 week. Prolactin levels are usually low.

Treatment with saline and stress doses of corticosteroids should be instituted immediately after drawing the blood tests. If later free thyroxine levels become low, then therapy with levothyroxine is indicated. Additional pituitary testing with subsequent therapy should be delayed until recovery. Diabetes insipidus may also occur [61].

When milder forms of infarction occur, the diagnosis may be delayed for months or even years [58, 59]. These women generally have a history of amenorrhea, decreased libido, failure to lactate, breast atrophy, loss of pubic and axillary hair, fatigue, and symptoms of secondary adrenal insufficiency with nausea, vomiting, diarrhea, and abdominal pain [58, 59]. Rarely, some women experience retained gonadotropin secretion and may have normal menses and fertility [58].

Lymphocytic hypophysitis

Lymphocytic hypophysitis is thought to be an autoimmune disease and pathologically there is infiltration and destruction of the parenchyma of the pituitary and infundibulum by lymphocytes and plasma cells [62–64]. It often manifests during pregnancy or the postpartum period [62–64]. Hypophysitis is associated with symptoms of hypopituitarism or an enlarging mass lesion with headaches and visual field defects and is suspected based on its timing and lack of association with an obstetric hemorrhage or prior history of menstrual difficulties or infertility [62–64]. Diabetes insipidus may also occur [62–64]. On MRI scans, there is usually diffuse, symmetric, enhancement rather than a focal lesion that might indicate a tumor [62–64]. The clinical picture often allows a clinical diagnosis to be made without invasive procedures.

Treatment is generally conservative and involves identification and correction of any pituitary deficits, especially of ACTH secretion which is particularly common in this condition [63, 64]. Data regarding the benefits of high dose corticosteroid treatment in reducing the size of the lesion are inconclusive [64]. Surgery to debulk but not remove the gland is indicated in the presence of uncontrolled headaches, visual field defects, and progressive enlargement on scan [63, 64]. Spontaneous regression and resumption of partial or normal pituitary function may occur, although most patients progress to chronic panhypopituitarism [63, 64]. In some cases, a late finding of an "empty" sella on MRI may be found [63, 64].

Posterior pituitary

The set point for plasma osmolality at which arginine vasopressin (AVP) is secreted and thirst is stimulated is reduced approximately 5–10 mOsm/kg in pregnancy; therefore, the normal serum sodium is reduced from about 140 to about 135 mEq/L [65–67]. The placenta produces vasopressinase, an enzyme that rapidly inactivates AVP thereby greatly increasing its clearance [66–68].

Standard water deprivation tests which require 5% weight loss should be avoided during pregnancy as they may cause uterine irritability and alter placental perfusion. Instead, desmopressin (DDAVP) is used to assess urinary concentrating ability [66]. Urinary concentrating ability in the pregnant patient should be determined in the seated position, as the lateral recumbent position inhibits maximal urinary concentration [65].

Diabetes insipidus

Central diabetes insipidus (DI) may newly develop in pregnancy due to an enlarging pituitary lesion, with lymphocytic hypophysitis or with hypothalamic disease. Due to the increased clearance of AVP by the vasopressinase, DI usually worsens during gestation and subclinical DI may become manifest [66, 67, 69]. Desmopressin is resistant to vasopressinase and provides satisfactory, safe treatment during gestation, although a higher dose may be required [66, 67, 70]. During monitoring of the clinical response, clinicians should remember that normal basal plasma osmolality and sodium concentration are 5 mEq/L lower during pregnancy [65–67]. The DDAVP transfers minimally into breast milk and is minimally absorbed from the intestine; therefore, there are no effects on the infant [67].

Transient AVP-resistant forms of DI secondary to placental production of vasopressinase may occur spontaneously in one pregnancy, but not in a subsequent one [71]. Some of these patients may respond to DDAVP therapy [71].

Acute fatty liver of pregnancy and other disturbances of hepatic function such as hepatitis may be associated with late onset transient DI of pregnancy in some patients [67, 72]. In some cases, this has been associated with the HELLP syndrome [67, 73]. It is presumed that the hepatic dysfunction is associated with reduced degradation of vasopressinase, further increasing vasopressinase levels and the clearance of AVP [67]. The polyuria may develop either prior to delivery or postpartum.

Diabetes insipidus that developing postpartum may be a result of Sheehan's syndrome or lymphocytic hypophysitis [67]. Transient DI of unknown etiology has been described postpartum, lasting only days to weeks [74].

References

1 Scheithauer BW, Sano T, Kovacs KT, et al. The pituitary gland in pregnancy. A clinicopathologic and immunohistochemical study of 69 cases. *Mayo Clin Proc.* 1990;65:461–474.

2 Elster AD, Sanders TG, Vines FS, et al. Size and shape of the pituitary gland during pregnancy and post-partum: measurement with MR imaging. *Radiology.* 1991;181:531–535.

3 Rigg LA, Lein A, Yen SSC. Pattern of increase in circulating prolactin levels during human gestation. *Am J Obstet Gynecol*. 1977;129:454–456.

4 Elster AD, Sanders TG, Vines FS, et al. Size and shape of the pituitary gland during pregnancy and post partum: measurement with MR imaging. *Radiology*. 1991;181:531–535.

5 Dinç H, Esen F, Demirci A, et al. Pituitary dimensions and volume measurements in pregnancy and post partum. MR assessment. *Acta Radiologica*. 1998;39:64–69.

6 Frankenne F, Closset J, Gomez F, et al. The physiology of growth hormones (GHs) in pregnant women and partial characterization of the placental GH variant. *J Clin Endocrinol Metab*. 1988;66:1171–1980.

7 Eriksson L, Frankenne F, Eden S, et al. Growth hormone 24-h serum profiles during pregnancy lack of pulsatility for the secretion of the placental variant. *Br J Obstet Gynaecol*. 1989;106:949–953.

8 Beckers A, Stevenaert A, Foidart J-M, et al. Placental and pituitary growth hormone secretion during pregnancy in acromegalic women. *J Clin Endocrinol Metab*. 1990;71:725–731.

9 Nolten WE, Lindheimer MD, Rueckert PA, et al. Diurnal patterns and regulation of cortisol secretion in pregnancy. *J Clin Endocrinol Metab*. 1980;51:466–472.

10 Lindsay JR, Nieman LK. The hypothalamic-pituitary-adrenal axis in pregnancy: challenges in disease detection and treatment. *Endocr Revs*. 2005;26:775–799.

11 Glinoer D. The regulation of thyroid function in pregnancy: pathways of endocrine adaptation from physiology to pathology. *Endocr Rev*. 1997;18:404–433.

12 Jeppsson S, Rannevik G, Liedholm P, et al. Basal and LHRH stimulated secretion of FSH during pregnancy. *Am J Obstet Gynecol*. 1977;127:32–36.

13 Casanueva FF, Molitch ME, Schlechte JA, et al. Guidelines of the Pituitary Society for the diagnosis and management of prolactinomas. *Clin Endocrinol*. 2006;65:265–273.

14 Gillam MP, Molitch MP, Lombardi G, et al. Advances in the treatment of prolactinomas. *Endocr Revs*. 2006;27:485–534.

15 Molitch ME. Prolactinoma in pregnancy. *Best Pract Res Clin Endocrinol Metab*. 2011;25:885–896.

16 Divers WA, Yen SSC. Prolactin-producing microadenomas in pregnancy. *Obstet Gynecol*. 1983;62:425–429.

17 Molitch ME. Medical treatment of prolactinomas. *Endocrinol Metab Clin North Am*. 1999;28:143–170.

18 Barkan AL, Stred SE, Reno K, et al. Increased growth hormone pulse frequency in acromegaly. *J Clin Endocrinol Metab*. 1989;69:1225–1233.

19 Grynberg M, Salenave S, Young J, et al. Female gonadal function before and after treatment of acromegaly. *J Clin Endocrinol Metab*. 2010;95:4518–1525.

20 Melmed S, Colao A, Barkan A, et al. Guideline for acromegaly management: an update. *J Clin Endocrinol Metab*. 2009;94;1509–1517.

21 Cheng V, Faiman C, Kennedy L, et al. Pregnancy and acromegaly: a review. *Pituitary*. 2012;15:59–63.

22 Cheng S, Grasso L, Martinez-Grozco JA, et al. Pregnancy in acromegaly: experience from two referral centers and systematic review of the literature. *Clin Endocrinol*. 2012;76:264–271.

23 Kupersmith MJ, Rosenberg C, Kleinberg D. Visual loss in pregnant women with pituitary adenomas. *Ann Intern Med*. 1994;121:473–477.

24 Okada Y, Morimoto I, Ejima K, et al. A case of active acromegalic woman with a marked increase in serum insulin-like growth factor-1 levels after delivery. *Endocr J*. 1997;44:117–120.

25 Cozzi R, Attanasio R, Barausee M. Pregnancy in acromegaly: a one-center experience. *Eur J Endocrinol*. 2006;155:279–284.

26 Caron P, Broussaud S, Bertherat J, et al. Acromegaly and pregnancy: a retrospective multicenter study of 59 pregnancies in 46 women. *J Clin Endocrinol Metab*. 2010;95:4680–4687.

27 Maffei P, Tamagno G, Nardelli GB, et al. Effects of octreotide exposure during pregnancy in acromegaly. *Clin Endocrinol*. 2010;72:668–677.

28 Brian SR, Bidlingmaier M, Wajnrajch MP, et al. Treatment of acromegaly with pegvisomant during pregnancy: maternal and fetal effects. *J Clin Endocrinol Metab*. 2007;92:3374–3377.

29 Bevan JS, Gough MH, Gillmer MD, et al. Cushings syndrome in pregnancy. The timing of definitive treatment. *Clin Endocrinol*. 1987;27:225–233.

30 Chico A, Manzanares JM, Halperin I, et al. Cushing's disease and pregnancy. *Eur J Obstet Gynecol Reprod Biol*. 1996;64:143–146.

31 Guilhaume B, Sanson ML, Billaud L, et al. Cushing's syndrome and pregnancy: aetiologies and prognosis in twenty-two patients. *Eur J Med*. 1992;1:83–89.

32 Amado JA, Pesquera C, Gonzalez EM, et al. Successful treatment with ketoconazole of Cushing's syndrome in pregnancy. *Postgrad Med J.* 1990;66:221–223.

33 Madhun ZT, Aron DC. Cushing's disease in pregnancy. In: Bronstein MD, ed. *Pituitary Tumors and Pregnancy.* Norwell, MA: Kluwer Academic Publishers, 2001; pp. 149–172.

34 Lindsay JR, Jonklaas J, Oldfield EH, et al. Cushing's syndrome during pregnancy: personal experience and review of the literature. *J Clin Endocrinol Metab.* 2005;90:3077–3083.

35 Vilar L, Freitas MDC, Lima LHC, et al. Cushing's syndrome in pregnancy. An overview. *Arq Bras Endocrinol Metab.* 2007;51:1293–1302.

36 Feelders RA, Hofland LJ. Medical treatment of Cushing's disease. *J Clin Endocrinol Metab.* 2013;98:425–438.

37 DeWilde JP, Rivers AW, Price DL. A review of the current use of magnetic resonance imaging in pregnancy and safety implications for the fetus. *Prog Biophys Mol Biol.* 2005;87:335–353.

38 Freda PU, Beckers AM, Katznelson L, et al. Pituitary incidentaloma: an endocrine society clinical practice guideline. *J Clin Endocrinol Metab.* 2011;96:894–904.

39 Kreines K, DeVaux WD. Neonatal adrenal insufficiency associated with maternal Cushings syndrome. *Pediatrics.* 1971;47:516–519.

40 Boronat M, Marrero D, López-Pascencia Y, et al. Successful outcome of pregnancy in a patient with Cushing's disease under treatment with ketoconazole during the first trimester of gestation. *Gynecol Endocrinol.* 2011;27:675–677.

41 Cohen-Kerem R, Railton C, Orfen D, et al. Pregnancy outcome following non-obstetric surgical intervention. *Am J Surgery.* 2005;190: 467–473.

42 Caron P, Gerbeau C, Pradayrol L, et al. Successful pregnancy in an infertile woman with a thyrotropin-secreting macroadenoma treated with the somatostatin analog (octreotide). *J Clin Endocrinol Metab.* 1996;81:1164–1168.

43 Blackhurst G, Strachan MW, Collie D, et al. The treatment of a thyrotropin-secreting pituitary macroadenoma with octreotide in twin pregnancy. *Clin Endocrinol.* 2002;56:401–404.

44 Chaiamnuay S, Moster M, Katz MR, et al. Successful management of a pregnant woman with a TSH secreting pituitary adenoma with surgical and medical therapy. *Pituitary.* 2003;6: 109–113.

45 Masding MG, Lees PD, Gawne-Cain ML, et al. Visual field compression by a non-secreting pituitary tumour during pregnancy. *J R Soc Med.* 2003;96:27–28.

46 Murata Y, Ando H, Nagasaka T, et al. Successful pregnancy after bromocriptine therapy in an anovulatory woman complicated with ovarian hyperstimulation caused by follicle stimulating hormone-producing plurihormonal pituitary microadenoma. *J Clin Endocrinol Metab.* 2003;88:1988–1993.

47 Sugita T, Seki K, Nagai Y, et al. Successful pregnancy and delivery after removal of gonadotrope adenoma secreting follicle-stimulating hormone in a 29-year-old amenorrheic woman. *Gynecol Obstet Invest.* 2005;59:138–143.

48 Hall R, Manski-Nankervis J, Goni N, et al. Fertility outcomes in women with hypopituitarism. *Clin Endocrinol.* 2006;65:71–74.

49 Overton CE, Davis CJ, West C, et al. High risk pregnancies in hypopituitary women. *Human Reprod.* 2002;17:1464–1467.

50 Hirshfeld-Cytron J, Kim HH. Treatment of infertility in women with pituitary tumors. *Expert Rev Anticancer Ther.* 2006;6(9 suppl):S55–S62.

51 Kübler K, Klingmüller D, Gembruch U, et al. High-risk pregnancy management in women with hypopituitarism. *J Perinatol.* 2009;29:89–95.

52 Mandel SJ, Larsen PR, Seely EW, et al. Increased need for thyroxine during pregnancy in women with primary hypothyroidism. *N Engl J Med.* 1990;323:91–96.

53 Beitins IZ, Bayard F, Ances IG, et al. The transplacental passage of prednisone and prednisolone in pregnancy near term. *J Pediatr.* 1972;81:936–945.

54 Kenny FM, Preeyasombat C, Spaulding JS, et al. Cortisol production rate: IV. Infants born of steroid-treated mothers and of diabetic mothers. Infants with trisomy syndrome and with anencephaly. *Pediatrics.* 1966;137:960–966.

55 McKenzie SA, Selley JA, Agnew JE. Secretion of prednisolone into breast milk. *Arch Dis Child.* 1975;50:894–896.

56 Curran AJ, Peacey SR, Shalet SM. Is maternal growth hormone essential for a normal pregnancy? *Eur J Endocrinol.* 1998;139:54–58.

57 Karaca Z, Kelestimir F. Pregnancy and other pituitary disorders (including GH deficiency). *Best Pract Res Clin Endocrinol Metab.* 2011;25:897–910.

58 Tessnow AH, Wilson JD. The changing face of Sheehan's syndrome. *Am J Med Sci.* 2010;340:402–406.

59 Gei-Guardia O, Soto-Herrera E, Gei-Brealey A, et al. Sheehan syndrome in Costa Rica: clinical experience with 60 cases. *Endocr Pract.* 2011;17:337–344.

60 Feinberg E, Molitch M, Endres L, et al. The incidence of Sheehan's syndrome after obstetric hemorrhage. *Fertil Steril.* 2005;84:975–979.

61 Iwasaki Y, Oiso Y, Yamauchi K, et al. Neurohypophyseal function in post-partum hypopituitarism: impaired plasma vasopressin response to osmotic stimuli. *J Clin Endocrinol Metab.* 1989;68:560–585.

62 Caturegli P, Newschaffer C, Olivi A, et al. Autoimmune hypophysitis. *Endocrine Reviews.* 2005;26:599–614.

63 Carpinteri R, Patelli I, Casanueva FF, et al. Inflammatory and granulomatous expansive lesions of the pituitary. *Best Pract Res Clin Endocrinol Metab.* 2009;23:639–650.

64 Foyouzi N. Lymphocytic adenohypophysitis. *Obstet Gynecol Surv.* 2011;66:109–113.

65 Lindheimer MD, Davison JM. Osmoregulation, the secretion of arginine vasopressin and its metabolism during pregnancy. *Eur J Endocrinol.* 1995;132:133–143.

66 Ananthakrishnan S. Diabetes insipidus in pregnancy: etiology, evaluation, and management. *Endo Pract.* 2009;15:377–382

67 Aleksandrov N, Audibert F, Bedard M-J, et al. Gestational diabetes insipidus: a review of an underdiagnosed condition. *J Obstet Gynaecol Can.* 2010;32:225–231.

68 Davison JM, Shiells EA, Barron WM, et al. Changes in the metabolic clearance of vasopressin and of plasma vasopressinase throughout human pregnancy. *J Clin Invest.* 1989;83:1313–1318.

69 Iwasaki Y, Oiso Y, Kondo K, et al. Aggravation of subclinical diabetes insipidus during pregnancy. *N Engl J Med.* 1991;324:522–526.

70 Ray JG. DDAVP use during pregnancy: an analysis of its safety for mother and child. *Obstet Gynecol Survey.* 1998;53:450–455.

71 Brewster UC, Hayslett JP. Diabetes insipidus in the third trimester of pregnancy. *Obstet Gynecol.* 2005;105:1173–1176.

72 Kennedy S, Hall PM, Seymour AE, et al. Transient diabetes insipidus and acute fatty liver of pregnancy. *Br J Obstet Gynaecol.* 1994;101: 387–391.

73 Ellidokuz E, Uslan I, Demir S, et al. Transient postpartum diabetes insipidus associated with HELLP syndrome. *J Obstet Gynaecol Res.* 2006;32: 602–604.

74 Raziel A, Rosenberg T, Schreyer P et al. Transient postpartum diabetes insipidus. *Am J Obstet Gynecol.* 1991;164:616–618.

CHAPTER 12

Movement disorders and pregnancy

Sathiji Nageshwaran[1], Marsha Smith[2], & Yvette M. Bordelon[3]

[1] Division of Brain Sciences, University College London School of Medicine, London, UK
[2] Department of Neurology, Southern Ohio Medical Center, Portsmouth, OH, USA
[3] Department of Neurology, David Geffen School of Medicine at UCLA, Los Angeles, CA, USA

Introduction

Disorders of movement are broadly characterized into those of predominantly decreased movement or hypokinetic and those of primarily excessive movement or hyperkinetic. Almost all movement disorders result from perturbation of basal ganglia circuitry, although precise mechanisms are not defined for all manifestations. Gender differences have been identified in the prevalence and expression of some movement disorders. In addition, hormonal state can influence the expression of neurologic signs and symptoms in women with certain disease processes and, as such, pregnancy may have a significant impact on disease manifestation and treatment. This is thought to be related to hormonal regulation of dopaminergic systems. Movement disorders are not commonly seen during pregnancy with few exceptions owing to the relatively late onset of most of these illnesses. As a result, there are few formal studies on whether disease manifestations are affected by the hormonal changes that occur during pregnancy or how treatment is affected given the potential deleterious effects of commonly used medications on the developing fetus. However, we will present the information currently known regarding: (1) movement disorders that are seen only during pregnancy (e.g., chorea gravidarum) or that may present during pregnancy (e.g., restless legs syndrome); (2) the effect that pregnancy has on movement disorder symptom manifestation and treatment (e.g., in Parkinson disease, essential tremor, dystonia, and others); and (3) the role of genetic testing for movement disorders in genetic counseling for pregnant women.

Movement disorders presenting during pregnancy

Chorea gravidarum

Chorea gravidarum was first described approximately four centuries ago, by Horstius in 1661 [1]. It is characterized clinically by the presence of chorea (defined as partially suppressible brief, irregular non-sustained movements flowing between muscle groups) that occurs during pregnancy. It is classified as either idiopathic or secondary to an underlying choreic disorder. Previously, in the pre-antibiotic era, the most common secondary cause was prior streptococcal infection with associated rheumatic fever. However, even currently it has been documented as a risk factor by Maia and colleagues who performed a retrospective study of patients diagnosed with Sydenham's chorea [2]. Of 66 patients, 20 became pregnant during the time of review and 75% of those that were pregnant had chorea gravidarum of varying severities [2].

Neurological Illness in Pregnancy: Principles and Practice, First Edition.
Edited by Autumn Klein, M. Angela O'Neal, Christina Scifres, Janet F. R. Waters and Jonathan H. Waters.
© 2016 John Wiley & Sons, Ltd. Published 2016 by John Wiley & Sons, Ltd.

More commonly now, chorea gravidarum has been linked to connective tissue disorders, including systemic lupus erythrematosus and antiphospholipid antibody syndrome, hyperthyroidism, medication-induced or related to a genetic disorder such as Huntington disease (HD) or Wilson disease. Chorea gravidarum is extremely rare with an estimated incidence in 1968 of 1 in 139,000 pregnancies [3]. More recent estimates are not documented.

If severe enough and unrelenting, chorea gravidarum can also cause hyperthermia, rhabdomyolysis, myoglobinuria, and eventually death [4, 5]. It typically begins after the first trimester (45% of cases) and can spontaneously abate after several months or after delivery [4, 6]. The severity of the chorea typically decreases as the pregnancy progresses [6]. Approximately one-third of patients go into remission before delivery, and another subset are essentially free of the illness after delivery [4]. There is a risk of recurrence in some patients during subsequent pregnancies.

The laboratory evaluation in a patient presenting with chorea during pregnancy should include screening tests: antinuclear antibody, thyroid and parathyroid function tests, lupus anticoagulant, 24 hour urine copper, and serum ceruloplasmin. A brain imaging study may be considered and documentation of family history of known choreic disorders and medication or drug exposure (neuroleptics, valproic acid, cocaine, amphetamines, and lithium).

Treatment should be reserved only for severe cases that may be jeopardizing the health of the mother or fetus [7]. Haloperidol is effective but carries risks of teratogenicity to the fetus or tardive dyskinesia to the mother and hyperkinetic movements in infants exposed *in utero* [8–11]. Dopamine depleters, reserpine and tetrabenazine, are effective for control of chorea but reserpine is teratogenic and contraindicated in pregnancy [12]. Tetrabenazine use was reported by Lubbe et al., in one case of chorea gravidarum secondary to lupus anticoagulant with

onset at 23 weeks gestation [13]. There were no complications during the pregnancy or delivery and the only reported incident was a small ventricular septal defect detected at birth. Clonazepam is not as effective as antidopaminergic medications but can also be considered. Treatment of the underlying problem if related to lupus or antiphospholipid syndrome may be indicated (steroids) [13].

Dystonia gravidarum

A newly recognized disorder is likely related to chorea gravidarum and is referred to as dystonia gravidarum [14–16]. These case reports describe the onset of cervical dystonia *de novo* in pregnancy in a total of three women with resolution of symptoms in the second trimester or soon after delivery. Although no underlying cause for dystonia was found, there was the suggestion of susceptibility based on a past history of oculogyric crisis in one woman and a family history of essential tremor in another. Two women received clonazepam as treatment with no adverse effect to pregnancy [14, 16].

Restless legs syndrome

Restless legs syndrome (RLS) is characterized by the presence of paresthesias or dysesthesia occurring predominantly in the legs with an irresistible urge to move the legs. The RLS is very common affecting 5–14.3% of the general population but has a 2-fold higher incidence in women compared to men [17]. Much of this gender effect is related to the higher incidence of RLS during pregnancy with estimates of 10–26% of pregnant women experiencing this [18–22]. It typically begins during the second or third trimester and improves or resolves after delivery and may be related to iron or folate deficiency, known risk factors for RLS. In women with preexisting RLS, symptoms may worsen during pregnancy as reported in 61% of women in a study by Manconi and colleagues [20]. Additionally, in women with the RLS during pregnancy, there is a greater risk of recurrence during subsequent pregnancies and a 4-fold greater risk of developing RLS in the future [23].

Treatment includes supplementing with iron or folate if indicated but otherwise should be avoided if possible unless symptoms are severe and detrimental to the health of the mother. Carbidopa/levodopa is effective and some case reports suggest it is relatively safe during pregnancy as discussed in the Parkinson disease section below. Doses as low as one tablet of 25/100 qhs should be tried and increased by $\frac{1}{2}$ tablets qhs if needed up to 2 tablets. Pramipexole, ropinirole, and rotigotine are effective in treating RLS but safety in pregnancy is not well established as yet. Dostal and colleagues performed a prospective study on 59 pregnancy outcomes in women taking medications for RLS and found that there was no significant increase above the general population in rates of major malformations or adverse outcomes with levodopa, pramipexole, ropinirole, or rotigotine [24]. Opiates (oxycodone), anticonvulsants (gabapentin, carbamazepine), and benzodiazepines (clonazepam) may also be considered with gabapentin being slightly preferable among these [25].

Spinocerebellar ataxia

Teive and colleagues reported the pregnancy-associated onset of disease symptoms in three family members with spinocerebellar ataxia (SCA) 10 [26]. The SCA10 is an autosomal dominant progressive disorder characterized by ataxia, dysarthria, dysphagia, eye movement abnormalities, and sometimes seizures. Onset is typically between the second-fifth decades. The symptoms that emerged according to the report were dysarthria and in one person both dysarthria and ataxia. Similar pregnancy-induced onset of symptoms has not yet been described in other adult-onset disorders but may be considered as discussed earlier regarding HD in cases of chorea gravidarum.

Dystonic reactions and tardive syndromes

Acute dystonic reactions and tardive syndromes may also be seen during pregnancy secondary to the use of dopamine receptor-blocking medications as anti-emetics such as prochlorperazine, metoclopramide, or promethazine. Dystonic reactions are not uncommon as indicated Tan and colleagues [27] who conducted a study in 73 women with hyperemesis gravidarum randomized to receive metoclopramide or promethazine and found an incidence of dystonia of 5.7% and 19.2%, respectively. Tardive syndromes include tardive akathisia, tardive dyskinesia, tardive dystonia, or tardive tics but there are no data of occurrence of these syndromes in the context of pregnancy. In severe cases where there is potential harm to mother and fetus, treatment with tetrabenazine may be considered or other agents as recommended for chorea gravidarum.

Influence of pregnancy on the signs, symptoms, and treatment of movement disorders

Parkinson disease

Parkinson disease (PD) is a neurodegenerative disease, characterized clinically by cogwheel rigidity, bradykinesia, and resting tremor. The pathologic hallmarks of the disease are degeneration of dopaminergic neurons in the substantia nigra pars compacta of the midbrain and the presence of cytoplasmic ubiquitinated inclusions, Lewy bodies, in the remaining neurons. The occurrence of pregnancy in patients with PD is extremely rare and because of this there are limited available data. This is attributable to a male predominance of PD and the typical onset of symptoms after the age of 50 [28]. In Rochester, Minnesota, and Northern California, a higher incidence of PD was observed in men than in women, with 13.0 and 19.0 per 100,000 in men compared with 8.8 and

9.9 per 100,000 in women, respectively [29, 30]. Data from a northern Manhattan population also support the male predominance of PD [31]. The reason for this gender difference is unclear, but it supports the hypothesis that estrogen is neuroprotective and enhances dopaminergic function. Animal studies have documented that estrogen increases dopamine concentrations in the brain by increasing tyrosine hydroxylase activity, enhancing dopamine release, and inhibiting dopamine reuptake [32–34]. Estrogen also exerts postsynaptic effects by modulating dopamine D2 receptors, thus increasing dopamine receptor density and sensitivity [35]. Neuroprotection by estrogen may be accomplished through its modulation of the dopaminergic system, antioxidant effects, and inhibition of neurotoxin uptake through the dopamine transporter [36].

The role that estrogen plays in modulating dopaminergic function is not firmly established. Studies have also shown the opposite effect, with a decrease in dopamine D2 receptors with estrogen treatment and increases in dopamine transporter density [37]. It has been suggested that these conflicting results are due to the biphasic effects of estrogen on dopamine modulation, but this has not been resolved [38].

It has been demonstrated that PD symptoms are influenced by the menstrual cycle such that symptoms peak just before the onset of menses when estrogen levels are lowest and are ameliorated at the time of ovulation, when estrogen levels are highest, supporting a dopaminergic effect of estrogen [38–40]. In addition, Saunders-Pullman et al. [41] found that women already diagnosed with PD who were on hormone replacement therapy had milder symptoms of disease than those who were not. Supporting the hypothesis of the beneficial effects of estrogen, treatment with estrogen versus placebo led to improvement in Unified Parkinson Disease Rating Scale motor scores [42] and a lower required dose of levodopa to treat symptoms [43]. Yet, conflicting data suggest that estrogen does not influence the expression of

PD [44, 45]. In fact, the few studies that have reported on pregnant women with PD when estrogen levels are high have found worsening or no change in parkinsonian symptoms [7, 46–48]. Golbe described that 8 of 14 pregnant women he interviewed reported worsening of their parkinsonism and that their PD symptoms did not fully return to baseline after delivery [7]. In a series of 35 pregnancies in 26 women diagnosed with PD, 46% (*n* = 16) had worsening or the appearance of new PD symptoms during or shortly after delivery [46]. Disease progression as a cause for worsening symptoms should be considered. Therefore, the role that estrogen plays in PD manifestation is not completely elucidated yet it appears to have a positive effect on PD. More research is needed to see whether the risks of hormone therapy outweigh the benefits to PD.

Treatments used in PD include the monoamine oxidase-B inhibitors, selegiline and rasagiline, the dopamine agonists, pramipexole and ropinirole, levodopa, amantadine, and entacapone all of which are FDA Pregnancy Category C. Older animal studies have failed to show teratogenic effects of levodopa but there are some reports of intrauterine growth retardation and malformations of the circulatory system [49]. Merchant et al. [50] demonstrated that levodopa does indeed cross the human placenta and is metabolized by the fetus. However, the few reports of the use of levodopa in humans during pregnancy all support its safety [7, 46, 47, 51].

Treatment with the dopamine agonists is contraindicated in breastfeeding mothers due to the prolactin inhibitory action of dopamine. Isolated case reports indicate that the dopamine agonists, bromocriptine, pergolide, cabergoline, and pramipexole, have been used without ill effect in pregnancy [48, 51–54].

Selegiline and rasagiline, inhibitors of monoamine oxidase B (MAO-B), are used both as monotherapy and as adjunctive therapy in the treatment of PD. There are no data as yet regarding the use of rasagiline during pregnancy. Kupsch and Oertel describe a patient that remained on both L-dopa and selegiline throughout her pregnancy, without any adverse effects on the fetus [55]. However, animal studies of MAO inhibitors have demonstrated mild to serious deleterious effects on neurobehavioral and functional fetal outcomes [56, 57].

Amantadine exposure during the first trimester has been demonstrated to cause cardiovascular maldevelopment [58]. In another study, amantadine exposure during the first trimester led to five major birth defects among 51 newborns [12].

Because of case reports of levodopa's safety in pregnancy, it should be considered preferable to the other agents if treatment must be undertaken during pregnancy although more data are accumulating to support safety of the dopamine agonists as well.

Essential tremor

Essential tremor (ET) is one of the most common movement disorders and is characterized by postural and kinetic tremor typically affecting the hands but also at times involving the head, voice, and lower extremities. Estimated prevalence is 1.7% of the general population and 5.5% in adults older than age 40 with equal frequency in men and women [59]. There are no data to suggest that pregnancy affects ET symptoms. The most commonly employed agents used to treat ET include primidone, propranolol, topiramate, and gabapentin. Primidone is known to have teratogenic potential and is FDA Pregnancy Category D, while all others are Category C. Thus, it is best to avoid medical therapy during pregnancy if possible.

Dystonia

Dystonia is characterized by abnormal sustained muscle contractions. These contractions can cause twisting and repetitive movements that can lead to abnormal postures. Dystonia can be classified based on etiology as idiopathic (primary) or symptomatic (secondary); or based on location: focal, segmental, multifocal, hemidystonia, and generalized. Idiopathic torsion dystonia typically begins before reproductive years and persists throughout adulthood and can therefore be a common finding in pregnant women. There is a bimodal age of onset, early onset (childhood) and late onset (fifth decade of life). During pregnancy, treating physicians should also be aware of symptomatic dystonia (as mentioned earlier, tardive dystonia) that may occur as a result of medications used to treat nausea, a common complaint during pregnancy [60].

Rogers and Fahn described 10 pregnant patients with dystonia [61]. Of 10 patients, 3 were noted to have partial or complete remission, 2 had exacerbation and the remaining patients had no notable change during pregnancy. Of the 10 patients studied, 1 had generalized dystonia, and the other patients had focal or segmental dystonia. Gwinn-Hardy and colleagues surveyed 279 women (62 premenopausal) with dystonia. They note that 4 of the 27 women that reported a pregnancy experienced a change in their dystonia symptoms but go on to add that no clear association was found [62]. In addition, we report the case of a woman with DYT1 dystonia who experienced deterioration in her symptoms throughout pregnancy. Yet this cannot be solely attributed to pregnancy by confounding medication withdrawal to reduce *in utero* exposure to the growing fetus [63].

Reports on dopa-responsive dystonia (DRD) and pregnancy have commented on the safe use of levodopa in these cases [64,65]. Oromandibular dystonia has been reported to recur and be exacerbated by pregnancy with episodes disappearing soon after delivery [66].

Treatment for dystonia includes oral agents such as trihexyphenidyl, baclofen (FDA Class C), and benzodiazepines (FDA Class D) as well as botulinum toxin (FDA Class C) injections of affected areas. There are no adequate human controlled studies with any of these treatments. One case report documents safety of high-dose trihexyphenidyl during two pregnancies in a woman with generalized dystonia [67]. There have also been recent reports of botulinum toxin type A being used without deleterious effects in pregnant women [68–70]. Deep brain stimulation therapy for the treatment of dystonia has been reported in very few cases in women who subsequently became pregnant but seems to be safe [71]. If during cesarean delivery diathermy is needed, bipolar diathermy should be used [72]. Medications used to treat dystonia should be avoided if possible, but when necessary there is some evidence to support the relative safety of botulinum toxin and trihexyphenidyl but benzodiazepines should be avoided.

Tics and Tourette syndrome

Tics are defined as sudden brief movements that are typically associated with a premonitory sensation that is only relieved by completion of the movement. Tics are classified as motor or vocal (phonic), and both must be present for a diagnosis of Tourette syndrome. Tourette syndrome typically begins in childhood and can be lifelong but as the person ages the severity of their symptoms decreases [73] It is often associated with obsessive-compulsive disorder (OCD) and attention deficit disorder. The etiology of Tourette syndrome is unknown but it is believed to be heritable and the search for gene mutations is ongoing [74]. Males are more often affected than females, but the reason for this gender dissociation is unclear. Studies have investigated whether women have fluctuations correlating with different hormonal states. Stern and colleagues reported in a study of 8 women with Tourette syndrome in a total of 11 pregnancies that 4 women felt an improvement in their symptoms, 2 felt no change, and 2 felt a worsening during pregnancy [75]. Schwabe et al. found that 26% of women reported an increase in tic frequency in the premenstrual cycle, but no consistent changes were associated with pregnancy, oral contraceptive use, or menopause [76–78].

Treatment for tics includes clonidine, guanfacine, and dopamine receptor-blocking agents (neuroleptics). Guanfacine (FDA Pregnancy Category B) is preferable to clonidine (Category C) in pregnancy. Neuroleptics as a class are generally contraindicated during pregnancy. However, depending on severity of tics, treatment benefits may outweigh risks and if necessary, high potency neuroleptics (haloperidol) are preferred [79]. Often the neurologist is treating the OCD component of Tourette syndrome as well which responds best to selective serotonin reuptake inhibitors (SSRIs). Guidelines published by the American Academy of Pediatrics recommend fluoxetine for the treatment of OCD during pregnancy [79].

Wilson disease

Wilson disease or hepatolenticular degeneration is an autosomal recessive neurodegenerative disorder associated with abnormal copper metabolism leading to copper accumulation in the liver, brain, and cornea. It is caused by a gene mutation in the ATP7b gene, a P-type copper-transporting ATPase [80].

There is a wide variability in age of onset of Wilson disease, ranging from 5 to 50 years of age [81]. The clinical picture consists of liver cirrhosis, chorea, tremor, psychiatric disturbances, and Kayser–Fleischer rings. Hepatic dysfunction usually predates neuropsychiatric symptoms in adolescents ages 10–13, whereas young adults ages 19–20 typically present with the neuropsychiatric illness [82]. Abnormal laboratory values include low total serum copper and ceruloplasmin levels.

There are limited data available on the effects of pregnancy on Wilson disease symptoms but Sinha and colleges reported that there was no change in clinical features in 16 women at their center with Wilson disease who became pregnant [82]. However, in this population, there were 24 spontaneous abortions and 3 stillbirths suggesting a high rate of pregnancy complications in Wilson disease, particularly untreated cases [83].

Treatment of Wilson disease typically involves chelation with penicillamine and the use of zinc.

Trientine or tetrathiomolybdate is also used. Data from case reports of pregnant women with Wilson disease suggest that the benefits of using chelation therapy with penicillamine during pregnancy far outweigh the risk of treatment to the fetus [84, 85]. Chelation therapy throughout pregnancy decreases the risk of possible fatal liver disease and hemolytic anemia to the mother and decreases the potential for liver damage and copper accumulation in the placenta of the fetus. It is therefore recommended that treatment be continued throughout the course of the pregnancy despite teratogenicity of penicillamine which is felt to increase in doses over 500 mg/day [12]. However, an alternative may include treatment with zinc alone during pregnancy, an agent known to be safe, as recent studies have suggested its efficacy as long as close follow-up of copper levels is performed to ensure adequate treatment is being delivered [86, 87].

Genetic testing issues during pregnancy

There has been a significant increase in our understanding of the genetic contributions to a variety of neurologic disorders in recent years with a number of gene mutations, deletions, triplications, and polymorphisms being identified at a rapid pace in Parkinson disease, Alzheimer disease, dystonia, Wilson disease, and adult-onset ataxias among others. As we gain a better understanding of the impact that these genetic mutations have on the manifestation of neurologic illness in regard to dominant or recessive patterns of inheritance, penetrance, variability of phenotype, etc., we then need to be able to communicate this to patients who may be at risk for passing these traits on to the next generation. The adult-onset, autosomal dominantly inherited neurodegenerative disorder, HD, can serve as a model for approaching genetic counseling in other disorders. The HD gene was identified in the early 1990s and

systematic approaches for discussing genetic testing issues have been implemented in clinical practice [88].

Huntington disease

Huntington disease is characterized by the triad of abnormal movements (typically chorea), cognitive impairment, and behavioral problems. It is caused by an expanded CAG repeat in the gene encoding the protein huntingtin on chromosome 4, making it a polyglutamine repeat disorder similar to several spinocerebellar ataxias and other adult-onset neurologic disorders. The usual age at presentation is in the fourth to fifth decade of life, when many people have already had children, each of whom then has a 50% chance of inheriting the mutant gene and developing HD.

There are no reports on the effects of pregnancy on HD symptoms although the prediction would be an increase in hyperkinetic movements due to hormonal shifts and increases in estrogen. Treatment for HD is symptomatic involving the use of antidopaminergic agents or dopamine depletors, such as typical and atypical neuroleptics, and tetrabenazine for chorea [89]. As mentioned previously in patients with chorea gravidarum and other movement disorders, tetrabenazine may be considered and the neuroleptics as a class are generally contraindicated but if warranted during pregnancy, the high potency agents are preferred [12, 79]. Benzodiazepines have also been tried and proven helpful for chorea and some of the behavioral aspects of HD [89]. Depression is a common occurrence in patients with HD. According to the American Academy of Pediatrics, there are insufficient data to recommend the use of bupropion, paroxetine, sertraline, venlafaxine, and monamine oxidase inhibitors in pregnant women. Fluoxetine, like the tricyclics are safe for use during pregnancy [79].

Presymptomatic and prenatal testing have been available since 1986 [90], with the HD locus being identified in 1983 and the gene in 1993. Now that HD genetic testing is available, this 'at-risk' population may choose to obtain testing to determine whether they have inherited the HD gene. Despite this technological advance, only a minority of at-risk people decide to obtain testing (estimated at 5% in the United States) as there are no known cures or treatments that delay the onset or progression of disease as yet [91]. Family planning issues are some of the major driving forces when persons at-risk for HD do decide to obtain genetic testing and studies have revealed that women more often than men seek predictive testing [92]. Women who are at-risk for HD who are pregnant or are thinking about becoming pregnant can meet with genetic counselors to discuss testing options that are currently available. The HD genetic testing can be obtained *in utero* through amniocentesis or chorionic villous sampling. Preimplantation genetic diagnosis (PGD) can be performed utilizing *in vitro* fertilization (IVF) technology [93]. Embryos are formed *in vitro* and tested for the HD gene at the 8-cell stage. Only those embryos not carrying the HD gene are implanted. This offers the advantage of not having to reveal the HD gene status to the at-risk parent. The downside is cost of the procedure and the failure rate of pregnancy with IVF techniques.

Despite advances in testing options, there are few reports available documenting reproductive decision-making in the HD at-risk population. Lesca et al. showed that in a group of 868 at-risk couples, 5% requested presymptomatic testing while pregnant [90]. The majority of the couples (73%) decided to continue their pregnancy, and only 9% decided to do prenatal testing on their current pregnancy. Decruyenaere and colleagues followed 89 subjects found to be carriers and 7 subjects with equivocal HD gene testing results for an average of 7 years after HD presymptomatic testing and reported on their reproductive decision-making [94]. They found that 48 subjects (46 gene positive and 2 equivocal) underwent gene testing for family planning reasons and 58% of them went on to have children with prenatal diagnosis or PGD. Thirty-five

percent decided not have children after receiving their results and 7% remained undecided or did not have children for other reasons.

Recently, ethical debates have arisen regarding the "right not to know." This has been heavily spurred by the Dutch government's stance on the exclusion testing and PGD for HD. Dutch policy in 2009 disallowed exclusion testing and required that PGD be permitted only in prospective parents who are willing to find out their own HD status. The government felt that unnecessary IVF and PGD could be avoided in this way, hence avoiding the extra costs and risks. This has raised an important counter argument suggesting that forcing people to know their HD status (with no cure currently available) as a prerequisite for IVF and PGD is immoral as knowing ones positive status can be psychologically detrimental [95]. Indeed, 32% of couples pursuing PGD for HD at three European centers requested exclusion testing over direct testing [96].

The state of knowledge of genetics of other neurologic disorders, such as PD, is in their infancy relative to HD, but in the future, similar counseling strategies and genetic testing options may be employed. Persons with strong family histories of a particular neurologic disease may choose to seek genetic counseling to discuss inheritance patterns, gene penetrance, and phenotypic correlations as they are planning their families.

Summary

Overall, movement disorders are not common during pregnancy with the exception of RLS. The high estrogen levels in pregnancy may influence disease manifestations in movement disorders (worsening hyperkinetic movements) as studies have documented estrogen's ability to modulate dopaminergic effects in the basal ganglia. Regarding the use of medications during pregnancy for movement disorders, it is advisable to avoid treatment if at all possible unless there is risk to the mother or fetus due to severity of symptoms. Based on case reports, levodopa and possibly dopamine agonist therapy is felt to be safe and can be maintained during pregnancy for the treatment of PD and RLS as is the case for botulinum toxin therapy and trihexyphenidyl for dystonia. Amantadine is contraindicated during pregnancy. Dopamine-receptor blocking agents (neuroleptics) are contraindicated but if necessary, the high potency drugs including haloperidol are preferred to treat symptoms in patients with tics, Tourette syndrome, or HD. Another safe alternative for treatment of tics during pregnancy is guanfacine. For those diseases with depressive symptoms such as PD, HD, and Tourette syndrome, tricyclic antidepressants and fluoxetine are felt to be relatively safe in pregnant women.

References

1 Wilson P, Preece AA. Chorea gravidarum. *Arch Intern Med*. 1932;49:471–533.

2 Maia DP, Fonseca PG, Camargos ST. et al. Pregnancy in patients with Syndenham's chorea. *Parkinsonism Relat Disord*. 2012;18:458–461.

3 Zegart KN, Schwarz RH. Chorea gravidarum. *Obstet Gynecol*. 1968;32:24–27.

4 Donaldson JO. Neurologic emergencies in pregnancy. *Obstet Gynecol Clin North Am*. 1991;18(2): 199–212.

5 Ichikawa K, Kim RC, Givelber H, et al. Chorea gravidarum. Report of a fatal case with neuropathological observations. *Arch Neurol*. 1980;37: 429.

6 Cardoso Francisco. Chorea gravidarum. *Arch Neurol*. 2002;59:868–870.

7 Golbe LI. Pregnancy and Movement disorders. *Neurol Clinics*. 1994;12(3):497–508.

8 Miller LJ. Clinical strategies for the use of psychotropic drugs during pregnancy. *Psychiatric Med*. 1991;9(2):275–298.

9 Altshuler LL, Szuba MP. Course of psychiatric disorders in pregnancy: dilemmas in pharmacologic management. *Neurol Clin* 1994;12(3):613–635.

10 Collins KO, Comer JB. Maternal haloperidol therapy associated with dyskinesia in a newborn. *Am J Health Syst Perinatol*. 2003;60:2253–2255.

11 Sexson WR, Barak Y. Withdrawal emergent syndrome in an infant associated with maternal haloperidol therapy. *J Perinatol*. 1989;9:170–172.

12 Briggs GG, Freeman RK, Yaffe SJ. *Drugs in Pregnancy and Lactation*, 4th ed. Baltimore, MD: Williams & Wilkins, 1994.

13 Lubbe WF, Walker EB. Chorea gravidarum associated with circulating lupus anticoagulant: successful outcome of pregnancy with prednisone and aspirin therapy. Case report. *Br J Obstet Gynaecol*. 1983;90:487–490.

14 Lim EC, Seet RC, Wilder-Smith EP et al. Dystonia gravidarum: a new entity? *Mov Disord*. 2006;21:69–70.

15 Fasano A, Elia AE, Guidubaldi A, et al. Dystonia gravidarum: a new case with a long-follow-up. *Mov Disord*. 2007;22:564–566.

16 Buccoliero R, Palmeri S, Malandrini A, et al. A case of dystonia with onset during pregnancy. *J Neurol Sci*. 2007;260:265–266.

17 Ohayon MM, O'Hara R, Vitiello MV. Epidemiology of restless legs syndrome. A synthesis of the literature. *Sleep Med Rev*. 2012;16(4):283–295.

18 Goodman JD, Brodie C, Ayida GA. Restless legs syndrome in pregnancy. *Br Med J*. 1988;297:1101–1102.

19 Suzuki K, Ohida T, Sone T, et al. The prevalence of restless legs syndrome among pregnant women in Japan and the relationship between restless legs syndrome and sleep problems. *Sleep*. 2003;26:673–677.

20 Manconi M, Govoni V, DeVito A, et al. Restless legs syndrome and pregnancy. *Neurology*. 2004;63:1065–1069.

21 Alves DA, Carvalho LB, Morais JF, et al. Restless legs syndrome during pregnancy in Brazilian women. *Sleep Med*. 2010;11:1049–1054.

22 Pantaleo NP, Hening WA, Allen RP, et al. Pregnancy accounts for most of the gender difference in prevalence of familial RLS. *Sleep Med*. 2010;11:310–313.

23 Cesnik E, Casetta I, Turri M, et al. Transient RLS during pregnancy is a risk factor for the chronic idiopathic form. *Neurol*. 2010;75:2117–2120.

24 Dostal M, Weber-Schoendorfer C, Sobesky J, et al. Pregnancy outcome following use of levodopa, pramipexole, ropinirole and rotigotine for restless legs syndrome during pregnancy: a case series. *Eur J Neurol*. 2013;20:1241–1246.

25 Djokanovic N, Garcia-Bournissen F, Koren G. Medications for restless legs syndrome during pregnancy. *J Obstet Gynaecol Can*. 2008;30:505–507.

26 Teive HA, Arruda WO, Raskin S, et al. Symptom onset of spinocerebellar ataxia type 10 in pregnancy and puerpium. *J Clin Neurosci.* 2011;18:437–438.

27 Tan PC, Khine PP, Vallikkannu N, et al. Promethazine compared with metoclopramide for hyperemesis gravidarum. A randomized controlled trial. *Obstet Gynecol.* 2010;115:975–981.

28 McKeigue PM, Marmot MG. Epidemiology of Parkinson's disease. In: Stern G, ed. *Parkinson's Disease.* London: Chapman and Hall, 1990; pp. 295–306.

29 Bower JH, Maraganore DM, McDonnell SK, Rocca WA. Incidence and distribution of parkinsonsism in Olmsted County, Minnesota, 1976–1990. *Neurology.* 1999;52:1214–1220.

30 Van Den Eeden SK, Tanner CM, Bernstein AL, et al. Incidence of Parkinson's disease: variation by age, gender and race/ethnicity. *Am J Epidemiol.* 2003;157:1015–1022.

31 Mayeux R, Marder K, Cote LJ, et al. The frequency of idiopathic Parkinson's disease by age, ethnic group and sex in northern Manhattan, 1988–1993. *Am J Epidemiol.* 1995;142:820–827.

32 Pasqualini C, Olivier V, Guibert B, Frain O, Leviel V. Acute stimulatory effect of estradiol on striatal dopamine synthesis. *J Neurochem.* 1995;65:1651–1657.

33 Xiao L, Becker JB. Effects of estrogen agonists on amphetamine-stimulated striatal dopamine release. *Synapse.* 1998;29:379–391.

34 Disshon KA, Boja JW, Dluzen DE. Inhibition of striatal dopamine transporter activity by 17 beta-estradiol. *Eur J Pharmacol.* 1998;345:207–211.

35 Levesque D, DiPaolo T. Modulation by estradiol and progesterone of the GTP effect on striatal D2 dopamine receptors. *Biochem Pharmacol.* 1993;45:723–733.

36 Dluzen DE. Neuroprotective effects of estrogen upon the nigrostriatal dopaminergic system. *J Neurocytol.* 2000;29:387–399.

37 Lammers CH, D'Souza U, Qin ZH, Lee SH, Yajima S, Mouradian MM. Regulation of striatal dopamine receptors by estrogen. *Synapse.* 1999;34:222–227.

38 Horstink MW, Strijks E, Dluzen DE. Estrogen and Parkinson's disease. *Adv Neurol.* 2003;91:107–114.

39 Quinn NP, Marsden CD. Menstrual-related fluctuations in Parkinson's disease. *Mov Disord.* 1986;1:85–87.

40 Sandyk R. Estrogens and the pathophysiology of Parkinson's disease. *Int J Neurosci.* 1989;45:119–122.

41 Saunders-Pullman R, Gordon-Elliott J, Parides M, Fahn S, Saunders HR, Bressman S. The effect of estrogen replacement on early Parkinson's disease. *Neurology.* 1999;52:1417–1421.

42 Tsang KL, Ho SL, Lo SK. Estrogen improves motor disability in parkinsonian postmenopausal women with motor fluctuations. *Neurology.* 2000;54:2292–2298.

43 Blanchet PJ, Fang J, Hyland K, et al. Short-term effects of high-dose 17beta-estradiol in postmenopausal PD patients: a crossover study. *Neurology.* 1999;53:91–95.

44 Kompoliti K, Comella CL, Jaglin JA, Leurgans S, Raman R, Goetz CG. Menstrual-related changes in motoric function in women with Parkinson's disease. *Neurology.* 2000;55:1572–1575.

45 Strijks E, Kremer JA, Horstink MW. Effects of female sex steroids on Parkinson's disease in postmenopausal women. *Clin Neuropharacol.* 1999;22:93–97.

46 Hagell P, Odin P, Vinge E. Pregnancy in Parkinson's disease: a review of the literature and a case report. *Mov Disord.* 1998;13:34–38.

47 Shulman LM, Minagar A, Weiner WJ. The effect of pregnancy in Parkinson's disease. *Mov Disord.* 2000;15:132–135.

48 Mucchiut M, Belgrado E, Cutuli D, Antonini A, Bergonzi P. Pramipexole-treated Parkinson's disease during pregnancy. *Mov Disord.* 2004;19:1114–1115.

49 Staples RE, Mattis PA. Teratology of L-dopa. *Teratology.* 1973;8:238.

50 Merchant CA, Cohen G, Mytilineou C, et al. Human transplacental transfer of carbidopa/levodopa. *J Neural Transm Park Dis Dement Sect.* 1995;9:239–242.

51 Scott M, Chowdhury M. Pregnancy in Parkinson's disease: unique case report and review of the literature. *Mov Disord.* 2005;20:1078–1079.

52 Benito-Leon Julian, Bermejo Felix. Pregnancy in Parkinson's Disease: a review of the literature and a case report. *Mov Disord.* 1999;14(1):194.

53 Mari M, De Zenzola A, Lamberti P. Antiparkinsonian treatment in pregnancy. *Mov Disord.* 2002;17:428–429.

54 Lamichhane D, Narayanan NS, Gonzalez-Alegre P. Two cases of pregnancy in Parkinson's disease. *Parkinsonism Relat Disord.* 2014;20(2):239–240.

55 Kupsch A, Oertel WH. Selegiline, pregnancy and Parkinson's disease. *Mov Disord.* 1998;13:175–176.

56 Whitaker-Azmita PM, Zhang X, Clarke C. Effects of gestational exposure to monamineoxidase

inhibitors in rats: preliminary behavioral and neurochemical studies. *Neuropsychopharmacology*. 1994;11:125–132.

57 Product information. *Eldepryl(selegiline)*. Tampa, FL: Somerset Pharmaceutical, 1996.

58 Nora JJ, Nora AH, Way GL. Cardiovascular maldevelopment associated with maternal exposure to amantadine. *Lancet*. 1975;2:607.

59 Tanner CM, Goldman SM. Epidemiology of movement disorders. *Curr Opin Neurol*. 1994;7(4):340–345.

60 Kranick S, Mowry EM, Colcher A et al. Movement disorders and pregnancy: a review of the literature. *Mov Disord*. 2010;25:665–671.

61 Rogers JD, Fahn S. Movement disorders and pregnancy. In: Devinsky O, Feldman E, Hainline B, eds., *Neurological Complications of Pregnancy*. New York: Raven Press, 1994; pp. 163–178.

62 Gwinn-Hardy KA, Adler CH, Weaver AL, et al. Effect of hormone variations and other factors on symptom severity in women with dystonia. *Mayo Clin Proc*. 2000;75:235–240.

63 Nageshwaran S, Nageshwaran S, Edwards MJ, Morcos M. Management of DYT1 dystonia throughout pregnancy. *BMJ Case Reports*. 2011; pii: bcr0520114214.

64 Nomoto M, Kaseda S, Iwata S, Osame M, Fukuda T. Levodopa in pregnancy. *Mov Disord*. 1997;12:261

65 Ball MC, Sagar HJ. Levodopa in pregnancy. *Mov Disord*. 1995;10:115.

66 Michelotti A, Silva R, Paduano S, et al. Oromandibular dystonia and hormonal factors: twelve years follow-up of a case report. *J Oral Rehabil*. 2009;36:916–921.

67 Robottom BJ, Reich SG. Exposure to high dosage trihexyphenidyl during pregnancy for treatment of generalized dystonia: case report and literature review. *Neurologist*. 2011;17:340–341.

68 Newman WJ, Davis TL, Padaliya BB, et al. Botulinum toxin type A therapy during pregnancy. *Mov Disord*. 2004;19:1384–1385.

69 Morgan JC, Iyer SS, Moser ET, Singer C, Sethi KD. Botulinum toxin A during pregnancy: a survey of treating physicians. *J Neurol Neurosurg Psychiatry*. 2006;77:117–119.

70 Li Yim JF, Weir CR. Botulinum toxin and pregnancy- a cautionary tale. *Strabismus*. 2010;18:65–66.

71 Paluzzi A, Bain PG, Liu X, et al. Pregnancy in dystonic women with in situ deep brain stimulators. *Mov Disord*. 2006;21:695–698.

72 http://www.medtronic.com/your-health/parkinsons-disease/important-safety-information/index.htm.

73 Bruun RD, Budman CL. The natural history of Tourette syndrome. *Adv Neurol*. 1992;58:1–6.

74 Keen-Kim D, Freimer NB. Genetics and epidemiology of Tourette syndrome. *J Child Neurol*. 2006;21:665–671

75 Stern JS, Orth M, Robertson MM. Gilles de la Tourette syndrome in pregnancy: a retrospective case series. *Obstet Med*. 2009;2:128–129.

76 Schwabe MJ, Konkol RJ. Menstrual cycle-related fluctuations of tics in Tourette's syndrome. *Pediatr Neurol*. 1992;8(1):43–46.

77 Robertson MM. The Gilles de la Tourette syndrome: the current status. *Br J Psychiatry*. 1989;154:147–169.

78 Shapiro AK, Shapiro E. Tourette syndrome: clinical aspects, treatment, and etiology. *Semin Neurol*. 1982;2:373–385.

79 American Academy of Pediatrics. Use of psychoactive medication during pregnancy and possible effects on the fetus and newborn. *Pediatrics*. 2000;105(4):880–887.

80 Tanzi RE, Petrukhin K, Chernov I, et al. The Wilson's disease gene is a copper transporting ATPase with homology to the Menke's disease gene. *Nat Genet*. 1993;5:344–350.

81 Pfeil SA, Lynn DJ. Wilson's disease: copper unfettered. *J Clin Gastroenterol*. 1999;29(1):22–31.

82 Bonne-Tamir B, Frydman M, Agger MS, et al. Wilson's disease in Israel: a genetic and epidemiological study. *Ann Hum Genet*. 1990;54:155–168.

83 Sinha S, Taly AB, Prashanth LK, Arunodaya GR, Swamy HS. Successful pregnancies and abortions in symptomatic and asymptomatic Wilson's disease. *J Neurol Sci*. 2004;15:37–40.

84 Berghella V, Steele D, Spector T, et al. Successful Pregnancy in a neurologically impaired woman with Wilson's disease: case report. *Am J Obstet Gynecol*. 1997;176(3):712–714.

85 Dupont P, Irion O, Beguin F. Pregnancy in a patient with treated Wilson's disease: a case report. *Am J Obstet Gynecol*. 1990;163:1527–1528.

86 Brewer GJ, Johnson VD, Dick RD, Hedera P, Fink JK, Kluin KL. Treatment of Wilson's disease with zinc. XVII: treatment during pregnancy. *Hepatology*. 2000;31:364–370.

87 Masciullo M, Modoni A, Bianchi ML, DeCarolis S, Silvestri G. Positive outcome in a patient with Wilson's disease treated with reduced zinc dosage

during pregnancy. *Eur J Obstet Gynecol Reprod Biol.* 2011;159:237–238.

88 Went L, Broholm J, Cassiman J-J, et al. Guidelines for the molecular genetics predictive test in Huntington disease. *J Med Genet.* 1994;31:555–559.

89 Quinn N, Schrag A. Huntington's disease and other choreas. *J Neurol.* 1998;245:709–716.

90 Lesca G, Goizet C, Durr A. Predictive testing in the context of pregnancy: experience in Huntington's disease and autosomal dominant cerebellar ataxia. *J Med Genet.* 2002;39:522–525.

91 Hayden MR. Predictive testing for Huntington's disease: a universal model? *Lancet Neurol.* 2003;2:141–142.

92 Goizet C, Lesca G, Durr A. Presymptomatic testing in Huntington's disease and autosomal dominant cerebellar ataxias. *Neurology.* 2002;59:1330–1336.

93 Moutou C, Gardes N, Viville S. New tools for preimplantation genetic diagnosis of Huntington's disease and their clinical applications. *Eur J Hum Genet.* 2004;12:1007–1014.

94 Decruyenaere M, Evers-Kiebooms G, Boogaerts A, et al. The complexity of reproductive decision-making in asymptomatic carriers of the Huntington mutation. *Eur J Hum Genet.* 2007;15:453–462.

95 Asscher E, Koops BJ. The right not to know and preimplantation genetic diagnosis for *Huntington's* disease. *J Med Ethics.* 2010;36:30–33.

96 Van Rij MC and the BruMaStra PGD Working Group. Preimplantation genetic diagnosis (PGD) for Huntington's disease: the experience of three European centres. *Eur J Hum Genetics.* 2012;20:368–375.

CHAPTER 13

Brain tumors and pregnancy

Soma Sengupta[1] & Elizabeth Gerstner[2]

[1] Division of Neuro-Oncology, Beth Israel Deaconess Medical Center, Harvard Medical School, Boston, MA, USA

[2] Department of Neurology, Massachusetts General Hospital, Harvard Medical School, Boston, MA, USA

Epidemiology of brain tumors in women

Primary tumors of the central nervous system (CNS) are a heterogeneous group of tumors. Gliomas and meningiomas represent about 75% of primary CNS tumors with an incidence of 6.3/100,000 in the United States [1]. The incidence of intracranial meningiomas is twice as high in women as in men, and intraspinal meningiomas are nine times more common in women than in men, suggesting that gender differences play a role [2, 3]. In contrast, most gliomas have a slight male predominance and an older age of onset; most high-grade gliomas present after the age of 50. Younger patients more commonly present with low-grade gliomas (WHO grade I) which tend to be slow growing. Metastatic brain tumors are much more common than primary brain tumors in both men and women. In a study carried out by Lentzsch et al. on breast cancer patients, the median age of diagnosis of brain metastases was 50 years (range 30–78 years) [4]. Eighty-one patients (50%) were pre-menopausal (including 15 patients under 40 years of age) and 81 patients (50%) were postmenopausal. The only type of brain metastasis that is more common in pregnant women is choriocarcinoma, which is exceedingly rare (~1/20,000 pregnancies in the United States) [5]. There is currently no strong scientific data on the influence of endogenous hormones in metastatic brain tumor development.

Tumors potentially influenced by pregnancy or hormonal changes

Meningiomas and pituitary adenomas are primary brain tumors that may be influenced by pregnancy or hormonal changes. Hormonal influence may be either endogenous or exogenous. Meningiomas may display accelerated growth during the luteal phase of the menstrual cycle and during pregnancy due to changes in progesterone levels and progesterone receptors [3]. According to a large European study by Michaud et al. [2], endogenous hormones in women did not seem to increase the risk of developing either a glioma or meningioma, whereas exogenous HRT or OCP use may predispose women to developing meningiomas. A higher risk of meningioma was observed among postmenopausal women who were on hormone replacement therapy (HRT) (HR, 1.79; 95% CI, 1.18–2.71) compared with women who never used HRT (Figure 13.1). Similarly, users of oral contraceptives (OCPs) were at a higher risk of developing meningiomas than those who had never used OCPs (HR, 3.61; 95% CI, 1.75–7.46) [2]. Considering the increased incidence of intracranial meningiomas in women as

Neurological Illness in Pregnancy: Principles and Practice, First Edition.
Edited by Autumn Klein, M. Angela O'Neal, Christina Scifres, Janet F. R. Waters and Jonathan H. Waters.
© 2016 John Wiley & Sons, Ltd. Published 2016 by John Wiley & Sons, Ltd.

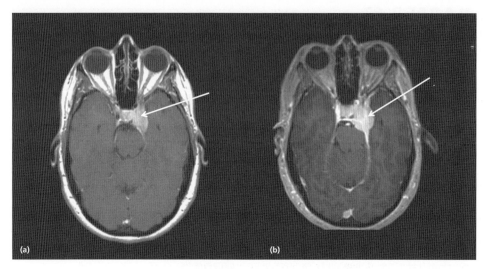

Figure 13.1 (a) T1 axial post contrast MRI showing an enhancing meningioma in the left cavernous sinus (white arrow). (b) T1 axial post contrast MRI 5 years later showing enlargement of the meningioma (white arrow). **Vignette 1:** A 47-year-old peri-menopausal woman presented to her primary care physician with pain in her left eye. A brain MRI with contrast revealed a meningioma in the left cavernous sinus (Figure 13.1a). Given the challenging surgical location, unknown growth rate of the meningioma, and mild symptoms that were not necessarily related to the meningioma, follow-up MRI was recommended. Unfortunately, the patient failed to follow-up until approximately 5 years later when she presented with progressive diplopia and was found to have a third nerve palsy. Repeat brain MRI showed an increase in the size of the meningioma (Figure 13.1b). Debulking surgery was recommended given the expansion of the meningioma close to the optic chiasm and pressure on surrounding normal brain. Although this growth happened during menopause, an association is hard to prove.

compared with men, these hormonal influences may be important.

Custer et al.'s [6] population-based study examined the association between exogenous hormone use and meningioma risk by compound type as well as by tumor estrogen and progesterone receptor status. They reported that in 142 meningioma tumor specimens: 2 (1%) expressed estrogen receptors and 130 (92%) expressed progesterone receptors. They also found a higher risk estimate for use of HRT preparations with both estrogen and progestin (OR, 1.3; 95% CI, 0.6, 2.8) than for compounds containing only estrogen (OR, 0.9, 95% CI, 0.5, 1.6). However, Claus et al. [7] point out that the confidence intervals are wide and not statistically significantly different. Importantly, the study [6] found no association between HRT use and progesterone receptor status but these

results are based on only 46 controls and 23 cases. This group, while noting an elevated but not statistically significant association with use of OCPs, did find an increased risk of meningiomas expressing less rather than more progesterone receptors, which is contradictory to their HRT data.

Pituitary adenomas are tumors that occur in the pituitary gland, and account for about 15% of intracranial neoplasms. These often remain undiagnosed, and are incidental findings during autopsy [8]. However, women who have pre-existing non-functional pituitary adenomas may have a small, undefined risk of developing pituitary apoplexy during pregnancy, due to the fact that the pituitary gland increases in size during pregnancy with a total increase of 3 mm by the end of pregnancy [9]. Interestingly, estrogens in a rat model cause hyperemia of the hypophysis

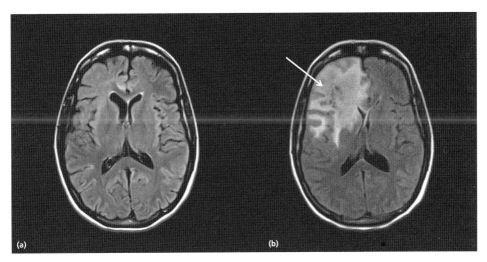

Figure 13.2 (a) FLAIR MRI showing no evidence of tumor. (b) FLAIR MRI 3 months later showing new hyperintensity in the right frontal lobe with significant mass effect and brain shift consistent with progressive glioma as shown by the white arrow. The patient was pregnant so did not receive gadolinium contrast.
Vignette 2: A 38-year-old woman with a known low-grade (WHO grade II) astrocytoma was being followed with surveillance MRIs (Figure 13.2a) when she presented with a seizure. She was 3 months pregnant at the time so a non-contrast MRI was done and revealed significant disease progression (Figure 13.2b). Given the degree of mass effect, she underwent a subtotal resection of the recurrence, and the pathology was consistent with a glioblastoma (WHO grade IV). She received involved field radiation without the standard chemotherapy regimen because of her pregnancy. At approximately 32 weeks, she had a successful caesarian section and delivered a healthy baby. Chemotherapy was started after delivery.

and this could theoretically contribute to the risk of pituitary apoplexy in pregnancy [10].

Coexistence of pregnancy and malignancy

The risk of any type of cancer complicating pregnancy is 1/1000 [11]. Approximately 89 pregnancies are complicated by the diagnosis of a maternal brain tumor in the United States each year [12]. The risk of developing a brain tumor is not altered either by age during the first pregnancy or the number of pregnancies [11]. The relative frequency of different primary brain tumor types (i.e., meningiomas, gliomas, pituitary tumors, vestibular schwannomas, etc.) is not changed by pregnancy, although basal meningiomas and vascular spinal tumors appear to be more common

in pregnant women [13, 14]. Interestingly, diagnosis of gliomas tends to cluster in the first trimester (Figure 13.2), whereas diagnosis of meningiomas is more prevalent in the second and third trimesters [12].

Symptoms of increased intracranial pressure including early morning headaches, nausea, and vomiting are similar to the symptoms of morning sickness, thus differentiating between these etiologies is challenging [15]. Diagnostic neuroimaging of the pregnant patient is a controversial subject, but MRI is the preferred imaging modality since there is no known risk to the fetus. Gadolinium contrast agent should be reserved for those patients whose benefit outweighs risk to the fetus. [12,16]. In an emergency setting, if CT must be used, then fetal exposure can be reduced by shielding the pregnant abdomen with a lead apron [17]. Fetal exposures less than 10 rads have been reported to reveal no adverse effects in excess of the background rate of spontaneous abnormalities in 3% of term pregnancies [15,17].

Treatment associated considerations in the pregnant patient

Management of brain tumors typically involves the use of corticosteroids, maximal safe surgical resection, radiation, and/or chemotherapy. Acute management of the complications of brain tumors such as cerebral edema and raised intracranial pressure during pregnancy, may necessitate the use of glucocorticoids and mannitol [18–21]. Fetal adrenal suppression may occur with glucocorticoids, but there is no evidence that mannitol harms the fetus [18–21]. Since low-grade gliomas are more common in younger women, there may be some flexibility in initiation of treatment in young pregnant women, thus, allowing the woman to near full term and deliver her baby before treatment needs to start. If treatment cannot be delayed, a careful discussion regarding the risks and benefits to the woman and the fetus needs to occur in conjunction with the obstetrical team. Given the rarity of primary brain tumors, their diagnosis in pregnancy is uncommon, making systematic study of the best treatment algorithm challenging.

Surgery

A retrospective review of neurosurgical management of pregnant women with intracranial lesions, including brain tumors, over a period of 36 years, found that surgical resection of intracranial lesions was generally well tolerated by both the mother and fetus. Pre-operative delivery by cesarean section of term or near-term babies was the preferred option because of concern over pushing raising intracranial pressure [22]. If a patient was deteriorating with an

intracranial lesion and the fetus was pre-term, a therapeutic abortion may be essential to save the life of the mother [23].

Radiation

Radiation exposure *in utero*, especially in the first trimester, can result in adverse fetal outcomes including: spontaneous abortion, anatomic malformation, growth and mental retardation, and possibly childhood cancer with the latter risk highest in the first trimester [15,17]. Due to these fetal outcomes, radiation is usually deferred until after the delivery. In a patient with a brain tumor, there would be internal scatter of radiation within the patient that cannot be shielded. However, if the use of radiation is essential, the following strategies may be employed: maximizing shielding with daily abdominal dose monitoring, the use of focal rather than whole brain irradiation (more applicable for brain metastasis), and radiation dose reduction [15]. There are no formal guidelines regarding proton therapy and pregnancy; thus it is indeterminate as to whether this provides a safer option.

Radiation therapy can disrupt the functioning of the hypothalamic–pituitary axis so cranial radiation sparing this axis should be performed in younger women. In addition, craniospinal radiation can directly cause ovarian failure, or, as is more commonly seen with abdominal or pelvic radiation, cause damage that later on makes the uterus unable to accommodate the growth of a fetus to full term [24, 25].

Chemotherapy

Chemotherapy for malignant brain tumors tends to be avoided during pregnancy since most of these agents are teratogenic and cross the placenta [26] (Table 13.1). 231 women were enrolled over 13 years in an international perinatal outcomes of pregnancy complicated

Table 13.1 Complications of chemotherapeutic and biological agents used in brain tumors on fertility and pregnancy

Class of drug and example	Effects on fertility or pregnancy
Anti-metabolite—methotrexate	Methotrexate can cause serious birth defects as well as pregnancy complications. Even after stopping methotrexate, contraception is required for 3 months. It is important to note that although a woman should not take methotrexate during pregnancy, taking the drug does not decrease the chance for future pregnancies, and it is used as a treatment for ectopic pregnancies.
Microtubule inhibitors—vincristine	Amenorrhea can occur in post-pubertal patients. It is a category D compound in pregnancy, and there are no proper studies in humans. However, there is plenty of evidence of teratogenicity in animal studies. Breast-feeding is also contraindicated on this medication.
Alkylating agents—temozolomide, Cyclophosphamide	Temozolomide impairs fertility. In addition, the FDA has assigned it to pregnancy category D. Animal studies have revealed evidence of embryolethality, and malformations of the external organs, soft tissues, and skeleton. Breast-feeding is also contraindicated on this medication.
	Cyclophosphamide has been assigned to pregnancy category D by the FDA. While normal newborns have been delivered to women who were exposed to cyclophosphamide during pregnancy, human data have revealed evidence of embryotoxicity and fetotoxicity.
	Cyclophosphamide is excreted into human milk. Neutropenia, thrombocytopenia, and immune suppression have been observed in infants whose mothers were receiving this drug during lactation. The drug also has an unacceptable risk of carcinogenesis. The American Academy of Pediatrics considers the use of cyclophosphamide to be contraindicated during breast-feeding.
Platinum agents—cisplatin/carboplatin	These compounds affect fertility. The FDA has assigned cisplatin to pregnancy category D. Animal studies have revealed evidence of embryotoxicity and teratogenicity in mice. Breast-feeding is also contraindicated on this medication.
Topoisomerase inhibitors—etoposide	The FDA has assigned etoposide to pregnancy category D. Animal studies have revealed evidence of teratogenicity in mice and rats even in tiny doses. Breast-feeding is also contraindicated on this medication.
Vascular endothelial growth factor inhibitor—cediranib	The FDA has assigned cediranib in pregnancy category D. This drug terminates fetal development in the rat, as expected for a process dependent on VEGF signaling. Breast-feeding is not recommended as the drug can be excreted in breast milk.
Anti-angiogenic agents—bevacizumab	The incidence of ovarian failure was higher (34% vs. 2%) in premenopausal women receiving bevacizumab in combination with mFOLFOX chemotherapy as compared to those receiving mFOLFOX.
	The FDA has assigned bevacizumab to pregnancy category C. Animal studies have revealed evidence of teratogenicity.
	Women should be advised to discontinue nursing during treatment with bevacizumab, since its half-life is approximately 20 days.
Epidermal growth factor receptor inhibitors—erlotinib	Erlotinib has been assigned to pregnancy category D by the FDA. Animal studies have shown embryo/fetal lethality and abortion.
	Although there is no data on breast-feeding, it is recommended that this is avoided, since many drugs are excreted in breast milk.
Immunomodulators—rituximab	The FDA has assigned rituximab to pregnancy category C. Animal studies have not been conducted. There are no controlled data in human pregnancy. There are no data on whether rituximab can cause fetal harm when administered to a pregnant woman or whether it can affect reproductive capacity. Because human IgG is known to cross the placental barrier, it may cause fetal B-cell depletion.
	In breast-feeding due to its IgG component, rituximab is thought to cross into breast milk; thus is contraindicated in breast-feeding.

Adapted from Reference 43.

by cancer registry. This registry also included neonatal outcome after *in utero* exposure to chemotherapy. The two main findings were that in pregnancies exposed to chemotherapy after the first trimester, congenital anomalies, pre-term delivery, and growth restriction were not increased as compared with the general population; and mean gestational age at delivery was not significantly different than neonates who were not exposed to chemotherapy [24]. However, a recent study about the long-term cognitive and cardiac effects due to pre-term chemotherapy exposure found that there may be subtle changes in cardiac and neurocognitive measurements emphasizing the need for long-term follow-up [27]. They also recommended avoiding iatrogenic pre-term delivery whenever possible because of the additional potential complications related to pre-term delivery.

Delivery considerations and post-partum setting

Cesarean section is the preferred method of delivery for a pregnant woman with a brain tumor if there is concern for increased intracranial pressure as pushing during vaginal delivery will only further increase intracranial pressure [15]. General anesthesia with intravenous propofol or inhalational gases, is preferred as opposed to epidural anesthesia. Epidural anesthesia has the potential of increasing intracranial pressure by compression on the dural sac, and complications such as subdural hematomas and subarachnoid hemorrhages have been reported [28]. Once the baby is delivered, the post-natal side effects of any medications that the mother has been on, need to be monitored. In addition, if the mother is receiving chemotherapy, the baby should not be breastfed due to the presence of these drugs in breast milk, and even after stopping the drug, it is unclear as to how long the effects of these agents persist in breast milk [29].

Impact of cancer treatment on fertility in female pediatric cancer survivors

Females have a fixed number of primordial follicles at birth that steadily decline with age, thus the risk for therapy-related ovarian failure and infertility is directly related to age. Pre-pubertal girls, having a greater reserve of follicles, are at lowest risk for these complications [26,30,31]. The Childhood Cancer Survivor Study cited a 10-fold greater cumulative incidence of nonsurgical premature menopause (before age 40) in survivors compared with siblings (8% vs. 0.8%), with survivors of Hodgkin's disease being the most affected group. Premature menopause was especially high in girls who received abdominopelvic irradiation, with a cumulative incidence approaching almost 30% [32–35]. Evaluation for gonadal failure and infertility centers on a good history focusing on the menstrual cycle, conception, and pregnancy. In addition, an annual physical examination with specific attention to Tanner staging is recommended. The Children's Oncology Group (COG) currently recommends baseline serum LH, FSH, and estradiol levels at the age of thirteen for girls who have undergone chemotherapy or radiation. The absence of signs of puberty by the age of 12 or lack of pubertal progression in girls over age 13 a year after cancer treatment warrants referral to an endocrinologist. Panhypopituitarism is also of concern post radiotherapy and can present with a variety of endocrine abnormalities contributing to infertility [30,31].

Impact of cancer treatment on fertility in women of child-bearing age

Chemotherapy agents destroy primordial follicles in the ovary by inducing apoptosis in the oocytes. This damages the ovarian reserves and interferes with follicle recruitment and maturation, thus often menses does not occur [35]. Alkylating agents, for example, temozolomide, which is a standard treatment of gliomas, are associated with the highest risk of ovarian failure. Ovarian failure has been reported as high as 90% in women older than 40 years who have received an alkylating agent as a combined agent in breast cancer treatment. In addition, tamoxifen, used in treating breast cancer, is associated with a high risk of ovarian failure [36].

Most of the clinical trials that look at effects of chemotherapy on fertility have been in the breast cancer setting. GnRH agonists have been studied to see if fertility can be preserved, but the results have been mixed. Nevertheless, these compounds may still be used to suppress ovarian function during chemotherapy [22]. International guidelines recommend that cryopreservation of unfertilized eggs or embryos is the most effective way of preserving fertility, and preconception planning should be offered to young women who are about to receive chemotherapy for curable cancers [22]. Although the preservation of fertility is an important consideration, it is also crucial to try and prevent premature menopause because this will accelerate premature osteoporosis. Finally, ovarian tissue preservation is a novel technique which is being explored in patients who have had chemotherapy [37–40].

The impact of newer targeted cancer drugs on fertility is still being discovered. For example, a substantially higher incidence of premature ovarian failure was found in pre-menopausal women receiving bevacizumab (Table 13.1), a monoclonal antibody to vascular endothelial growth factor, when given with mFOLFOX (34%) compared to mFOLFOX alone (2%). Premature ovarian failure was defined as amenorrhea lasting 3 or more months, a follicle-stimulating hormone (FSH) level of at least 30 mIU/mL, and a negative serum β-HCG pregnancy test. Once bevacizumab was discontinued, ovarian function returned to normal in 22% of women [41]. Thus, women need to be

carefully counseled on the risks—known and unknown—related to the evolving field of cancer treatment.

Hereditary tumor syndromes necessitating prenatal counseling

Phakomatoses or neurocutaneous syndromes such as neurofibromatosis (NF) I and II, tuberous sclerosis complex, von Hippel–Lindau (VHL) syndrome, Turcot syndrome, Li–Fraumeni cancer syndrome, and Gorlin syndrome are associated with brain tumors and are autosomal dominant. NF I is associated with a variety of tumors, including: CNS tumors (gliomas, optic or vestibular schwannoma, meningiomas), carcinoids, pheochromocytomas, neuroblastomas, ependymomas, primitive neuroectodermal tumors, rhabdomyosarcomas, plexiform neurofibromas and approximately 10% of these can transform into malignant peripheral nerve sheath tumors (MPNSTs). NF II is associated with bilateral vestibular schwannomas, gliomas, meningiomas, and intradermal neurofibromas. Tuberous sclerosis has variable penetrance and is associated with subependymal giant cell astrocytomas, epilepsy, tubers, and autism. Thus, a mother with the disorder may be highly functional but may produce offspring who are severely affected by the disorder. Neurological sequelae of VHL syndrome can occur due to cerebellar and spinal hemangioblastomas. Li–Fraumeni syndrome is associated with the formation of an array of cancers, including rhabdomyosarcoma, osteogenic sarcoma, brain tumors (gliomas, primary neuroectodermal tumors, choroid plexus carcinomas, and medulloblastomas), breast cancer, leukemia, adrenal cortical carcinoma, and radiation-induced cancers. Approximately half of the individuals with Li–Fraumeni syndrome will develop cancer by the age of 30 [42]. Gorlin syndrome is more commonly associated with nevoid basal cell carcinoma, medulloblastoma, and benign boney tumors in the jaw.

For people with these genetic disorders, genetic counseling needs to be offered to couples. Individuals with Li–Fraumeni syndrome also carry the added risk of fertility being affected because they develop cancers early in life, and hence would have undergone treatments for cancer including chemotherapy and radiotherapy. This is the precise population where assisted reproductive methods need to be discussed and efforts for fertility preservation optimized. Recent advances in *in vitro* fertilization techniques offer promise to families carrying these mutations. Pre-implantation genetic testing is a technique by which eggs can be harvested, fertilized *ex vivo*, and then tested for the specific genetic mutation carried by the affected parent. Only those embryos without the deleterious mutation are implanted in the uterus. This technique is an alternative to amniocentesis or chorionic villus sampling which often leads to emotionally challenging decisions regarding pregnancy termination.

Summary

There is surprisingly a huge gap in our scientific knowledge regarding the actual mechanisms by which hormones may affect various brain tumors. The rarity of primary brain tumors in pregnancy makes systematic study challenging. As data from more genomic sequencing projects on the various tumor types is produced, perhaps there will be clues as to why there may be epidemiological data favoring certain kinds of tumors in women. Genetic syndromes associated with cancer and cancer survivors who have undergone chemotherapy and radiation suffer from significant fertility issues, and the techniques by which fertility may be preserved are constantly evolving. The move to more targeted therapies in cancer treatment is promising but the long-term effects of these drugs on women and fertility will need to be explored.

Acknowledgements

We would like to thank Dr. H. Shih, MD (Radiation Oncology, MGH) for information about radiation and pregnancy, and Dr. T. Batchelor, MD, MPH (Neuro-oncology, MGH) for imaging studies and for invaluable information regarding brain tumors in women.

References

1 CBTRUS. CBTRUS Statistical Report: primary brain and central nervous system tumors diagnosed in the United States in 2004–2006 central brain tumor registry of the United States, Hinsdale, IL; 2010; Available at: http://www.cbtrus.org/2010-NPCR-SEER/CBTRUS-WEBREPORT-Final-3-2-10.pdf

2 Michaud DS, Gallo V, Schlehofer B, et al. Reproductive factors and exogenous hormone use in relation to risk of glioma and meningioma in a large European cohort study. *Cancer Epidemiol Biomarkers Prev.* 2010;19(10):2562–2569.

3 Carroll RS, Zhang J, Dashner K, et al. Androgen receptor expression in meningiomas. *J Neurosurg.* 1995;82:453–460.

4 Lentzsch S, Reichardt P, Weber F, et al. Brain metastases in breast cancer: prognostic factors and management. *Eur J Cancer.* 1999;35(4): 580–585.

5 Brinton LA, Bracken MB, Connelly RR. Choriocarcinoma Incidence in the US. *Am J Epidemiol.* 1986;123(6):1094–1100.

6 Custer B, Longstreth WT Jr, Phillips LE, et al. Hormonal exposures and the risk of intracranial meningioma in women: a population-based case-control study. *BMC Cancer.* 2006;6:152.

7 Claus EB, Black PM, Bondy ML, et al. Exogenous hormone use and meningioma risk: what do we tell our patients? *Cancer.* 2007;110(3):471–476.

8 Ezzat S, Asa SL, Couldwell WT, et al. The prevalence of pituitary adenomas: a systematic review. *Cancer.* 2004;101(3):613–619.

9 de Heide LJ, van Tol KM, Doorenbos B. Pituitary apoplexy presenting during pregnancy. *Neth J Med.* 2004;62(10):393–396.

10 Tiboldi T, Nemessanyi Z, Csernay I, Kovacs K. Effect of oestrogen on pituitary blood flow in rats. *Endocrinol Exp.* 1967;1:73–77.

11 Pavlidis NA. Coexistence of pregnancy and malignancy. *The Oncologist.* 2002;7(4):279–287.

12 Simon RH. Brain tumors in pregnancy. *Semin Neurol.* 1988;8(3):214–221.

13 Schlehofer B, Blettner M, Wahrendorf J. Association between brain tumors and menopausal status. *J Natl Cancer Inst.* 1992;84(17):1346–1349.

14 Roelvink NC, Kamphorst W, van Alphen HA, Rao BR. Pregnancy-related primary brain and spinal tumors. *Arch Neurol.* 1987;44:209–215.

15 Glick RP, Penny D, Hart A. The pre-operative and post-operative management of the brain tumor patient. In: Morantz RA, Walsh JW, eds. *Brain Tumors.* New York: Marcel Dekker, 1994; pp. 345–366.

16 The national radiological protection board ad hoc advisory group on nuclear magnetic resonance clinical imaging. Revised guidelines on acceptable limits of exposure during nuclear magnetic resonance clinical imaging. *Br J Radiol.* 1983;56:974–977.

17 Doll DC, Ringenberg S, Yarbro JW. Management of cancer during pregnancy. *Arch Intern Med.* 1988;148:2058–2064.

18 Collaborative group on antenatal steroid therapy. Effects of antenatal dexamethasone administration in the infant: long-term follow-up. *J Pediatr.* 1984;104:259–267.

19 Evans MJ, Chrausas GP, Mann DW, et al. Pharmacologic suppression of the fetal adrenal gland in utero. *JAMA.* 1985;253:1015–1020.

20 Bain MD, Copas DK, Landon MJ, et al. In vivo permeability of the human placenta to inulin and mannitol. *J Physiol.* 1988;399:313–319.

21 Basso A, Fernandez A, Althabe O, et al. Passage of mannitol from mother to amniotic fluid and fetus. *Obstet Gynecol.* 1977;49(5):628–631.

22 Rugo HS, Mitchell MP. Reducing the long-term effects of chemotherapy in young women with early-stage breast cancer. *JAMA.* 2011;306(3):312–314.

23 Cohen-Gadol AA, Friedman JA, Friedman JD, et al. Neurosurgical management of intracranial lesions in the pregnant patient: a 36-year institutional experience and review of the literature. *J Neurosurg.* 2009;111(6):1150–1157.

24 Cardonick E, Usmani A, Ghaffar S. Perinatal outcomes of a pregnancy complicated by cancer, including neonatal follow-up after in utero exposure to chemotherapy: results of an international registry. *Am J Clin Oncol.* 2010;33(3):221–228.

25 Terry AR, Barker FG 2nd, Leffert L. Outcomes of hospitalization in pregnant women with CNS neoplasms: a population-based study. *Neuro Oncol.* 2012;14(6):768–776.

26 Sklar CA, Mertens AC, Mitby P, et al. Premature menopause in survivors of childhood cancer: a report from the childhood cancer survivor study. *J Natl Cancer Inst.* 2006;98:890–896.

27 Amant F, Van Calsteren K, Halaska MJ, et al. Long-term cognitive and cardiac outcomes after prenatal exposure to chemotherapy in children aged 18 months or older: an observational study. *Lancet Oncol.* 2012;13(3):256–264.

28 Wang LP, Paech MJ. Neuroanesthesia for the pregnant woman. *Anesth Analg.* 2008;107(1):193–200.

29 Leslie KK, Koil C, Rayburn WF, et al. Chemotherapeutic drugs in pregnancy. *Obstet Gynecol Clin N Am.* 2005;32:627–640.

30 Oberfield SE, Sklar CA. Endocrine sequelae in survivors of childhood cancer. *Adolesc Med.* 2002;13:161–169.

31 Winther JF, Olsen JH. Adverse reproductive effects of treatment for cancer in childhood and adolescence. *Eur J Cancer.* 2011;47(Suppl 3):S230–S238.

32 Green DM, Kawashima T, Stovall M, et al. Fertility of female survivors of childhood cancer: a report from the childhood cancer survivor study. *J Clin Oncol.* 2009;27(16):2677–2685.

33 Oktay K, Oktem O. Fertility preservation medicine: a new field in the care of young cancer survivors. *Pediatr Blood Cancer.* 2009;53(2):267–273.

34 Green DM, Whitton JA, Stovall M, et al. Pregnancy outcome of female survivors of childhood cancer: a report from the Childhood Cancer Survivor Study. *Am J Obstet Gynecol.* 2002;187(4):1070–1080.

35 Warne GL, Fairley KF, Hobbs JB, et al. Cyclophosphamide-induced ovarian failure. *N Engl J Med.* 1973;289(22):1159–1162.

36 Bines J, Oleske DM, Cobleigh MA. Ovarian function in premenopausal women treated with adjuvant chemotherapy for breast cancer. *J Clin Oncol.* 1996;14(5):1718–1729.

37 Demeestere I, Simon P, Emiliani S, et al. Fertility preservation: successful transplantation of cryopreserved ovarian tissue in a young patient previously treated for Hodgkin's disease. *The Oncologist.* 2007;12(12):1437–1442.

38 Fabbri R, Vicenti R, Macciocca M, et al. Cryopreservation of ovarian tissue in pediatric patients. *Obstet Gynecol Int.* 2012;2012:910698.

39 Wo JY, Viswanathan AN. Impact of radiotherapy on fertility, pregnancy, and neonatal outcomes in female cancer patients. *Int J Radiat Oncol Biol Phys.* 2009;73(5):1304–1312.

40 Batchelor T. Neurooncologic Diseases. In Cudkowicz M, Irizarry M, eds. *Neurologic Disorders In Women.* Issue 491, 1997.

41 Avastin Prescribing Information. Genentech, Inc. http://www.avastin.com/avastin/hcp/index.html. September 2011

42 Shinagare AB, Giardino AA, Jagannathan JP. Hereditary cancer syndromes: a radiologist's perspective. *AJR Am J Roentgenol.* 2011;197(6): W1001–W1007.

43 www.drugs.com/pregnancy/

CHAPTER 14

Neuro-ophthalmology in pregnancy

Linda P. Kelly, Nancy J. Newman, & Valérie Biousse

Emory University School of Medicine, Atlanta, GA, USA

Introduction

Pregnancy creates a unique situation of physiologic changes to support a growing fetus which include alterations that affect the mother's ophthalmologic and neurologic systems. For example, the physiologic increase in corneal thickness and alteration in the shape of the cornea can cause decreased vision and contact lens discomfort. Enlargement of the pituitary gland during pregnancy is usually asymptomatic, but has been reported to cause compression of the optic apparatus, and also sets the stage for potential pituitary apoplexy with postpartum hemorrhage (Sheehan's syndrome) [1–3]. Although cerebrospinal fluid pressure does not change during pregnancy, it can become elevated to over 700 mm of water with Valsalva during labor [1]. There are also systemic changes in pregnancy that could potentially cause neuro-ophthalmologic complications. Fibrinogen and factors VII, VIII, IX, X, and XII and von Willebrand factor increase, protein S decreases and there is decreased fibrinolysis in preparation to manage blood loss during delivery. These changes lead to increased risk of thrombosis. Immunologic changes also occur so the mother's body accepts the immunologically distinct fetus, and immune-mediated problems such as multiple sclerosis may become more quiescent during pregnancy, only to flare postpartum [1].

This chapter reviews the approach to visual signs and symptoms in pregnancy and the puerperium, and highlights specific neuro-ophthalmologic complications of pregnancy and the postpartum period.

Visual signs and symptoms during pregnancy and postpartum

General approach to visual complaints

The general approach to visual complaints should be the same for patients who are pregnant and those who are not. However, the differential diagnosis should be tailored to the specific population, in this case young women. In addition, there are specific conditions that occur only in the setting of pregnancy, such as preeclampsia, that must be given special consideration. Furthermore, the stage of pregnancy plays a role in both diagnosis and management. For example, the risk of venous thrombosis is greater in the third trimester and postpartum period compared to early pregnancy, whereas the teratogenic risks of various medications are most concerning in the first trimester.

Blurry vision/visual loss

The first step in evaluating a patient with vision loss is to determine if the symptom is present in one or both eyes. Monocular vision loss is due to a problem in the ipsilateral eye or optic nerve, whereas binocular symptoms are due to bilateral

Neurological Illness in Pregnancy: Principles and Practice, First Edition.
Edited by Autumn Klein, M. Angela O'Neal, Christina Scifres, Janet F. R. Waters and Jonathan H. Waters.
© 2016 John Wiley & Sons, Ltd. Published 2016 by John Wiley & Sons, Ltd.

lesions anterior to the chiasm or conditions affecting the chiasm or retrochiasmal pathways. Key features on history are the time course and severity of the visual disturbance and other associated symptoms. Patients with blurry vision need to have a comprehensive ophthalmologic examination and visual field testing must be obtained when there is no obvious ocular cause.

Vision loss is often due to problems in the eye itself, such as changes in refractive error or progression of diabetic retinopathy associated with pregnancy. Decreased visual acuity associated with abnormal color vision, a relative afferent pupillary defect (if the defect is unilateral or asymmetric) and a swollen or pale optic disc (although the optic nerve might be normal acutely) suggests an optic neuropathy. A bitemporal visual field defect suggests a chiasmal lesion such as from pituitary enlargement or tumor. A homonymous hemianopia indicates retrochiasmal disease such as stroke [2].

Refractive changes

Physiologic changes in corneal thickness and curvature during pregnancy induce refractive errors. The increase in corneal thickness is thought to be due to changes in the fluid content of the cornea caused by progesterone. This can cause a myopic shift and consequently blurry vision at distance and at night. The alteration in the shape of the cornea can also cause contact lens discomfort, since the lenses no longer fit properly as they did prior to pregnancy [4]. Because these changes are reversible, it is better not to obtain new prescription eyewear during pregnancy and to delay any refractive surgery until at least 1 year after delivery.

Progression of diabetic retinopathy

Patients who have type I or II diabetes prior to pregnancy are at risk for development or worsening of diabetic retinopathy during pregnancy (Figure 14.1). Longer duration of diabetes and poor glycemic control prior to conception and during pregnancy are risk factors for worsening of retinopathy. Additionally, severity of diabetic retinopathy at baseline is a strong predictor of progression during pregnancy. Although pregnancy itself is an independent risk factor for progression of diabetic retinopathy, this can be further accelerated by pregnancy-associated hypertension and preeclampsia. Rapidly improved metabolic control during pregnancy also increases the risk of progression of retinopathy. Close monitoring of diabetic retinopathy needs to occur

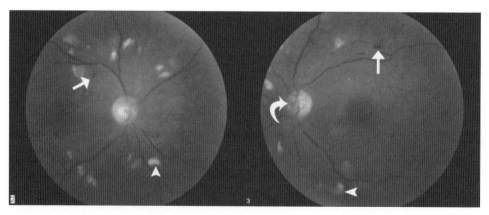

Figure 14.1 Worsening of diabetic retinopathy during pregnancy. Retinal hemorrhages (straight white arrows) and cotton wool spots (white arrowheads) are present in both eyes. The right eye (left panel) also has retinal exudates nasal to the optic disc (gray arrow). The left eye (right panel) has neovascularization on the optic nerve (curved arrow).

during the entire pregnancy and for 1 year postpartum, as there can be continued progression after delivery. On the other hand, women with only gestational diabetes are not at risk for the development of diabetic retinopathy and do not require funduscopic examination during pregnancy [4, 5].

Compressive optic neuropathy from pituitary enlargement

The physiologic enlargement of the pituitary during pregnancy does not usually cause any visual compromise. However, vision loss has been described in patients with pituitary adenomas who become pregnant. This may be partly due to normal enlargement of the gland during pregnancy or tumor growth. Additionally, prolactinomas previously treated with bromocriptine may enlarge when treatment is necessarily discontinued during pregnancy. This can cause uni- or bilateral optic neuropathies and chiasmal visual field defects such as bitemporal hemianopia. These often improve after delivery and medical management is often preferred to surgery during pregnancy unless the visual loss is profound. Vision loss can also occur from enlargement of anterior visual pathway meningiomas during pregnancy, especially if they are progesterone receptor-positive.

Optic disc edema

Optic disc edema can occur in the setting of an anterior optic neuropathy or can be due to elevated intracranial pressure. Disc edema due to optic neuropathy is more often unilateral, but can be bilateral, and is usually associated with central visual acuity loss. Papilledema (disc edema due to raised intracranial pressure) is almost always bilateral, and often associated with symptoms of intracranial hypertension, such as headaches, nausea and vomiting, tinnitus and transient visual obscurations. With papilledema, visual acuity is normal (at least initially) and there is often progressive constriction of the visual field.

The differential diagnosis of anterior optic neuropathies is similar in pregnant and nonpregnant patients. However, optic neuritis occurs less commonly during pregnancy and there is a subsequent increase in the rate of demyelinating events postpartum.

Hypertension

Optic disc edema is present in stage IV hypertensive retinopathy and is usually bilateral. Other signs of hypertensive retinopathy such as hemorrhages, attenuated arteries and cotton wool spots are classically present, but disc edema can be isolated (Figure 14.2).

Preeclampsia/eclampsia

Preeclampsia and eclampsia are specific to pregnancy and can manifest with optic disc edema. Diagnosis of preeclampsia includes blood pressure elevation ≥140/90 mmHg and proteinuria ≥300 mg/24 hours. Eclampsia is the development of seizure and/or coma in a woman with preeclampsia. In addition to disc edema, there are many neuro-ophthalmologic manifestations associated with these conditions (see preeclampsia/eclampsia section below).

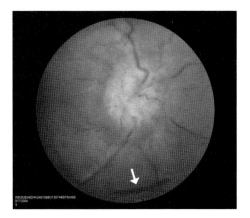

Figure 14.2 Hypertensive retinopathy. There is optic disc edema, blood vessel tortuosity, and pre-retinal hemorrhage (arrow).

Elevated intracranial pressure

Bilateral optic nerve edema always raises concern for elevated intracranial pressure. The differential diagnosis of elevated intracranial pressure is the same in pregnant women as in non-pregnant patients and includes intracranial masses (e.g., tumor, abscess, hemorrhage), hydrocephalus, a meningeal process (e.g., infectious, inflammatory, or neoplastic), cerebral venous thrombosis or idiopathic intracranial hypertension. If there is clinical concern for increased intracranial pressure, a brain MRI should be obtained. If the MRI is normal or only shows signs of increased intracranial pressure, an MRV should be obtained to rule out venous sinus thrombosis. This is a particularly important consideration for women in the third trimester and postpartum when the risk of venous thrombosis is higher. If there is no thrombosis, lumbar puncture to assess cerebrospinal fluid opening pressure and constituents will reveal whether the intracranial pressure is truly elevated and if the cerebrospinal fluid constituents are normal, suggesting idiopathic intracranial hypertension. The lumbar puncture also begins therapy for elevated intracranial pressure from any cause.

Cerebral venous sinus thrombosis

Cerebral venous sinus thrombosis is a critical entity to consider in all patients with elevated intracranial pressure, even when papilledema is isolated. The incidence of cerebral venous sinus thrombosis in pregnancy is in the range of 1/1000–1/10,000 [1]. It can mimic idiopathic intracranial hypertension and this is why MRI (and often MRV) need to be obtained in all pregnant patients with isolated raised intracranial pressure (Figure 14.3). Alternatively, patients may present with focal neurological deficits such as aphasia, hemiparesis, hemianopia, seizure, or altered mental status. It is especially important to consider cerebral venous sinus thrombosis in women in the third trimester and postpartum period.

Idiopathic intracranial hypertension

Idiopathic intracranial hypertension is a syndrome of isolated elevated intracranial pressure. Patients present with signs and symptoms that are attributable to elevated intracranial pressure (headaches, transient visual obscurations, tinnitus, papilledema (Figure 14.4), sometimes with unilateral or bilateral sixth nerve palsy). Cerebrospinal fluid opening pressure must be 25 cm of water or higher, and the constituents should be normal. Any other cause of elevated intracranial pressure should be ruled out with appropriate neuroimaging [6].

It is important to emphasize that idiopathic intracranial hypertension is not more common in pregnant compared to non-pregnant women; however, because it is a disease which predominantly affects young women of childbearing age, it is often seen in pregnant women. Idiopathic intracranial hypertension can be diagnosed at any time during pregnancy, but most new cases occur in the first or second trimester. Signs and symptoms are the same as in non-pregnant patients with idiopathic intracranial hypertension [7].

The management of idiopathic intracranial hypertension can be challenging during pregnancy. Goals of therapy are to alleviate symptoms and preserve vision; therefore, not all patients require treatment. Weight gain should be limited to recommended healthy levels. If medical therapy is deemed necessary, consideration must be given to potential teratogenicity of medications. Acetazolamide is commonly employed for treatment of idiopathic intracranial hypertension and has shown adverse effects in animals, including limb anomalies. However, this medication has not been documented to cause any adverse effect on pregnancy in humans, or to cause congenital malformations, including when started in the first trimester [8]. Loop diuretics can be used with caution for a short period during pregnancy but thiazide diuretics are contraindicated. A short course of corticosteroids can be used in pregnancy, but should be reserved for patients with rapidly

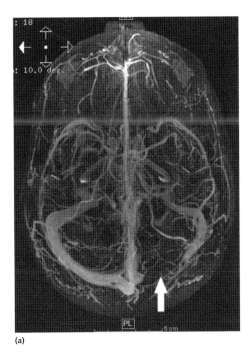

(a)

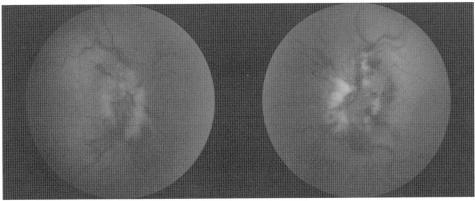

(b)

Figure 14.3 Cerebral venous sinus thrombosis in the immediate postpartum period. (a) Magnetic resonance venogram with contrast showing a filling defect consistent with thrombosis from the torcula to the mid left transverse sinus (arrow). (b) Severe bilateral papilledema secondary to raised intracranial pressure from venous sinus thrombosis. Both optic discs are elevated and there are bilateral hemorrhages and exudates.

progressive visual loss (so-called fulminant idiopathic intracranial hypertension) and should not be prescribed chronically.

More invasive measures are necessary when severe papilledema results in visual field deficits (Figure 14.5) or for intractable headaches. Serial lumbar punctures are often performed in pregnancy. Indeed, it is usually best to try to delay any surgical intervention until after delivery, or at least until the third trimester. Optic nerve sheath fenestration can be performed without difficulty in pregnant patients, as long as the risk

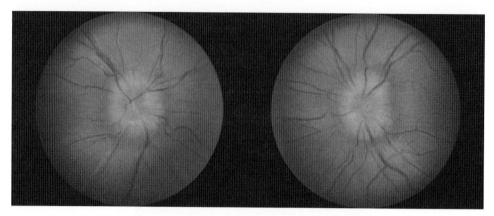

Figure 14.4 Moderate bilateral papilledema in idiopathic intracranial hypertension. The disc margins are blurred and elevated, and the vessels are obscured.

directly related to anesthesia is deemed minimal by the obstetrical team. Cerebrospinal fluid shunting procedures (lumboperitoneal or ventriculoperitoneal shunts) are usually avoided during pregnancy. However, it is usually safe to leave indwelling shunts in place when a woman with idiopathic intracranial hypertension becomes pregnant.

Idiopathic intracranial hypertension does not interfere with pregnancy and these patients have the same rate of spontaneous abortion as the general population. Method of delivery, anesthesia, and analgesia should be based only on obstetrical considerations [9]. Indeed, although vaginal delivery is associated with a severe increase in intracranial pressure, even in normal patients, it is transient and does not alter the prognosis of idiopathic intracranial hypertension.

Diplopia

The first step in evaluation of a patient with diplopia is to determine if it is monocular or binocular in nature by instructing the patient to cover each eye individually. If the diplopia does

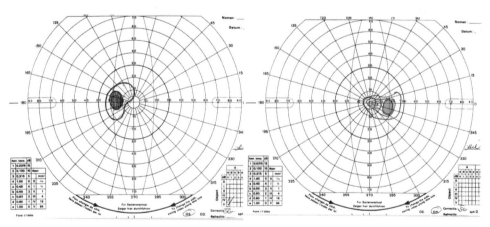

Figure 14.5 Goldmann visual fields showing severe peripheral visual field constriction due to idiopathic intracranial hypertension.

not resolve with covering one eye, it is monocular and due to a problem with the eye itself, such as a refractive error (e.g., astigmatism). If the diplopia resolves with covering either eye, it is binocular and the underlying problem is a misalignment of the eyes.

A logical approach in the evaluation of binocular diplopia is to follow the anatomic course from the eye to the brain and localize the cause of the ocular misalignment. In general, many conditions will be the same in pregnant and non-pregnant patients, although pregnant patients are young, so many etiologies of diplopia are not considered. For example, there may be dysfunction of the extraocular muscles due to an orbital process such as thyroid eye disease, a neuromuscular junction problem, such as myasthenia gravis, or dysfunction of cranial nerves III, IV, or VI anywhere along their course. In the cavernous sinus, one or more ocular motor nerves can be compressed by a lesion in the sinus itself or by external compression from an enlarging pituitary tumor or pituitary apoplexy (Figure 14.6). Cranial nerves can also be affected by aneurysms, such as a posterior communicating artery aneurysm causing a third nerve palsy. In the subarachnoid space, increased intracranial pressure may cause unilateral or bilateral sixth nerve palsies, and meningeal processes (whether infectious, inflammatory, or neoplastic) can affect any of the ocular motor nerves. Cranial nerves, internuclear, or supranuclear pathways may also be affected in the brainstem. Systemic diseases must also be considered for their neuro-ophthalmologic manifestations: a demyelinating lesion of multiple sclerosis affecting the medial longitudinal fasciculus causing internuclear ophthalmoplegia, thiamine deficiency causing bilateral sixth nerve palsies in Wernicke encephalopathy, or the Miller Fisher variant of Guillain–Barré syndrome with its triad of ophthalmoplegia, ataxia, and areflexia. Congenital issues might become manifest, such as decompensation of a congenital fourth nerve palsy.

In any patient who presents with new onset binocular diplopia, there are two entities of greatest concern because of their life-threatening nature: third cranial nerve palsy due to aneurysm and pituitary apoplexy. Careful examination must be performed to assess for features of third nerve palsy, including limitation of adduction, elevation and depression, ptosis and pupil dilation. Pituitary apoplexy often presents with headache, ocular motor nerve palsies, and visual deficits.

Rarely, hyperemesis gravidarum can cause thiamine deficiency and Wernicke encephalopathy (see section Wernicke–Korsakoff syndrome with hyperemesis gravidarum). The classic symptoms include ophthalmoplegia, confusion, and ataxia, but the presence of the complete triad is found in less than half of patients with Wernicke encephalopathy.

Specific neuro-ophthalmologic complications of pregnancy and postpartum

Wernicke–Korsakoff syndrome with hyperemesis gravidarum

Wernicke encephalopathy occurs due to a deficiency of thiamine (vitamin B1). This is an essential vitamin obtained from the diet which acts as a coenzyme in various pathways, including glucose-energy using pathways. Because thiamine requirements are higher during pregnancy and because hyperemesis can cause overall nutritional deficiency, pregnant women are at greater risk of thiamine deficiency and Wernicke encephalopathy. Mean gestational age when this usually occurs is about 14 ± 3 weeks. The onset of Wernicke encephalopathy can be precipitated by intravenous administration of glucose without thiamine [10].

The clinical features of Wernicke encephalopathy are ophthalmoplegia, confusion, and ataxia. However, this classic triad is found in less than half of patients. Visual symptoms are found in a majority of patients,

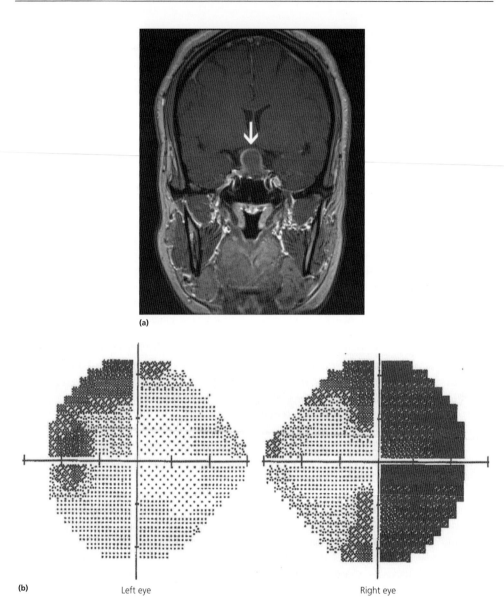

(a)

(b) Left eye Right eye

Figure 14.6 Pituitary apoplexy in the postpartum period (Sheehan syndrome). (a) Coronal T1 MRI with gadolinium shows a sellar/suprasellar mass with peripheral rim enhancement. The optic chiasm is draped over the mass lesion (arrow). This patient presented with acute onset of headache, diplopia, and visual loss. (b) Automated visual field (24–2 SITA standard) showing a bitemporal hemianopia worse in the right eye (the dark areas are not seen).

most commonly diplopia; a few have blurred vision or visual loss. Ocular signs are present in almost all patients, most commonly nystagmus or ophthalmoplegia, especially bilateral sixth nerve palsies. A high level of suspicion should result in empiric treatment with thiamine supplementation [10]. However, full recovery is not achieved in most patients even after treatment. Ocular symptoms usually improve within hours to days, and nystagmus, ataxia, and confusion in days to weeks, but approximately 60% of patients continue to have residual nystagmus or ataxia. In one review of 49 case reports, complete remission was documented in only 29% of patients [10]. In the same study, the overall pregnancy loss rate directly and indirectly related to Wernicke encephalopathy was 48%, with 16 spontaneous abortions, 2 fetal deaths and 5 elective abortions due to the severity of the symptoms, highlighting the importance of prevention.

Preeclampsia/eclampsia

Diagnosis of preeclampsia includes blood pressure elevation ≥140/90 mmHg and proteinuria ≥300 mg/24 hours. Eclampsia is the development of seizure and/or coma in a woman with preeclampsia. Hemolysis, elevated liver enzymes, and low platelets (HELLP syndrome) frequently accompanies preeclampsia.

Visual disturbances occur in about 25% of patients with severe preeclampsia and eclampsia and consist mainly of "spots" in vision, blurry vision, photopsias, color deficits, and visual field defects [1, 5, 11]. The underlying etiologies of visual symptoms associated with preeclampsia include retinal and choroidal ischemia, serous retinal detachment, Purtscher retinopathy, and optic neuropathy. Patients with HELLP syndrome have been reported to have visual dysfunction from retinal vein occlusion, retinal detachment, retinal hemorrhage, vitreous hemorrhage, and homonymous hemianopia or cerebral blindness from intracerebral hemorrhage or occipital infarction. Most visual symptoms of preeclampsia, eclampsia, and HELLP fully resolve within several weeks but permanent loss of vision can occur [5].

Cerebral blindness occurs in about 15% of cases of preeclampsia/eclampsia and may last for hours to a few days, but is classically reversible [5, 11]. This may be due to cerebral vasospasm with ischemic injury or vasogenic edema,

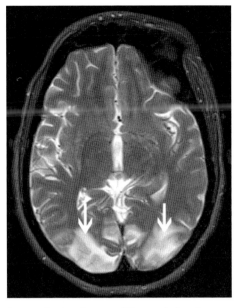

Figure 14.7 Posterior reversible encephalopathy syndrome in a patient with preeclampsia and cerebral blindness. Axial T2 MRI reveals hyperintense areas in the occipital lobes bilaterally (arrows). The patient's vision was normal within a few days after delivery and three weeks later, the MRI abnormalities had resolved.

so-called posterior reversible encephalopathy syndrome (PRES) (Figure 14.7). Disorders of higher cerebral visual function also occur in eclampsia, including simultanagnosia and ocular apraxia, which are features of Bálint's syndrome. Alexia or Anton's syndrome (denial of cortical blindness) might also occur in the setting of eclampsia [1, 11].

Abnormalities on MRI are more common in patients with eclampsia than preeclampsia. The abnormalities in preeclampsia consist predominantly of foci of increased signal on T2-weighted studies in the deep white matter, mainly in the frontal and parietal lobes. In eclampsia, MRI lesions are in the white matter and at the gray–white matter junction, especially in the parietal and occipital lobes, the high posterior frontal region, as well as in the external capsule or basal ganglia [11, 12].

Complications of obstetrical anesthesia

Anesthesia for labor and delivery can be accomplished by several different methods. One is epidural anesthesia, in which a catheter is placed in the epidural space and anesthetic agent diffuses across the dura. Alternatively, spinal analgesia can be used, which involves entry into the intrathecal or subarachnoid space. A combination of epidural and spinal anesthesia is sometimes used.

Horner's syndrome

Uni- or even bilateral Horner's syndrome can occur with epidural anesthesia. It usually occurs on the dependent side on which the patient lay in the lateral decubitus position when the epidural anesthetic was injected and is most likely caused by the effect of the anesthetic agent on the oculosympathetic pathway where the preganglionic neurons exit the spinal cord.

This is usually a benign and transient condition and in most cases spontaneously resolves in an average of 215 minutes (range of a few minutes to 24 hours) [13]. The epidural does not need to be discontinued as long as there is no hemodynamic instability or respiratory compromise to suggest that there is a higher level of sympathetic block.

Cranial neuropathies

Cranial neuropathies can also occur in conjunction with epidural and spinal anesthesia. Transient trigeminal nerve palsy has been documented in association with Horner's syndrome, especially with high cephalad spread of epidural block [13]. Impairment of the sixth cranial nerve can also occur, either in spinal anesthesia or in accidental dural puncture during attempted epidural anesthesia.

Intracranial hypotension

Intracranial hypotension can result from unrecognized dural puncture during epidural placement, occurring in up to 3% of obstetric epidurals [14, 15]. Cerebrospinal fluid leakage through the breached dura causes a postural headache worse in the upright position, and is associated with caudal displacement of the brain. The sixth cranial nerves may be "stretched." Characteristic MRI findings include diffuse meningeal enhancement, subdural effusions, caudal displacement of the brain and optic chiasm, flattening of the pons against the clivus and cerebellar ectopia [16, 17]. Sixth nerve palsies usually resolve, but recovery can take weeks to several months [18].

Orbital hemorrhage with emesis or in labor

Orbital hematoma can rarely occur during labor or with emesis. It can present as an acute orbital syndrome with pain, proptosis, diplopia, and visual loss. Urgent decompression is required when vision is threatened.

Valsalva retinopathy

Valsalva retinopathy describes retinal and preretinal hemorrhages occurring during a Valsalva maneuver. A sudden increase in intrathoracic or intra-abdominal pressure results in a rapid elevation in venous pressure, which may result in intraocular hemorrhage (Figure 14.8) [19].

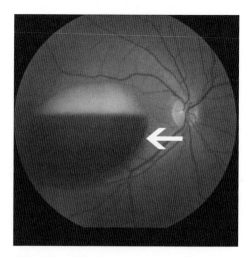

Figure 14.8 Valsalva retinopathy in the right eye. There is a large boat-shaped pre-retinal hemorrhage obscuring the macula (arrow).

Several features of pregnancy make this more likely to occur, including the enlarged uterus causing both increased intra-abdominal pressure and venous compression, and the Valsalva maneuver of labor. Hematologic changes in pregnancy such as thrombocytopenia also increase the risk of hemorrhage. In most cases, the hemorrhages resolve spontaneously and visual acuity recovers with no intervention, but this can take several months. It is also possible to be left with permanently reduced visual acuity if the hemorrhage involved the fovea [19].

Sheehan's syndrome

During pregnancy, there is physiologic enlargement of the pituitary gland. If the woman experiences severe postpartum hemorrhage, compromised blood flow due to hypovolemia can cause pituitary infarction and/or hemorrhage, so-called pituitary apoplexy. Sheehan's syndrome is the term classically used to describe this condition when the underlying cause is specifically enlargement of the pituitary during pregnancy. It may present with acute onset of headache or diplopia or may manifest as isolated pituitary dysfunction in the postpartum period, such as amenorrhea, inability to lactate, hypothyroidism or hypoadrenalism [20].

Reversible cerebral vasoconstriction syndrome

Reversible cerebral vasoconstriction syndrome is a syndrome of segmental cerebral artery vasoconstriction which is by definition reversible when the condition resolves. Patients most frequently present with thunderclap headache, sometimes with focal neurological deficits and seizures. About a third have visual impairment, often elements of Bálint's syndrome. This may occur spontaneously in the postpartum period or with the use of vasoconstrictive drugs [21].

Vascular imaging shows multiple areas of arterial narrowing followed by segments of normal-caliber or distended arteries. While the majority of patients eventually develop ischemic stroke, subarachnoid or intracerebral hemorrhage, or cerebral edema, most patients recover [21].

Postpartum increased risk of cerebral venous sinus thrombosis

Although cerebral venous sinus thrombosis can occur during pregnancy, the overwhelming majority of cases occur in the postpartum period (Figure 14.3). Approximately 35% of cases occur in the first week postpartum, and 60% in the second and third weeks after delivery [22]. It is important to consider this condition when evaluating any postpartum patient with headaches with or without papilledema.

Acknowledgements

This work was supported in part by an unrestricted departmental grant (Department of Ophthalmology) from Research to Prevent Blindness, Inc., New York, and by NIH/NEI core grant P30-EY06360 (Department of Ophthalmology). Dr. Newman is a recipient of the Research to Prevent Blindness Lew R. Wasserman Merit Award.

The authors have no conflict of interest to disclose.

References

1 Digre KB. Neuro-ophthalmology and pregnancy: what does a neuro-ophthalmologist need to know? *J Neuro-ophthalmol.* 2011;31:381–387.

2 Biousse V, Newman NJ. *Neuro-ophthalmology Illustrated.* New York: Thieme, 2009.

3 Inoue T, Hotta A, Awai M, Tanihara H. Loss of vision due to a physiologic pituitary enlargement during normal pregnancy. *Graefe's Arch Clin Exp Ophthalmol.* 2007;245:1049–1051.

4 Dinn RB, Harris A, Marcus PS. Ocular changes in pregnancy. *Obstet Gynecol Surv.* 2003;58:137–144.

5 Schultz KL, Birnbaum AD, Goldstein DA. Ocular disease in pregnancy. *Curr Opin Ophthalmol.* 2005;16:308–314.

6 Biousse V, Bruce BB, Newman NJ. Update on the pathophysiology and management of idiopathic intracranial hypertension. *J Neurol Neurosurg Psychiatry.* 2012;83:488–494.

7 Huna-Baron R, Kupersmith MJ. Idiopathic intracranial hypertension in pregnancy. *J Neurol.* 2002;249:1078–1081.

8 Lee AG, Pless M, Falardeau J, Capozzoli T, Wall M, Kardon RH. The use of acetazolamide in idiopathic intracranial hypertension during pregnancy. *Am J Ophthalmol.* 2005;139:855–859.

9 Digre KB, Varner MW, Corbett JJ. Pseudotumor cerebri and pregnancy. *Neurology.* 1984;34:721–729.

10 Chiossi G, Neri I, Cavazzuti M, Basso G, Facchinetti F. Hyperemesis gravidarum complicated by Wernicke encephalopathy: background, case report, and review of the literature. *Obstet Gynecol Surv.* 2006;61:255–268.

11 Shah AK, Rajamani K, Whitty JE. Eclampsia: a neurological perspective. *J Neurol Sci.* 2008; 271:158–167.

12 Digre KB, Varner MW, Osborn AG, Crawford S. Cranial magnetic resonance imaging in severe preeclampsia vs eclampsia. *Arch Neurol.* 1993; 50:399–406.

13 Biousse V, Guevara RA, Newman NJ. Transient Horner's syndrome after lumbar epidural anesthesia. *Neurology.* 1998;51:1473–1475.

14 MacArthur C, Lewis M, Knox EG. Accidental dural puncture in obstetric patients and long term symptoms. *BMJ.* 1993;306:883–885.

15 Norris MC, Leighton BL, DeSimone CA. Needle bevel direction and headache after inadvertent dural puncture. *Anesthesiology.* 1989;70:729–731.

16 Corbonnois G, O'Neill T, Brabis-Henner A, Schmitt E, Hubert I, Bouaziz H. Unrecognized dural puncture during epidural analgesia in obstetrics later confirmed by brain imaging. *Ann Fr Anesth Reanim.* 2010;29:584–588.

17 Hejazi N, Al-Witry M, Witzmann A. Bilateral subdural effusion and cerebral displacement associated with spontaneous intracranial hypotension: diagnostic and management strategies. *J Neurosurg.* 2002;96:956–959.

18 Loo CC, Dahlgren G, Irestedt L. Neurological complications in obstetric regional anaesthesia. *Int J Obstet Anesth.* 2000;9:99–124.

19 Deane JS, Ziakas N. Valsalva retinopathy in pregnancy. *Eye (Lond).* 1997;11:137–138.

20 Vaphiades MS, Simmons D, Archer RL, Stringer W. Sheehan syndrome: a splinter of the mind. *Surv Ophthalmol.* 2003;48:230–233.

21 Singhal AB, Hajj-Ali RA, Topcuoglu MA, et al. Reversible cerebral vasoconstriction syndromes: analysis of 139 cases. *Arch Neurol.* 2011;68:1005–1012.

22 Cantú C, Barinagarrementeria F. Cerebral venous thrombosis associated with pregnancy and puerperium: review of 67 cases. *Stroke.* 1993;24:1880–1884.

CHAPTER 15

Neurological infections in pregnancy

Shibani S. Mukerji[1] & Jennifer L. Lyons[2]

[1] *Department of Neurology, Massachusetts General Hospital, Harvard Medical School, Boston, MA, USA*
[2] *Department of Neurology, Brigham and Women's Hospital, Harvard Medical School, Boston, MA, USA*

Introduction

Infections of the nervous system are of special interest during pregnancy. This is due to differing epidemiology in this population and also to effects of both the infection and the treatments on the developing fetus. By far, the most important steps to take are preventive, thus obviating the need for concern about these issues. In most cases, simple measures can be employed to achieve this, fortunately, as with many neurological infections, the outcomes otherwise can be dire. Herein we detail the risks, manifestations, treatments, and prevention measures for some of the most common neurological infections occurring in pregnancy.

Listeria monocytogenes

Pregnancy is not generally associated with an increased risk of bacterial meningitis or meningoencephalitis with the exception of *Listeria monocytogenes* [1]. *L. monocytogenes* is a small, facultative, intracellular, Gram-positive bacterium that infects humans via gastrointestinal phagocytosis to disseminate hematogenously after ingesting contaminated foods [1–3]. *L. monocytogenes* contamination of food is difficult to prevent because the bacteria can continue to slowly multiply despite being in a properly refrigerated environment, acidic conditions, or under high salt concentrations [2, 4].

The Centers for Diseases Control and Prevention (CDC) estimates 1660 invasive *L. monocytogenes* occur annually in the United States resulting in 266 related deaths. Of 758 reported Listeria cases in the United States from 2004–2008, 128 (16.9%) were pregnancy-associated [4]. In outbreaks between 1998–2008, deli meats, frankfurters, Mexican-style cheese (queso fresco or queso blanco) involving both pasteurized and unpasteurized milk were determined to be culprits. *L. monocytogenes* serotype 4b is associated with the largest number of outbreak-associated cases with the highest hospitalization rate (70%) and highest case related fatalities (13%) [2]. New research on virulence mechanisms demonstrates that certain mutations in the *inl*A gene encoding for a membrane-anchored protein called internalin can attenuate *L. monocytogenes* virulence. These mutations are prevalent in serotypes that are less virulent but not observed in the serotype 4b isolates.

L. monocytogenes is the most common cause of an infectious rhombencephalitis. Common symptoms of *L. monocytogenes* meningitis/meningoencephalitis are fever, headache, and a depressed level of consciousness. Meningismus is not as common in *L. monocytogenes* meningitis as with other bacterial meningitis or meningoencephalitis. In those with cranial neuropathies, the third, sixth, and seventh are the most affected [5, 6]. In a series of 43 patients with CNS listeriosis, 12% had seizures [6]. The

Neurological Illness in Pregnancy: Principles and Practice, First Edition.
Edited by Autumn Klein, M. Angela O'Neal, Christina Scifres, Janet F. R. Waters and Jonathan H. Waters.
© 2016 John Wiley & Sons, Ltd. Published 2016 by John Wiley & Sons, Ltd.

average duration of symptoms before admission was 3 days and 15% of patients had symptoms for more than 5 days before hospitalization [6].

Clinical presentations in pregnancy vary considerably with fever as the most common symptom. Women may have influenza-like symptoms or be entirely asymptomatic [1, 6]. Maternal infections with *L. monocytogenes* predominantly occur during the third trimester of pregnancy when maternal T-cell immunity is most impaired [1]. In a case series of eleven pregnant women with listeriosis, nine were in their third trimester and two were in their seventeenth and eighteenth week of gestation. The latter two pregnancies ended in spontaneous abortion and early death of a preterm infant. In the remaining cases, six pregnancies resulted in preterm delivery and developed signs and symptoms consistent with listeriosis soon after birth. Three pregnancies did not have evidence of *L. monocytogenes* infection. In eight cases, including infants without evidence of listeriosis, the placenta revealed acute chorioamnionitis [5]. Maternal listeriosis can result in amnionitis, preterm labor, or fetal loss if there is maternal bacteremia, meningitis, or encephalitis. In these cases, the fetus may be stillborn or die within hours as a result of a disseminated form of *L. monocytogenes* called granulomatosis infantiseptica, which results in microabscesses and granulomas in the fetus [1, 5, 7–9].

Cerebral spinal fluid (CSF) analysis will typically demonstrate an elevated white blood cell count (median > 500 cells/mm3) with the majority of cases having a predominance of polymononuclear neutrophils. In most forms of bacterial meningitis, neutrophils account for more than 80% of the inflammatory cellular response. However, in *L. monocytogenes* meningitis, up to 70% of patients had less than 80% neutrophils in the CSF with elevated monocytes counts. The CSF protein concentration is elevated in almost all cases and hypoglycorrhachia was noted in 33% of patients in a series of 43 patients. Gram stain is frequently negative and in some cases may initially point to another

organism, typically Gram-positive cocci. A diagnosis can be made by either CSF, amniotic fluid, or blood cultures and PCR is useful when antibiotic treatment has already been started in cases of preterm labor [1, 3, 6].

Empiric therapy should be immediately started when there is concern for meningitis and in pregnant women should cover for *L. monocytogenes*. This includes a third- or fourth-generation cephalosporin, vancomycin, and ampicillin. High-dose ampicillin is the treatment of choice for CNS *Listeria* infections in pregnancy (200 mg/kg/day or 2 g every 4 hours) for 3–6 weeks [1, 4, 6]. The synergistic and bactericidal effects of adding gentamicin may be desirable in patients with underlying diseases; however, its use in pregnancy is controversial. There is some concern of gentamycin and fetal ototoxicity with a few case reports, while several small cohort studies have not borne out this association [8]. In non-pregnant patients, trimethoprim/sulfamethoxazole is a second-line agent for listeriosis. In pregnancy, its safety to the fetus is unknown and is listed as FDA category C. In cases of bacterial meningitis due to *L. monocytogenes*, allergy testing and/or penicillin desensitization should strongly be considered.

The use of dexamethasone in pregnancy has not been well studied and there is some concern of an association of isolated cleft lip with or without cleft palate or isolated cleft palate if steroids are administered in the first trimester [8]. In late pregnancy, there are few side effects and steroids are used effectively to improve fetal lung maturation for preterm births. The beneficial effect of dexamethasone in meningitis is most apparent in adult patients with pneumococcal meningitis (Class III evidence) and is recommended in adult bacterial meningitis [10–13].

Given the severity of disease, diagnostic difficulty, and poor fetal and maternal outcomes, careful attention to preventive measures for listeriosis is paramount. Two primary strategies for reducing *L. monocytogenes* exposure are decreasing contamination in food supply and health education for high-risk groups, particularly pregnant women. In all trimesters of pregnancy, but particularly in the third, expectant mothers should take care to thoroughly rinse all fresh produce and scrub firm fruits and vegetables (i.e., cantaloupe) with a produce brush, thoroughly cook all meats and keep uncooked meat separated from ready-to-eat foods, and avoid unpasteurized milk and soft cheeses. As *L. monocytogenes* can thrive in low temperatures, refrigerator walls should be kept disinfected and spills, especially from processed meats and/or cheeses, should be promptly cleaned [14, 15].

Mycobacterium tuberculosis

In 2011, there were an estimated 8.7 million new cases of tuberculosis (TB) (13% co-infected with HIV), and 1.4 million people died from TB worldwide. In the United States, a total of 9945 TB cases were reported in 2012 [16]. The disease is one of the top killers of women and is among the three leading causes of death among women aged 15–45 years in high burden areas [17, 18]. TB lesions form in the brain or meninges likely early in infection via hematogenous dissemination of bacilli as part of the primary infection or less commonly as part of chronic disease. CNS TB manifests itself primarily as TB meningitis and less commonly as tubercular encephalitis, intracranial tuberculoma, or a TB brain abscess. TB meningitis develops when *Mycobacterium* lesions communicating with the meninges called Rich's foci rupture and release massive amounts of acid fact bacilli into the subarachnoid space (Figure 15.1) [19, 20].

The diagnosis of TB in pregnancy is challenging as the symptoms can be ascribed to or

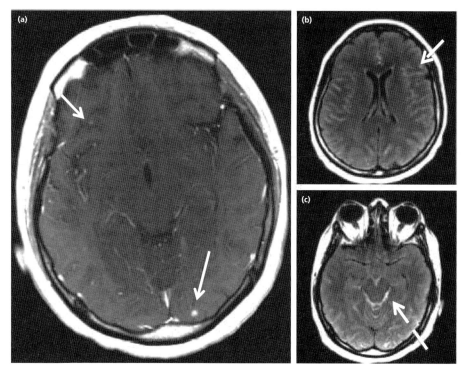

Figure 15.1 Tuberculous meningitis. (a) Axial T1-weighted post contrast MRI demonstrating multiple nodular enhancing regions (arrows) throughout the cerebral hemisphere. (b, c) Axial T2 FLAIR MRI demonstrating diffuse sulcal and cisternal hyperintensities, respectively (dashed arrows).

masked by pregnancy. The weight loss associated with the disease can be hidden by the normal weight gain in pregnancy [21, 22]. Other symptoms include night sweats, evening pyrexia, and protracted cough. In TB meningitis, recurrent headaches and drowsiness with persistent nausea and vomiting can be cardinal signs. The strongest clinical feature of TB meningitis across multiple studies is symptom duration greater than 5 days [20]. Neurological consequences such as paralysis, seizures, hydrocephalus, vasculitis, and strokes are poor prognostic factors [21, 23, 24]. A history of prior exposure or latent TB should be elicited and a heightened awareness should be given to patients with a history of ineffective attempts at antibiotics for viral or bacterial meningitis or refractory headaches [21, 22].

The medical viewpoint on how pregnancy affects TB and vice versa has been widely debated and opinions have varied dramatically throughout the centuries. At one time, recommendations included therapeutic abortions for women with TB [21, 25]. A recent large study found an increased risk in developing TB in the 6 months after pregnancy, but numbers did not reach significance during pregnancy [26]. Other reports have not shown an increased association between pregnancy and active TB [25, 27]. There is strong evidence that mortality is decreased when patients present within 3 weeks of symptom onset and increases with later presentations. However, despite effective antituberculous therapy and younger patient population, between 32% and 68% of pregnant or puerperal women with TB meningitis die [23]. A low index of suspicion is a major reason for delay of diagnosis. The worst prognosis is recorded in women with advanced disease and those with HIV co-infection [21, 23].

The diagnosis of tuberculous meningitis remains the same in pregnant populations as in the general public. CSF findings demonstrate an elevated opening pressure (>25 cm H2O) in 50% of cases, mixed pleocytosis, elevated total protein, and CSF:plasma glucose ratio <0.5 in 95% of cases [20]. CSF Ziehl–Neelsen staining and microscopy for acid-fast bacilli is variable and while larger CSF volumes improve sensitivity, it rarely exceeds 60% [28]. Commercial nucleic acid amplification techniques (NAAT) can be used to rule-in tuberculous meningitis, but is not sufficient to rule out the disease given 56% sensitivity and 98% specificity rates. There is recent evidence to indicate that real-time PCR improves sensitivity with the commercially available Xpert MTB/RIF assay reaching 80% sensitivity compared with cultures from extrapulmonary TB in some studies. However, larger scale studies are required to determine its utility [20]. Magnetic resonance imaging (MRI) is superior to computed tomography (CT) at defining neuroradiological features of tuberculous meningitis. Gadolinium-enhanced MRI enhances visualization of leptomeningeal tubercles, which are present in approximately 70% of adults with the disease [20]. Tuberculomas have variable appearances on MRI depending on its pathological maturation. Non-caseating tuberculomas are usually hypointense on T1-weighted images and hyperintense on T2-weighted images with homogeneous enhancement after contrast administration. Caseating tuberculomas appear isointense to hypointense on T2-weighted images with rim enhancement. Liquefied caseating tuberculomas have a T2-weighted hyperintense core with rim enhancement after contrast administration. Tuberculous abscesses are typically larger than tuberculomas (>3 cm in diameter), solid, thin-walled, multiloculated with rim enhancement after contrast administration.

Pregnancy does not preclude the use of anti-TB drugs as isoniazid, ethambutol, and rifampin are relatively safe to use during pregnancy and are Food and Drug Administration (FDA) pregnancy category C. Little is known about the fetal effects of pyrazinamide. Current guidelines for initial TB therapy should include a four-drug 2-month regimen consisting of isoniazid (5–10 mg/kg orally daily), rifampin (10–20 mg/kg orally daily), ethambutol (15–20 mg/k daily), and pyrazinamide (15–30 mg/kg daily). Breastfeeding should be avoided when on anti-tuberculous therapies [29]. Similar to all neurological infections in pregnancy, diagnostic and management challenges make prevention key. Utilization of droplet protection when traveling to endemic areas or in close approximation to carriers is prudent if overall avoidance is impossible.

HIV-1

HIV-1 (HIV) infection in the United States disproportionately affects men. In 2011, fewer than one-third of new HIV diagnoses in the United States were in women [30]. Given this epidemiology, most study cohorts are predominated by men. However, there have been studies into the relationship between estrogen and HIV, and it has been shown that women with HIV tend to have higher CD4 counts and lower viral loads at seroconversion and have a higher incidence of developing AIDS at similar CD4 counts to male counterparts [31]. Additionally, pregnancy seems to influence HIV progression [32, 33].

In brain estrogen is known to be neurotrophic and neuroprotective as evidenced by its ability to curb multiple mechanisms of neuronal excitotoxicity [34]. As CNS HIV infection involves bystander neuronal damage due to multiple mechanisms including several that lead to excitotoxicity [35], it follows that estrogen may have an impact on neuronal cell death [36]. Additionally, *Tat* and gp-120, viral proteins that are shed from productively and non-productively infected cells such as microglia and astrocytes, respectively, are both directly and indirectly (through provocation of chronic immune activation) toxic to neurons [37, 38]. *In vitro* studies have demonstrated a protective role for estrogen against these toxicities [39–42]. Indeed, there is some clinical evidence to support this in humans, as low estrogen levels seem to increase the risk of HIV dementia [43].

Although clinical neurological disease associated with HIV infection is common [44], acute neurological disease occurring during pregnancy by and large is secondary to opportunistic infection and as such covered elsewhere in this chapter. In one report from 1995 of two cases of peripartum seizure in the setting of undiagnosed HIV, however, Finelli et al. postulated there may be heightened risk during this time [45]. This has been the only report of such an occurrence, although prenatal HIV testing has become routine in the United States since.

HIV-associated neurocognitive disorders (HAND) and distal sensory polyneuropathy (DSPN), the most common neurological manifestations of HIV, are generally indolent. Neuropathic pain relating to DSPN can be managed similar to any pain disorder in pregnancy. There is no evidence that these diseases worsen in the setting of pregnancy, and control of plasma viral load should adequately address these complications. That said, there is increasing recognition of an escape phenomenon in the CNS whereby HIV replication in this immune privileged compartment is disparate from that in the periphery. Manifestations are that of encephalopathy and/or focal neurological deficit [46], and the management approach is to increase the CNS penetration effectiveness (CPE) score [47] and subsequently repeat the CSF viral load to assess resolution. There have been no reports of this entity in pregnancy, but in the scenario where it could arise, management should ostensibly be similar.

Herpes simplex viruses

Herpes simplex virus encephalitis (HSE) is the most common cause of acute, sporadic encephalitis in western countries. The herpes simplex virus (HSV) is a common viral agent with two closely related types, HSV-1 and HSV-2. In a German study, the prevalence of HSV-1 and HSV-2 antibodies in the adult population are 90% and 15%, respectively [48]. Approximately one-third of cases are caused by a primary HSV-1 infection and two-thirds stem from viral reactivation [49]. The clinical manifestations of HSV infections can be more severe in pregnancy and there is a higher risk for dissemination, especially during the third trimester, resulting in skin and genital lesions, encephalitis, cerebral edema, and hepatitis [1, 50].

HSE clinical presentation in pregnancy is similar to the general population with headache, confusion, fevers, seizures, or paralysis. MRI is the superior imaging modality, demonstrating abnormalities 24–48 hours earlier than CT. It can be used safely during pregnancy, and contrast is not required. The diagnosis of HSE is supported by T2 hyperintensities in cortical and subcortical regions of the medial temporal lobes, insula, orbitofrontal, and cingulate gyri. There may be additional evidence of subacute hemorrhages within edematous brain tissue. Restricted diffusion correlates with cytotoxic edema and is present early in disease [51]. EEG typically demonstrates periodic lateralized epileptiform discharges or seizures. CSF HSV PCR is a rapid, reliable test with 98% sensitivity and 94% specificity [52].

The early use of IV acyclovir has produced favorable outcomes for the mother and fetus in HSV infections. Sellner et al. reviewed HSE reports from 1986 to 2006 documenting five published and one unpublished cases [49]. All patients received IV acyclovir, and for the outcomes reported, all mothers and neonates survived. Prior to the advent of IV acyclovir for HSE, high maternal and fetal deaths were reported as seen in the general population with rates exceeding 70% [49, 50, 53]. Acyclovir crosses the placenta and while transplacental intrauterine HSV infection is rare, it has been reported during maternal viremia. Among HSV infections acquired *in utero*, 90% of those identified type are due to HSV-2 [1]. Disseminated infection of the fetus is characterized by skin lesions, cataracts, intracerebral calcifications, and seizures [48].

Mainstay treatment for HSE in the general population and in pregnancy is acyclovir 10 mg/kg every 8 hours for 14–21 days. Resistance to acyclovir is very uncommon in treatment naïve patients with overall prevalence of resistant HSV-1 in immunocompetent hosts estimated to be about 0.3% [53, 54]. Acyclovir resistance stems from viral thymidine kinase mutations in 95% of cases or in viral DNA polymerase genes. These mutations result in decreased or absent HSV thymidine kinase production, altered affinity of the thymidine kinase or HSV DNA polymerase for the active phosphorylated acyclovir.

Varicella zoster virus

Varicella zoster virus (VZV) causes two clinically distinct diseases: a primary, highly contagious infection (primary VZV or chickenpox) and reactivation of latent VZV in the dorsal root ganglia (shingles). VZV is transmitted via direct contact, respiratory droplets or aerosolization of vesicular fluid from skin eruptions, resulting in primary disease [1]. Shingles, or reactivation VZV, is usually limited to a dermatomal rash, often in the thoracic spine. Those with compromised immune systems have a higher proclivity to reactivation VZV.

The incidence of neurological complications associated with varicella is 1–3 per 10,000 cases of primary infection [55] The CNS complications that occur most frequently are cerebellar ataxia and encephalitis, with other less common manifestations including transverse myelitis, meningitis, and Guillian–Barre syndrome. Neurological symptoms include headache, fever, vomiting, and behavioral changes typically one week after a varicella rash, although rash is not required. The CSF is abnormal with an elevated opening pressure, lymphocytic pleocytosis (usually <100 cells/uL), elevated protein and normal glucose. Long-term sequelae include epilepsy and is present in 10–20% survivors. IV acyclovir is warranted in these cases.

Reactivation of varicella can include CNS signs and symptoms, including myelitis, meningitis, encephalitis, and acute or delayed vasculitis with or without stroke; these CNS manifestations may occur regardless of manifest dermatomal shingles. During pregnancy, VZV infections can lead to maternal and intrauterine infection. The latter can result in fetal loss, congenital varicella syndrome, or a perinatal infection when the primary disease occurs in the mother at the time of delivery [56]. The primary neurological features of infants with congenital varicella syndrome include cortical and spinal cord atrophy, limb paresis, seizures, microcephaly, Horner's syndrome, and encephalitis [57].

Varicella infections are rare in pregnancy as 90% of women are protected by virus-specific IgG antibodies [57]. The average incidence of varicella is approximately 2–3 per 1000 pregnancies. In adults, primary VZV infections are associated with pneumonitis, hepatitis, and encephalitis and in pregnancy, there appears to be a higher risk of fatality associated with primary VZV infections. As in herpes virus, the disease is more often to occur in the third trimester with higher morbidity and a greater risk of transmission to the fetus in this trimester [56, 57].

Recommendation for VZV prevention is that seronegative women receive the varicella vaccine before pregnancy. The VZV vaccine is a live, attenuated virus vaccine and is contraindicated in pregnant women, and pregnancy has to be avoided for at least 4 weeks following vaccination. If a non-immune pregnant woman has been exposed to VZV (household contact, face-to-face contact for greater than 5 minutes, or indoor contact for greater than 15 minutes), the VZV IgG antibodies should be measured immediately. If no antibodies are detected or there is an indeterminate response, the intramuscular or intravenous application of VZV immunoglobulin within 72–96 hours is recommended [57].

Lymphocytic choriomeningitis virus

Lymphocytic choriomeningitis virus (LCMV) is a prevalent human pathogen and a cause of meningitis, encephalitis, and neurological birth defects [58]. LCMV is a member of the Arenaviridae family of viruses. These viruses are single-stranded RNA viruses and like all arenaviruses, rodents are their principal reservoir. The common house mouse, *Mus musculus*, is a natural host for LCMV, which is vertically transmitted between generations via intrauterine infection. Hamsters and other pet rodents are also competent reservoirs [58]. LCMV-positive rodents infected transplacentally can be heavily infected but remain asymptomatic because the virus is not cytolytic and there is immunologic tolerance.

Rodents infected with LCMV shed the virus through saliva, urine, feces, and nasal secretions. Humans then typically acquire LCMV by direct contact with contaminated fomites or inhalation of aerosolized virus from rodents. The prevalence of LCMV in humans living within urban areas in the United States is approximately 5% with risk of congenital infections throughout the continental United States [59]. Acquisition of LCMV occurs during any season, most commonly during late autumn and early winter, reflecting the movement of mice into homes during the cold season. Direct human-to-human transmission of LCMV is highly unusual and has been associated with organ transplantation. There have been four clusters of organ-transplant-associated LCMV transmissions identified in the United States in 2003, 2006, 2008, and 2011 resulting in the deaths of most organ recipients [60–62]. Each cluster received tissue from a common donor and it is believed that the severity of the LCMV infection stemmed from significant T-cell depletion due to immunosuppression following transplantation resulting in unimpeded LCMV viral replication [58].

Another more common human-to-human acquisition is through vertical transmission from a pregnant woman to her fetus resulting in congenital LCMV. In LCMV infections in adults, the virus typically enters via an aerosolized form and is deposited into a patient's lung where initial viral replication occurs. When the virus enters the bloodstream and enters other organs, further replications occur. LCMV reaches the meninges, choroid plexus, and ventricular ependymal linings where viral titers are high, and an ensuing inflammatory response occurs [58]. In clinically apparent infections, the incubation period is 5–13 days and is followed by fever typically ranging from 100–104°F, headache, photophobia, and myalgias. Abdominal pain, diarrhea, and rash have been described [58, 61, 63]. Resolution of symptoms is the predominant outcome in most cases. Rarely, after 5–9 days of a convalescence period, a second phase of CNS illness occurs with meningitis or encephalomyelitis, transverse myelitis, parotitis, orchitis, pneumonitis, myocarditis, or arthritis [64]. In those with meningitis, a CSF lymphocytic pleocytosis is seen with cell counts often exceeding 1000 cells/uL, hypoglycorrhachia and mild protein elevation [65]. Diagnostic testing can be performed with CSF samples using LCMV PCR. The typical outcome of this second phase is good, with mortality rate of less than 1%, with patients returning to normal neurological function [61]. Effective antiviral therapy for LCMV has not been identified, and while ribavirin has been used with some success, there is substantial toxicity. In general, it is not recommended during pregnancy due to unknown effects on the fetus.

Unfortunately, it is increasingly apparent that LCMV is an under-recognized abortifacient and fetal teratogen. The incidence of congenital LCMV infection is unknown due to lack of epidemiological studies. As it is not commonly diagnosed, infections during pregnancy may go unnoticed. Congenital LCMV occurs primarily via transplacental transmission and rarely during the intrapartum period through exposure to maternal vaginal secretions or blood. Early first trimester illness with LCMV is associated with an increased risk of spontaneous abortion [66]. Late first trimester and second trimester infections can cause result in congenital LCMV. The virus exhibits tropism for the brain and principal signs are visual impairment and brain dysfunction. In a survey of children in a group home for mental retardation by Mets et al., 4 of the 96 patients examined had chorioretinal scars, 2 of which had positive serum titers for LCMV. In the same study of 14 cases of chorioretinal scars seen in a children's hospital, 4 had positive serum titers for LCMV, suggesting a higher incidence of LCMV infection than previously documented (in 2000, there were 10 documented cases in the United States and 32 cases in world literature) [67].

Cerebral abnormalities due to congenital LCMV infections can produce microcephaly, periventricular calcifications, hydrocephalus, cerebellar hypoplasia, gyral dysplasia, and chorioretinitis. Animal models of LCMV demonstrate infection perturbs neuronal migration in developing rats and the virus infects neuroblasts present in periventricular regions of the fetal brain. LCMV can infect brain parenchyma in fetuses, a factor not seen in postnatal infections. These models demonstrate LCMV infections trigger a profound T-lymphocytic response that further produces tissue destruction and ependymal inflammation leading to blockage of CSF and hydrocephalus [68].

Other infectious pathogens that cross the placenta should be included in the differential of LCMV, including *Toxoplasma gondii*, rubella, CMV, herpetic viruses, syphilis, and HIV. In LCMV and CMV, intracranial calcifications primarily occur in periventricular regions as compared to diffuse calcifications in toxoplasmosis. CMV infection is associated with hearing loss, which is rarely noted in LCMV [66]. The diagnosis of congenital LCMV is either an immunofluorescent antibody test or an enzyme immunoassay to detect specific antibody in blood or cerebrospinal fluid [66]. The mortality rate in a meta-analysis of reported cases of congenital LCMV is as high as 35% by 21 months [69]. As there are no specific treatments, pregnant women should reduce their risk of contracting the virus by minimizing exposure to mice and pet rodents. Pregnant women who work at animal care facilities or laboratories with rodents are at risk for LCMV infections and should wear gloves, gowns, and face masks to avoid aerosolized or secreted LCMV [70].

Influenza virus

Influenza-associated neurological complications affect multiple levels of the nervous system with a wide spectrum of severity ranging between mild to aggressive disease with fatality. Influenza A subtypes are identified by two surface proteins, hemagglutinin (H) and neuraminidase (N), and several of these subtypes have caused several large-scale pandemics worldwide [71]. The single most fatal pandemic was the "Spanish flu" in 1918–1919 resulting from the H1N1 subtype. Isolated virulent strains include H1N1, H3N2, and H5N1 subtypes, with most reported cases originating from Japan and Taiwan [72–74]. However, outside of pandemics, the incidence of neurological complications from influenza in adults is low.

The most common clinical neurological syndromes include influenza-associated encephalopathy, myopathy, movement disorders with extrapyramidal features, transverse myelitis, Guillain–Barre syndrome, myositis, and a post-infectious acute disseminated encephalomyelitis. Acute necrotizing encephalopathy (ANE) is the most commonly reported neurological complication affecting both pediatrics and adult populations. The presentation typically includes a fever with respiratory tract infection followed by a rapid decline in consciousness. On average, neurological symptoms arise within 1–5 days of symptom onset. Multiple other viral illnesses present in a similar fashion, including West Nile, Japanese encephalitis, Eastern equine encephalitis, acute measles encephalitis, and rabies, and as such ANE is not a defining clinical feature for influenza.

Influenza viral RNA is rarely detected in CSF and a negative result does not rule out the possibility of influenza as the inciting cause. MRI findings suggestive of ANE include primarily symmetric diffusion restriction in bilateral putamen and thalami, midbrain, tegmentum, and cerebellar hemispheres [74]. On autopsy, hemorrhagic necrosis with severe edema is seen. There is expansion of perivascular spaces with leukocytes but no other evidence of inflammatory infiltrate. Mortality rates in case series of influenza-associated ANE are 30% with significant morbidity occurring in another 33% of patients.

In April 2009, a novel H1N1 influenza A outbreak started in Mexico which spread throughout the world accounting for six million cases, 270,000 hospitalizations, and over 12,000 deaths [75,76]. This strain was particularly devastating to pregnant and postpartum women [77]. The primary complication in these women was adult respiratory distress syndrome, occurring principally in the second or third trimester. Perez-Padilla et al. reviewed 18 cases of confirmed 2009 H1N1, reporting 100% of patients tested had elevated lactate dehydrogenase, 61% with lymphopenia, 11% with mild thrombocytopenia, and 61% with elevated transaminases [75]. In the first two months of the outbreak alone, six of the 46 deaths in the United States occurred in pregnant women with confirmed or probable H1N1 infection [77].

The diagnosis of H1N1 in pregnancy is typically made by enzyme immunoassay from nasopharyngeal swabs. The sensitivity of the rapid influenza test is 10–70% and negative results do not rule out influenza [78]. Viremia is rare with H1N1, limiting transplacental infections [1]. The majority of fetal morbidity or mortality is secondary to maternal morbidity and mortality. First-line treatment options are neuraminidase inhibitors such as oseltamivir or zanamivir–oseltamivir is preferred. These are category C medications in pregnancy indicating there are no clinical studies to assess their safety [78]. In the case of neurological complications from influenza, these drugs have limited CSF penetration and thus likely limited activity for CNS infections. Additionally, there is increasing evidence of NA inhibitor resistance in several influenza strains. Recent investigation of H7N9 influenza A detected in early 2013 in China revealed evidence of oseltamivir-resistance mutation in the neuraminidase protein in some patients infected with the strain [79]. The high mortality rate of influenza during pregnancy highlights the importance of preventative measures including immunization and early use of neuraminidase inhibitors [80]. The seasonal influenza vaccination in all trimesters is strongly recommended by multiple organizations [78, 81, 82].

West Nile virus

West Nile virus (WNV) is a mosquito-borne flavivirus commonly found in Africa, Europe, Middle East, and Asia and is becoming an increasingly important pathogen in North America. In 1999, a WNV strain circulating in Israel and Tunisia was imported to New York, producing a large and severe outbreak that spread throughout the continental United States in the following years [83]. WNV was first isolated in 1937 from a Ugandan woman and eventually identified in birds where the virus can cause encephalitis and paralysis. Human infection is most often the result of infected mosquito bites and typical outbreaks are on major bird migratory routes. Since its introduction in 1999 into the United States, the virus is now widely established from Canada to Venezuela and has resulted in the largest epidemic of arboviral neuroinvasive disease in US history [1, 83]. In 2012, there were 5674 cases of symptomatic WNV cases in the United States reported to the CDC, but the true number of infections is unknown, as most are asymptomatic and as such not reported [84].

WNV infection is asymptomatic in 80% of infected people. The remaining typically develop fever, headache, fatigue, nausea, vomiting, and occasionally an erythematous, macular, papular or morbilliform rash on the trunk [83, 85]. A small proportion of patients (<1%) develop a neuroinvasive disease characterized by encephalitis, meningitis, poliomyelitis, and/or radiculitis. WNV encephalitis can additionally present with movement disorders including myoclonus, tremor, parkinsonism, as well as seizures [86]. The preferred method of WNV diagnosis is through an enzyme-linked immunosorbent assay (ELISA) of IgM in CSF and serum or IgG antibody seroconversion in two serial specimens collected at a one-week interval. Alternative methods but typically less sensitive (<60% sensitive) than ELISA in immunocompetent hosts for viral RNA detection include reverse transcription polymerase chain reaction or virus isolation by culture [52]. WNV IgM can be detected in CSF and serum of infected patients with neuroinvasive disease at the time of their clinical presentation; however, once positive, serum IgM may persist for more than a year [83]. Finally, there is emerging evidence to support WNV RNA detection in urine as a diagnostic test [87].

Mother-to-infant transmission has been described both prenatally and through breast milk, although the latter is extremely rare [88, 89]. In 2002, a 20-year-old woman was diagnosed with WNV 2 months before delivery. The mother was admitted with flu-like symptoms that progressed to paraparesis. She had serum and CSF WNV-specific IgM antibodies. Her infant was born at 38 weeks gestation with Apgar scores of 6 and 8. The child's ocular exam revealed a large chorioretinal scar in the right eye involving the macula and MRI brain demonstrated lissencephaly, white matter loss in the temporal and occipital lobes, and mild-to-moderate enlargement of ventricles. Serological tests were negative for toxoplasmosis, rubella, cytomegalovirus, LCMV, and HSV. Cord blood, heel stick, and CSF were positive for WNV-specific IgM antibodies [90, 91]. This index case of congenital WNV prompted a WNV surveillance system for pregnant women. In 2003–2004, 83 pregnant women were identified with WNV. Three possible congenital cases of infection were identified, but intrauterine transmission was not confirmed, as there was possibility of intrapartum or immediate postpartum transmission [71]. As such, the CDC recommends that mothers with febrile illness suspicious of WNV infection should be counseled regarding possible risk of transmission during pregnancy and via breast milk [90, 92]. There is no definitive data to suggest that WNV infection during pregnancy results in a higher risk for neuroinvasive disease for the mother.

There are no approved treatments for WNV infection. Ribavirin is sometimes used in WNV, but this has not been validated nor is it recommended, and the drug is contraindicated in pregnancy. The use of intravenous immunoglobulin (IVIg) to dampen viral injury and subsequent inflammatory reaction remains controversial in WNV. There are several case studies of using nonspecific IVIg in WNV, and experimental results from pooled IVIg obtained from Israeli donors who have higher titers of WNV-specific antibodies due to natural exposure exist in the literature [93–95]. To date, there are no consensus guidelines on IVIg use in any arboviral infection.

Preventive measures of using mosquito repellant on skin and wearing protective clothing are the most important recommendations for WNV infection. Pregnant women should be cautious when outdoors during peak season, which is traditionally June through October but can occur in December in warmer climates. If WNV illness is diagnosed during pregnancy, a detailed ultrasound of the fetus evaluating for structural abnormalities should be considered. Amniotic fluid and chorionic villi can be tested for WNV but the sensitivity and specificity are unknown. Infants born to mothers with WNV infection should have serologic ELISA testing within 2 days of birth and repeat testing in 2 weeks if the maternal illness was less than or equal to 8 days before delivery. Infants with evidence of a WNV infection should undergo neuroimaging, CSF studies, ophthalmologic exam at time of infection and 6 months later, hearing screen at 6 months, and pathological examination of the placenta and umbilical cord [96].

Borrelia burgdorferi (Lyme neuroborreliosis)

Lyme disease is the most common tick-borne infectious disease in North America. Lyme borreliosis is caused by a group of related spirochetes named *Borrelia burgdorferi* sensu lato (*B. burgdorferi*), all of which are transmitted by *Ixodes* species of ticks. The burden of disease is concentrated in Northeast and Midwest territories around the Great Lakes but has been documented in Canadian territories of Manitoba, Ontario, southern Quebec, New Brunswick, Nova Scotia and British Columbia, and in Mexico [97, 98]. In Europe, at least five species of Lyme can cause the disease, leading to a wider variety of possible clinical manifestations. *Borrelia afzelii* and *Borrelia garinii* account for most infections in Europe, and *B. garinii* is dominant in Asia. *B. afzelii* is mostly associated with skin manifestations. *B. garinii* is the most neurotropic, and *B. burgdorferi* appears to be the most arthrogenic [99].

Transmission of Lyme borrelia occurs through injection of tick saliva during its feeding, and typically a feeding period of greater than 36 hours is required for transmission of *B. burgdorferi* [99]. Infection of humans elicits immune responses that result in macrophage and antibody-mediated targeting of spirochetes. The same *Ixodes* species of ticks may also transmit *Anaplasma phagocytophilum*, the cause of human granulocytic anaplasmosis, and *Babesia microti*, the etiologic agent of babesiosis. As many as 2–12% of patients with early Lyme are co-infected with *Anaplasma*, and approximately 2–40% of patients are co-infected with *Babesia* [100–102].

Nervous system involvement in Lyme borrelia occurs most commonly as part of the acute phase, affecting 10–15% of individuals [99, 103]. Neuroborreliosis pathogenesis can involve both the peripheral and CNS. The acute phase is associated typically with meningitis, cranial neuritis (primarily affecting the facial nerve), and radiculitis [103–106]. A lymphocytic pleocytosis with mildly elevated protein is typically present in the CSF, along with a history of systemic symptoms attributable to Lyme disease and/or appropriate serology.

Serum abnormalities including elevated white blood cell count, low hemoglobin, and low platelet counts are not typically seen in Lyme unless co-infected with *Anaplasma phagocytophilum*, *B. microti* or tick-borne encephalitis virus. Elevated liver enzymes are seen in approximately 35% of patients in the United States and 20% in Europe [99]. For non-EM presentations, diagnostic testing is enzyme-linked immunosorbent assay (ELISA). If equivocal or positive, a confirmatory IgM/IgG immunoblot is performed. If symptoms have been present for at least 4 weeks, then there should be IgG antibodies present. However, the presence of Lyme-specific IgG antibodies does not mean a patient has active Lyme borreliosis. Rates of seropositivity in endemic areas of the United States and Europe can exceed 4%. Additionally, intrathecal synthesis of antibodies persists for moths to years after successful antibiotic treatment [99]. Thus, treatment is based on clinical features and not solely on laboratory testing.

Adverse events during pregnancy have been frequently cited with other spirochete infections, such as *Treponema pallidum*, the etiologic agent of syphilis, *Leptospira canicola*, the cause of leptospirosis, and *Borrelia recurrentis*, the cause of relapsing fever [107, 108]. Transplacental transmission of *B. burgdorferi* was first documented in a 28-year-old woman who had headache, stiff neck, and arthralgia and was later found to have increased *B. burgdorferi* titers. She remained untreated and gave birth to an infant who died 39 hours later with autopsy revealing severe cardiovascular defects. On histological examination, rare *B. burgdorferi* were found in fetal tissue [109]. In a case study by Markowitz et al., 19 women with Lyme disease during pregnancy were identified between 1976 and 1984. In this case series, 89% of women had erythema migrans (EM), one woman had EM and meningoencephalitis and one woman had facial palsy with fever and without EM. In the case of Lyme meningoencephalitis, the patient was in her third trimester and delivered a healthy infant except for a generalized petechial, vesicular rash, and hyperbilirubinemia. The infant was treated with penicillin G despite no identified pathogen and remained well. In the case of the woman with a facial palsy, she was in her first trimester and had not received antibiotic therapy. At 36 weeks gestation, she

prematurely delivered a 2100 g infant with hyperbilirubinemia but was otherwise normal. In all 19 cases, there was one case of fetal demise in the second trimester. There was no evidence of *B. burgdorferi* infection, but given that one second-trimester abortion in 19 pregnancies was more than expected, the authors could not rule out a complication due to maternal Lyme disease [108]. Several subsequent larger studies have been performed evaluating the effects of Lyme borrelia during pregnancy and pregnancy outcomes. To date, there is no definitive data to suggest that Lyme infection in pregnancy results in a higher risk for neuroinvasive disease for the mother. There remains inconsistent data as to the precise effects of *B. burgdorferi* on pregnancy outcomes [99, 107, 110, 111].

The choices for oral treatment of Lyme borreliosis are doxycycline, amoxicillin, or cefuroxime axetil for 14 days with early localized or early disseminated Lyme or uncomplicated facial palsy in the absence of other neurological deficits [101, 112]. In the United States, parenteral treatment is the strategy adopted for neuroborreliosis with numerous data supporting the efficacy of ceftriaxone, cefotaxime, and penicillin [113–115]. In Europe, studies have demonstrated the efficacy of oral doxycycline for primary manifestations of early Lyme neuroborreliosis with comparable treatment success as intravenous ceftriaxone [113, 116, 117]. As there is no class I clinical trial determining whether oral doxycycline is as effective as parenteral treatment especially in patients infected with US strains of *B. burgdorferi*, the US guidelines continue to recommend parenteral treatment for neuroborreliosis [113]. Doxycycline is contraindicated in pregnancy or during breastfeeding. Thus, alternative oral agents such as amoxicillin are sufficient for EM or isolated cranial nerve palsies during pregnancy while the use of parenteral antibiotics is recommended for evidence of neuroborreliosis [118]. Lyme borreliosis can be prevented by use of tick repellents or avoiding known tick-infested environments. Bathing within 2 hours of tick exposure decreases the risk of contracting Lyme disease. Inspection of the entire skin surface along with the scalp and gently removing ticks close to the mouth with tweezers reduces the likelihood of contracting the disease [99].

Cryptococcal disease

CNS cryptococcal disease ranges from meningitis (CM), which is most common, to focal abscesses (cryptococcomas) often in the deep grey structures, to stroke. A disease of immune compromise and specifically of T-cell immune deficiency, the relative immunosuppressed state of pregnancy may increase susceptibility to this disease independent of concomitant HIV infection, although no definitive evidence for this exists [119]. The most common manifestations in pregnancy mirror those outside of pregnancy and include headaches almost invariably along with varying degrees of altered vision, altered mental status, nausea, and fever. In CM, imaging is often unremarkable but should be included in the diagnostic work up to look for mass lesions and assess safety for lumbar puncture. Definitive diagnosis is by detection of cryptococcal antigen in the CSF; lymphocytic pleocytosis with high protein, low glucose, and high opening pressure are the standard CSF findings.

Treatment during pregnancy is with amphotericin B with or without flucytosine [120]. Amphotericin B is a pregnancy category B drug, but as flucytosine is category C, its use in pregnancy should be individualized based on a careful risk assessment [120–122]. Fluconazole treatment follows, but this may be deferred until postpartum and should be avoided in the first trimester. Serial lumbar punctures may be required for to alleviate symptomatic elevated CSF pressures of >24 cm H2O [120]. Outcomes have been studied retrospectively; in a literature review of 27 patients with CM diagnosed at varying stages of gestation, there were 9 maternal deaths and 4 definite fetal deaths, with the delivery outcomes not reported in 7 cases. Most cases of successful delivery seemed not to have

demonstration of vertical transmission to the child, although this does occur [119, 123].

Molds and dimorphic fungi

A handful of case reports on infections in pregnancy caused by endemic dimorphic fungi and molds pepper the literature [124–128]. The most common mold is *Aspergillus fumigatus*, and although it is an invasive mold in the CNS, which often results in tissue damage and stroke, reports in pregnancy are fortunately limited to meningitis. Dimorphic fungi include environmental molds *Histoplasma capsulatum, Coccidioides immitis, Blastomyces dermatitidis*, and *Paracoccidioides brasiliensis*, which become yeast-like *in vivo*. Infections occur after exposure in endemic areas for the pathogens: histoplasmosis and blastomycosis in the Ohio River Valley; coccidioidomycosis in arid parts of California, New Mexico, Nevada, and Arizona; and paracoccidioidomycosis in South America. The most common neurological presentation is a subacute to chronic, sometimes basilar meningitis in the setting of immune compromise; pregnancy at any gestational age seems to suffice for immune deficiency. Definitive diagnosis if no systemic signs/symptoms are present can be difficult; CSF will show a neutrophilic pleocytosis with very low glucose, but cultures are often negative. (1,3) β-d-glucan from blood and more recently from CSF promises utility, but the latter is an unvalidated test, and notably *B. dermatitidis* sheds very little (1,3) β-d-glucan. Blood or CSF galactomannan is specific for *Aspergillus* and can be helpful in this diagnosis [129].

Management differs in pregnancy than otherwise, as for *Aspergillus* infection, voriconazole is the treatment of choice. This drug is category D, though, and amphotericin B (category B) is instead recommended for all fungal infections. Similar to *Cryptococcus*, adjunctive flucytosine (category C) can be considered in severe cases. Hydrocephalus, when present, must be addressed.

Prevention of these rare neurological infections in pregnancy comes by avoidance of endemic areas. *Aspergillus* is ubiquitous, however. Good hand-washing practices after handling soil is also always prudent.

Toxoplasmosis

Toxoplasma gondii is a parasite that is ubiquitous throughout the world. As such, exposure is common, but cell-mediated immunity protects from devastating infection. However, once exposed, the organism encysts and lies dormant; if cell-mediated immunity wanes—most commonly in the setting of advanced HIV infection—*T. gondii* is able to re-emerge and cause a severe encephalitis characterized by rim-enhancing lesions with often impressive surrounding edema preferentially involving the basal ganglia. Diagnosis is made essentially by imaging characteristics, epidemiology, and response to treatment; also on the differential are bacterial abscesses, metastases, CNS lymphoma, and neurocysticercosis, but biopsy is rarely necessary. Detection of IgG antibodies specific for toxoplasma from plasma is helpful, but polymerase chain reaction on CSF is of low sensitivity [130]. IgM antibodies indicate primary infection, which is important in pregnancy as it can be vertically transmitted to the fetus.

Management of CNS toxoplasmosis in pregnancy is with pyrimethamine, sulfadiazine, and supplemental folate; it also involves addressing concomitant HIV infection. Alternatives for treatment include clindamycin and spiramycin; the latter has poor CNS but high placental penetration, which may be desirable for prevention of vertical transmission in primary infection [130, 131].

Prevention of CNS toxoplasmosis during pregnancy depends on history of CNS toxoplasmosis. Primary prophylaxis is not standard regardless of immune status given the potential for teratogenicity of pyrimethamine and low risk of new toxoplasmic encephalitis. However, secondary prophylaxis is recommended in HIV-infected patients because the risk in this population is much higher [130]. Additionally, pregnant women with baseline immune suppression or HIV should be screened for infection, and anyone with primary or reactivation of toxoplasmosis should be counseled to wait 6 months prior to attempting conception [131]. In counseling for prevention of primary (systemic) infection by toxoplasmosis during pregnancy, patients should be educated not to handle or consume undercooked meat, to avoid handling cat excrement, and to thoroughly wash hands after exposure to soil [132].

Neurocysticercosis

Neurocysticercosis (NCC) is a major cause of seizures worldwide, and so it comes as no surprise that it can pose a problem during pregnancy. This infection is caused by ingestion of *Taenia solium* (pork tapeworm) eggs via a fecal/oral route. Ingestion of infested undercooked pork causes CNS infection only indirectly through fecal/oral autoinfection after establishment of the tapeworm in the intestine of the host. Seizures caused by NCC are typically easier to control in pregnancy than are seizures due to other etiologies [133], and similar guidelines apply regarding antiepileptic drugs (AEDs) in this population as in other pregnancy populations [134–136]. NCC can present during pregnancy and has been reported as being confused with eclampsia [137, 138]. Diagnosis depends largely on epidemiology and imaging (Figure 15.2), as CSF studies and serologies are of variable utility aside from assessing other etiologies of the clinical picture.

Antihelminthic treatment in the nonpregnant population depends on location and stage of disease. Parenchymal lesions are more common than cisternal or subarachnoid cysts, and for calcific parenchymal lesions without enhancement or surrounding edema (implying nonviable organisms), utility of antihelminthic agents is unclear [139]. Rim-enhancing parenchymal lesions with surrounding edema are typically treated with albendazole and steroids [139], in addition to

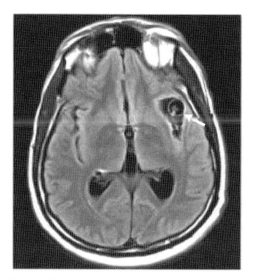

Figure 15.2 Neurocysticercosis. Axial T2 FLAIR image demonstrates cystic lesion with scolex in the left Sylvian fissure (arrow).

AEDs when seizures are present. However, antihelminthic drugs are contraindicated at least in the first trimester of pregnancy and are to be avoided until after delivery. Although these agents are pregnancy class C, they have been associated with increased incidence of infantile eczema [140–142]. This may actually be related to eradication of the helminths, however, as these infections are inversely correlated with development of allergic diseases. Severe or life-threatening cases of NCC can additionally require neurosurgical intervention for hydrocephalus or impending herniation [143].

NCC is rarely contracted in the United States. When traveling to developing countries, NCC can be prevented by avoidance of foods and beverages that could potentially be contaminated with infected fecal material and by stringent hand-washing practices. Raw fruits and vegetables should be washed and peeled or cooked and only sealed, bottled beverages without ice should be consumed.

Acknowledgment

This chapter is dedicated to Dr. Autumn Marie Klein, a phenomenal clinician, esteemed mentor, and wonderful friend. Her demeanor, grace, and intelligence will forever be remembered and remain an inspiration.

References

1 Baldwin KJ, Roos KL. Neuroinfectious diseases in pregnancy. *Semin Neurol.* 2011;31(4):404–412.

2 Baud D, Greub G. Intracellular bacteria and adverse pregnancy outcomes. *Clin Microbiol Infect.* 2011;17(9): 1312–1322.

3 Southwick FS, Purich DL., Intracellular pathogenesis of listeriosis. *N Engl J Med.* 1996;334(12):770–776.

4 Cartwright EJ, Jackson KA, Johnson SD, Graves LM, Silk BJ, Mahon BE. Listeriosis outbreaks and associated food vehicles, United States, 1998–2008. *Emerg Infect Dis.* 2013;19(1):1–9; quiz 184.

5 Mylonakis E, Paliou M, Hohmann EL, Calderwood SB, Wing EJ. Listeriosis during pregnancy: a case series and review of 222 cases. *Medicine.* 2002;81(4):260–269.

6 Mylonakis E, Hohmann EL, Calderwood SB. Central nervous system infection with Listeria monocytogenes. 33 years' experience at a general hospital and review of 776 episodes from the literature. *Medicine.* 1998;77(5):313–336.

7 Bubonja-Sonje M, Mustac E, Brunn A, Deckert M, Abram M. Listeriosis in pregnancy: case report and retrospective study. *J Matern Fetal Neonatal Med.* 2013;26(3):321–323.

8 Chan BT, Hohman E, Barshak MB, Pukkila-Worley R. Treatment of listeriosis in first trimester of pregnancy. *Emerg Infect Dis.* 2013;19(5):839–841.

9 Chaudhuri K, Chang QC, Tan EK, Yong EL. Listeriosis in pregnancy with placental abruption. *J Obstet Gynaecol.* 2012;32(6):594.

10 Fritz D, Brouwer MC, van de Beek D. Dexamethasone and long-term survival in bacterial meningitis. *Neurology.* 2012;79(22):2177–2179.

11 Heckenberg SG, Brouwer MC, van der Ende A, van de Beek D. Adjunctive dexamethasone in adults with meningococcal meningitis. *Neurology.* 2012;79(15):1563–1569.

12 Greenwood BM. Corticosteroids for acute bacterial meningitis. *N Engl J Med*. 2007;357(24):2507–2509.

13 Tunkel AR, Hartman BJ, Kaplan SL, et al. Practice guidelines for the management of bacterial meningitis. *Clin Infect Dis*. 2004;39(9):1267–1284.

14 McCollum JT, Cronquist AB, Silk BJ, et al. Multistate outbreak of listeriosis associated with cantaloupe. *N Engl J Med*. 2013;369(10):944–953.

15 CDC. *Listeria (Listeriosis) Prevention*. 2013. Available from: http://www.cdc.gov/listeria/prevention.html (last accessed 24 October 2013).

16 CDC. *Trends in Tuberculosis, 2012*. 2013. Available from: http://www.cdc.gov/tb/publications/factsheets/statistics/TBTrends.htm (last accessed 15 October 2013).

17 World Health Organisation. *Global Tuberculosis Report 2012*. France: WHO, 2012; p. 1.

18 Mathad JS, Gupta A. Tuberculosis in pregnant and postpartum women: epidemiology, management, and research gaps. *Clin Infect Dis*. 2012;55(11):1532–1549.

19 Prevost MR, Fung Kee Fung KM. Tuberculous meningitis in pregnancy–implications for mother and fetus: case report and literature review. *J Matern Fetal Neonatal Med*. 1999;8(6):289–294.

20 Thwaites GE, van Toorn R, Schoeman J. Tuberculous meningitis: more questions, still too few answers. *Lancet Neurol*. 2013;12(10):999–1010.

21 Loto OM, Awowole I. Tuberculosis in pregnancy: a review. *J Pregnancy*. 2012;2012:379271.

22 Kingdom JC, Kennedy DH. Tuberculous meningitis in pregnancy. *Br J Obstet Gynaecol*. 1989;96(2):233–235.

23 Brandstetter RD, Murray HW, Mellow E. Tuberculous meningitis in a puerperal woman. *JAMA*. 1980;244(21):2440.

24 Ersoz M, Yildirmark MT, Gedik H, et al. Tuberculous meningitis: a report of 60 adult cases. *West Indian Med J*. 2012;61(6):592–597.

25 Snider D. Pregnancy and tuberculosis. *Chest*. 1984;86(3 Suppl):10S–13S.

26 Zenner D, Kruijshaar ME, Andrews N, Abubakar I. Risk of tuberculosis in pregnancy: a national, primary care-based cohort and self-controlled case series study. *Am J Respir Crit Care Med*. 2012;185(7):779–784.

27 Espinal MA, Reingold AL, Lavandera M. Effect of pregnancy on the risk of developing active tuberculosis. *J Infect Dis*. 1996;173(2):488–491.

28 Thwaites GE, Chau TT, Farrar JJ. Improving the bacteriological diagnosis of tuberculous meningitis. *J Clin Microbiol*. 2004;42(1):378–379.

29 CDC. *Tuberculosis and Pregnancy Fact Sheets*. 2012. Available from: http://www.cdc.gov/tb/publications/factsheets/specpop/pregnancy.htm (last accessed 15 October 2013).

30 CDC. *HIV Surveillance Report*. 2011;23.

31 Farzadegan H, Hoover DR, Astemborski J, et al. Sex differences in HIV-1 viral load and progression to AIDS. *Lancet*. 1998;352(9139):1510–1514.

32 Hewitt RG, Parsa N, Gugino L. The role of gender in HIV progression. *BETA*. 2001;14(1):13–16.

33 Hewitt RG, Parsa N, Gugino L. Women's health. The role of gender in HIV progression. *AIDS Read*. 2001;11(1):29–33.

34 Simpkins JW, Singh M. More than a decade of estrogen neuroprotection. *Alzheimers Dement*. 2008;4(1 Suppl 1):S131–136.

35 Bell JE. An update on the neuropathology of HIV in the HAART era. *Histopathology*. 2004;45(6):549–559.

36 Wilson ME, Dimayuga FO, Reed JL, et al. Immune modulation by estrogens: role in CNS HIV-1 infection. *Endocrine*. 2006;29(2):289–297.

37 Gonzalez-Scarano F, Martin-Garcia J. The neuropathogenesis of AIDS. *Nat Rev Immunol*. 2005;5(1):69–81.

38 Yadav A, Collman RG. CNS inflammation and macrophage/microglial biology associated with HIV-1 infection. *J Neuroimmune Pharmacol*. 2009;4(4):430–447.

39 Turchan J, Anderson C, Hauser KF, et al. Estrogen protects against the synergistic toxicity by HIV proteins, methamphetamine and cocaine. *BMC Neurosci*. 2001;2:3.

40 Kendall SL, Anderson CF, Nath A, et al. Gonadal steroids differentially modulate neurotoxicity of HIV and cocaine: testosterone and ICI 182,780 sensitive mechanism. *BMC Neurosci*. 2005;6:40.

41 Howard SA, Brooke SM, Sapolsky RM. Mechanisms of estrogenic protection against gp120-induced neurotoxicity. *Exp Neurol*. 2001;168(2):385–391.

42 Zemlyak I, Brooke SM, Sapolsky RM. Protection against gp120-induced neurotoxicity by an array of estrogenic steroids. *Brain Res*. 2002;958(2):272–276.

43 Clark RA, Bessinger R. Clinical manifestations and predictors of survival in older women infected with HIV. *J Acquir Immune Defic Syndr Hum Retrovirol*. 1997;15(5):341–345.

44 McArthur JC, Steiner J, Sacktor N, Nath A. Human immunodeficiency virus-associated neurocognitive disorders: Mind the gap. *Ann Neurol.* 2010;67(6):699–714.

45 Finelli PF, Gonzalez JA. Peripartum seizure and HIV infection. *Pediatr AIDS HIV Infect.* 1995;6(6):354–355.

46 Peluso MJ, Ferretti F, Peterson J, et al. Cerebrospinal fluid HIV escape associated with progressive neurologic dysfunction in patients on antiretroviral therapy with well controlled plasma viral load. *AIDS.* 2012;26(14): 1765–1774.

47 Letendre SL, Ellis RJ, Ances BM, McCutchan JA. Neurologic complications of HIV disease and their treatment. *Top HIV Med.* 2010;18(2): 45–55.

48 Sauerbrei A, Wutzler P. Herpes simplex and varicella-zoster virus infections during pregnancy: current concepts of prevention, diagnosis and therapy. Part 1: herpes simplex virus infections. *Med Microbiol Immunol (Berl).* 2007;196(2):89–94.

49 Sellner J, Buonomano R, Nedeltchev K, et al. A case of maternal herpes simplex virus encephalitis during late pregnancy. *Nat Clin Pract Neurol.* 2009;5(1):51–56.

50 Sappenfield E, Jamieson DJ, Kourtis AP. Pregnancy and susceptibility to infectious diseases. *Infect Dis Obstet Gynecol.* 2013;2013: 752–852.

51 Duckworth JL, Hawley JS, Riedy G, Landau ME. Magnetic resonance restricted diffusion resolution correlates with clinical improvement and response to treatment in herpes simplex encephalitis. *Neurocritical care.* 2005;3(3):251–253.

52 Debiasi RL, Tyler KL. Molecular methods for diagnosis of viral encephalitis. *Clin Microbiol Rev.* 2004;17(4):903–925, table of contents.

53 Schulte EC, Sauerbrei A, Hoffmann D, Zimmer C, Hemmer B, Mühlau M. Acyclovir resistance in herpes simplex encephalitis. *Ann Neurol.* 2010;67(6):830–833.

54 Sauerbrei A, Bohn K, Heim A, et al. Novel resistance-associated mutations of thymidine kinase and DNA polymerase genes of herpes simplex virus type 1 and type 2. *Antivir Ther.* 2011;16(8):1297–1308.

55 Gnann JW Jr. Varicella-zoster virus: atypical presentations and unusual complications. *J Infect Dis.* 2002;186(Suppl 1):S91–S98.

56 Daley AJ, Thorpe S, Garland SM., Varicella and the pregnant woman: prevention and management. *Aust N Z J Obstet Gynaecol.* 2008;48(1):26–33.

57 Sauerbrei A, Wutzler P. Herpes simplex and varicella-zoster virus infections during pregnancy: current concepts of prevention, diagnosis and therapy. Part 2: Varicella-zoster virus infections. *Med Microbiol Immunol (Berl).* 2007;196(2):95–102.

58 Bonthius DJ. Lymphocytic choriomeningitis virus: an underrecognized cause of neurologic disease in the fetus, child, and adult. *Semin Pediatr Neurol.* 2012;19(3):89–95.

59 Centers for Disease Control and Prevention. Lymphocytic choriomeningitis virus infection in organ transplant recipients–Massachusetts, Rhode Island, 2005. *MMWR Morb Mortal Wkly Rep.* 2005;54(21):537–539.

60 Macneil A, Ströher U, Farnon E, et al. Solid organ transplant-associated lymphocytic choriomeningitis, United States, 2011. *Emerg Infect Dis.* 2012;18(8):1256–1262.

61 Fischer SA, Graham MB, Kuehnert MJ, et al. Transmission of lymphocytic choriomeningitis virus by organ transplantation. *N Engl J Med.* 2006;354(21):2235–2249.

62 Centers for Disease Control and Prevention. Brief report: Lymphocytic choriomeningitis virus transmitted through solid organ transplantation–Massachusetts, 2008. *MMWR Morb Mortal Wkly Rep.* 2008;57(29):799–801.

63 Armstrong D, Fortner JG, Rowe WP, Parker JC. Meningitis due to lymphocytic choriomeningitis virus endemic in a hamster colony. *JAMA.* 1969;209(2):265–267.

64 Baum SG, Lewis AM Jr, Rowe WP, Huebner RJ. Epidemic nonmeningitic lymphocyticchoriomeningitis-virus infection. An outbreak in a population of laboratory personnel. *N Engl J Med.* 1966;274(17):934–936.

65 Asnis DS, Muana O, Kim do G, et al. Lymphocytic choriomeningitis virus meningitis, New York, NY, USA, 2009. *Emerg Infect Dis.* 2010;16(2):328–330.

66 Jamieson DJ, Kourtis AP, Bell M, Rasmussen SA. Lymphocytic choriomeningitis virus: an emerging obstetric pathogen? *Am J Obstet Gynecol.* 2006;194(6):1532–1536.

67 Mets MB, Barton LL, Khan AS, Ksiazek TG. Lymphocytic choriomeningitis virus: an underdiagnosed cause of congenital chorioretinitis. *Am J Ophthalmol.* 2000;130(2):209–215.

68 Bonthius DJ, Perlman S. Congenital viral infections of the brain: lessons learned from lymphocytic choriomeningitis virus in the neonatal rat. *PLoS Pathog.* 2007;3(11):e149.

69 Wright R, Johnson D, Neumann M, et al. Congenital lymphocytic choriomeningitis virus syndrome: a disease that mimics congenital toxoplasmosis or Cytomegalovirus infection. *Pediatrics.* 1997;100(1):E9.

70 Centers for Disease Control and Prevention. Notes from the field: lymphocytic choriomeningitis virus infections in employees of a rodent breeding facility–Indiana, May-June 2012. *MMWR Morb Mortal Wkly Rep.* 2012;61(32):622–623.

71 Theiler RN, Rasmussen SA, Treadwell TA, Jamieson DJ. Emerging and zoonotic infections in women. *Infect Dis Clin North Am.* 2008;22(4):755–772, vii–viii.

72 Glaser CA, Winter K, DuBray K, et al. A population-based study of neurologic manifestations of severe influenza A(H1N1)pdm09 in California. *Clin Infect Dis.* 2012;55(4):514–520.

73 Okumura A, Nakagawa S, Kawashima H, et al. Severe form of encephalopathy associated with 2009 pandemic influenza A (H1N1) in Japan. *J Clin Virol.* 2013;56(1):25–30.

74 Tsai JP, Baker AJ. Influenza-associated neurological complications. *Neurocritical care.* 2013;18(1):118–130.

75 Perez-Padilla R, de la Rosa-Zamboni D, Ponce de Leon S, et al. Pneumonia and respiratory failure from swine-origin influenza A (H1N1) in Mexico. *N Engl J Med.* 2009;361(7):680–689.

76 CDC. *H1N1 flu.* 2009. Available from: http://www.cdc.gov/h1n1flu/general_info.htm (last accessed 11 September 2013).

77 Mangtani P, Mak TK, Pfeifer D. Pandemic H1N1 infection in pregnant women in the USA. *Lancet.* 2009;374(9688):429–430.

78 CDC. Updated interim recommendations for obstetric health care providers related to use of antiviral medications in the treatment and prevention of influenza for the 2009–2010 season. 2009. Available from: http://www.cdc.gov/h1n1flu/pregnancy/antiviral_messages.htm (last accessed 11 September 2013).

79 Hu Y, Lu S, Song Z, et al. Association between adverse clinical outcome in human disease caused by novel influenza A H7N9 virus and sustained viral shedding and emergence of antiviral resistance. *Lancet.* 2013;381(9885):2273–2279.

80 Jamieson DJ, Honein MA, Rasmussen SA, et al. H1N1 2009 influenza virus infection during pregnancy in the USA. *Lancet.* 2009;374(9688):451–458.

81 American College of Obstetricians and Gynecologists Committee on Obstetric Practice. ACOG Committee Opinion No. 468: Influenza vaccination during pregnancy. *Obstet Gynecol.* 2010;116(4):1006–1007.

82 Advisory Committee on Immunization, P. Prevention and control of influenza with vaccines: interim recommendations of the Advisory Committee on Immunization Practices (ACIP), 2013. *MMWR Morb Mortal Wkly Rep.* 2013;62(18):356.

83 WHO. *West Nile Virus.* 2011. Available from: http://www.who.int/mediacentre/factsheets/fs354/en/ (last accessed 15 October 2013).

84 CDC. West Nile virus disease cases and presumptive viremic blood donors reported to ArboNET, United States, 2012. 2012. Available from: http://www.cdc.gov/westnile/statsMaps/finalMapsData/data/2012WNVHumanInfectionsbyState.pdf (last accessed 15 October 2015).

85 Tsai J, Nagel MA, Gilden D. Skin rash in meningitis and meningoencephalitis. *Neurology.* 2013;80(19):1808–1811.

86 Sejvar JJ, Haddad MB, Tierney BC, et al. Neurologic manifestations and outcome of West Nile virus infection. *JAMA.* 2003;290(4):511–515.

87 Barzon L, Pacenti M, Franchin E, et al. Excretion of West Nile virus in urine during acute infection. *J Infect Dis.* 2013;208(7):1086–1092.

88 Centers for Disease Control and Prevention. Possible West Nile virus transmission to an infant through breast-feeding–Michigan, 2002. *MMWR Morb Mortal Wkly Rep.* 2002;51(39):877–878.

89 Hinckley AF, O'Leary DR, Hayes EB. Transmission of West Nile virus through human breast milk seems to be rare. *Pediatrics.* 2007;119(3):e666–e671.

90 Centers for Disease Control and Prevention. Intrauterine West Nile virus infection–New York, 2002. *JAMA.* 2003;289(3):295–296.

91 Alpert SG, Fergerson J, Noel LP. Intrauterine West Nile virus: ocular and systemic findings. *Am J Ophthalmol.* 2003;136(4):733–735.

92 Centers for Disease Control and Prevention. Intrauterine West Nile virus infection–New York, 2002. *MMWR Morb Mortal Wkly Rep.* 2002;51(50):1135–1136.

93 Haley M, Retter AS, Fowler D, Gea-Banacloche J, O'Grady NP. The role for intravenous

immunoglobulin in the treatment of West Nile virus encephalitis. *Clin Infect Dis.* 2003;37(6):e88–e90.

94 Ben-Nathan D, Gershoni-Yahalom O, Samina I, et al. Using high titer West Nile intravenous immunoglobulin from selected Israeli donors for treatment of West Nile virus infection. *BMC Infect Dis.* 2009;9:18.

95 Makhoul B, Braun E, Herskovitz M, Ramadan R, Hadad S, Norberto K. Hyperimmune gammaglobulin for the treatment of West Nile virus encephalitis. *Isr Med Assoc J.* 2009;11(3):151–153.

96 Centers for Disease Control and Prevention. Interim guidelines for the evaluation of infants born to mothers infected with West Nile virus during pregnancy. *MMWR Morb Mortal Wkly Rep.* 2004;53(7):154–157.

97 Gordillo-Perez G, Torres J, Solórzano-Santos F, et al. Borrelia burgdorferi infection and cutaneous Lyme disease, Mexico. *Emerg Infect Dis.* 2007;13(10):1556–1558.

98 Aenishaenslin C, Hongoh V, Cissé HD, et al. Multi-criteria decision analysis as an innovative approach to managing zoonoses: results from a study on Lyme disease in Canada. *BMC Public Health.* 2013;13(1):897.

99 Stanek G, Wormser GP, Gray J, Strle F. Lyme borreliosis. *Lancet.* 2012;379(9814):461–473.

100 Wormser GP. Clinical practice. Early Lyme disease. *N Engl J Med.* 2006;354(26):2794–2801.

101 Wormser GP, Dattwyler RJ, Shapiro ED, et al. The clinical assessment, treatment, and prevention of lyme disease, human granulocytic anaplasmosis, and babesiosis: clinical practice guidelines by the Infectious Diseases Society of America. *Clin Infect Dis.* 2006;43(9):1089–1134.

102 Steere AC, McHugh G, Suarez C, Hoitt J, Damle N, Sikand VK. Prospective study of coinfection in patients with erythema migrans. *Clin Infect Dis.* 2003;36(8):1078–1081.

103 Pachner AR, Steiner I. Lyme neuroborreliosis: infection, immunity, and inflammation. *Lancet Neurol.* 2007;6(6):544–552.

104 Zajkowska J, Lewczuk P, Strle F, Stanek G. Lyme borreliosis: from pathogenesis to diagnosis and treatment. *Clin Dev Immunol.* 2012;2012:231657.

105 Miklossy J. Chronic or late lyme neuroborreliosis: analysis of evidence compared to chronic or late neurosyphilis. *Open Neurol J.* 2012;6:146–157.

106 Pachner AR. Do we need to broaden the spectrum of Lyme neuroborreliosis? *J Neurol Sci.* 2010;295(1–2):8–9.

107 Elliott DJ, Eppes SC, Klein JD. Teratogen update: Lyme disease. *Teratology.* 2001;64(5):276–281.

108 Markowitz LE, Steere AC, Benach JL, Slade JD, Broome CV. Lyme disease during pregnancy. *JAMA.* 1986;255(24):3394–3396.

109 Schlesinger PA, Duray PH, Burke BA, Steere AC, Stillman MT. Maternal-fetal transmission of the Lyme disease spirochete, Borrelia burgdorferi *Ann Intern Med.* 1985;103(1):67–68.

110 Lakos A, Solymosi N. Maternal Lyme borreliosis and pregnancy outcome. *Int J Infect Dis.* 2010;14(6):e494–498.

111 Strobino BA, Williams CL, Abid S, Chalson R, Spierling P. Lyme disease and pregnancy outcome: a prospective study of two thousand prenatal patients. *Am J Obstet Gynecol.* 1993;169(2 Pt 1):367–374.

112 Halperin JJ, Shapiro ED, Logigian E, et al. Practice parameter: treatment of nervous system Lyme disease (an evidence-based review): report of the Quality Standards Subcommittee of the American Academy of Neurology. *Neurology.* 2007;69(1):91–102.

113 Halperin JJ, Shapiro ED, Logigian E, et al. Practice parameter: treatment of nervous system Lyme disease (an evidence-based review): report of the Quality Standards Subcommittee of the American Academy of Neurology. *Neurology.* 2007;69(1):91–102.

114 Pfister HW, Preac-Mursic V, Wilske B, Schielke E, Sörgel F, Einhäupl KM. Randomized comparison of ceftriaxone and cefotaxime in Lyme neuroborreliosis. *J Infect Dis.* 1991;163(2):311–318.

115 Pfister HW, Preac-Mursic V, Wilske B, Einhäupl KM. Cefotaxime vs penicillin G for acute neurologic manifestations in Lyme borreliosis. A prospective randomized study. *Arch Neurol.* 1989;46(11):1190–1194.

116 Borg R, Dotevall L, Hagberg L, et al. Intravenous ceftriaxone compared with oral doxycycline for the treatment of Lyme neuroborreliosis. *Scand J Infect Dis.* 2005;37(6–7):449–454.

117 Dotevall L, Hagberg L. Successful oral doxycycline treatment of Lyme disease-associated facial palsy and meningitis. *Clin Infect Dis.* 1999;28(3):569–574.

118 Alexander JM, Cox SM, Lyme disease and pregnancy. *Infect Dis Obstet Gynecol.* 1995;3(6):256–261.

119 Costa ML, Souza JP, Oliveira Neto AF, Pinto E Silva JL. Cryptococcal meningitis in HIV negative pregnant women: case report and

review of literature. *Rev Inst Med Trop Sao Paulo*. 2009;51(5):289–294.

120 Perfect JR, Dismukes WE, Dromer F, et al. Clinical practice guidelines for the management of cryptococcal disease: 2010 update by the infectious diseases society of America. *Clin Infect Dis*. 2010;50(3):291–322.

121 Jarvis JN, Govender N, Chiller T, et al. Cryptococcal antigen screening and preemptive therapy in patients initiating antiretroviral therapy in resource-limited settings: a proposed algorithm for clinical implementation. *J Int Assoc Physicians AIDS Care (Chic)*. 2012;11(6): 374–379.

122 Nayak SU, Talwani R, Gilliam B, Taylor G, Ghosh M. Cryptococcal meningitis in an HIV-positive pregnant woman. *J Int Assoc Physicians AIDS Care (Chic)*. 2011;10(2):79–82.

123 Sirinavin S, Intusoma U, Tuntirungsee S. Mother-to-child transmission of cryptococcus neoformans. *Pediatr Infect Dis J*. 2004;23(3):278–279.

124 Pagliano P, Attanasio V, Fusco U, Rossi M, Scarano F, Faella FS. Pulmonary aspergillosis with possible cerebral involvement in a previously healthy pregnant woman. *J Chemother*. 2004;16(6):604–607.

125 Wack EE, Ampel NM, Galgiani JN, Bronnimann DA. Coccidioidomycosis during pregnancy. An analysis of ten cases among 47,120 pregnancies. *Chest*. 1988;94(2):376–379.

126 Peterson CM, Johnson SL, Kelly JV, Kelly PC. Coccidioidal meningitis and pregnancy: a case report. *Obstet Gynecol*. 1989;73(5 Pt 2):835–836.

127 Patel S, Lee RH. The case of the sinister spores: the patient was hospitalized for a menacing infection in the second trimester of pregnancy. *Am J Obstet Gynecol*. 2013;208(5):417 e1.

128 Whitt SP, Koch GA, Fender B, Ratnasamy N, Everett ED. Histoplasmosis in pregnancy: case series and report of transplacental transmission. *Arch Intern Med*. 2004;164(4):454–458.

129 De Pauw B, Walsh TJ, Donnelly JP, et al. Revised definitions of invasive fungal disease from the European Organization for Research and Treatment of Cancer/Invasive Fungal Infections Cooperative Group and the National Institute of Allergy and Infectious Diseases Mycoses Study Group (EORTC/MSG) Consensus Group. *Clin Infect Dis*. 2008;46(12): 1813–1821.

130 Nath A, Sinai AP. Cerebral Toxoplasmosis. *Curr Treat Options Neurol*. 2003;5(1):3–12.

131 Paquet C, Yudin MH. Toxoplasmosis in pregnancy: prevention, screening, and treatment. *J Obstet Gynaecol Can*. 2013;35(1):78–79.

132 Di Mario S, Basevi V, Gagliotti C, et al. Prenatal education for congenital toxoplasmosis. *Cochrane Database Syst Rev*. 2013;2:CD006171.

133 Pandian JD, Venkateswaralu K, Thomas SV, Sarma PS. Maternal and fetal outcome in women with epilepsy associated with neurocysticercosis. *Epileptic Disord*. 2007;9(3):285–291.

134 Harden CL, Hopp J, Ting TY, et al. Practice parameter update: management issues for women with epilepsy–focus on pregnancy (an evidence-based review): obstetrical complications and change in seizure frequency: report of the Quality Standards Subcommittee and Therapeutics and Technology Assessment Subcommittee of the American Academy of Neurology and American Epilepsy Society. *Neurology*. 2009;73(2):126–132.

135 Harden CL, Meador KJ, Pennell PB, et al. Practice parameter update: management issues for women with epilepsy–focus on pregnancy (an evidence-based review): teratogenesis and perinatal outcomes: report of the Quality Standards Subcommittee and Therapeutics and Technology Assessment Subcommittee of the American Academy of Neurology and American Epilepsy Society. *Neurology*. 2009;73(2): 133–141.

136 Harden CL, Pennell PB, Koppel BS, et al. Practice parameter update: management issues for women with epilepsy–focus on pregnancy (an evidence-based review): vitamin K, folic acid, blood levels, and breastfeeding: report of the Quality Standards Subcommittee and Therapeutics and Technology Assessment Subcommittee of the American Academy of Neurology and American Epilepsy Society. *Neurology*. 2009;73(2):142– 149.

137 Grondin L, D'Angelo R, Thomas J, Pan PH. Neurocysticercosis masquerading as eclampsia. *Anesthesiology*. 2006;105(5):1056–1058.

138 Singhal SR, Nanda S, Singhal SK. Neurocysticercosis as an important differential of seizures in pregnancy: two case reports. *J Med Case Rep*. 2011;5:206.

139 Baird RA, Wiebe S, Zunt JR, Halperin JJ, Gronseth G, Roos KL. Evidence-based guideline: treatment of parenchymal neurocysticercosis: report of the Guideline Development Subcommittee of the American Academy of Neurology. *Neurology*. 2013;80(15):1424–1429.

140 Webb EL, Mawa PA, Ndibazza J, et al. Effect of single-dose anthelmintic treatment during pregnancy on an infant's response to immunisation and on susceptibility to infectious diseases in infancy: a randomised, double-blind, placebo-controlled trial. *Lancet.* 2011;377(9759): 52–62.

141 Mpairwe H, Webb EL, Muhangi L, et al. Anthelminthic treatment during pregnancy is associated with increased risk of infantile eczema: randomised-controlled trial results. *Pediatr Allergy Immunol.* 2011;22(3):305–312.

142 Elliott AM, Ndibazza J, Mpairwe H, et al. Treatment with anthelminthics during pregnancy: what gains and what risks for the mother and child? *Parasitology.* 2011;138(12):1499–1507.

143 Ramus RM, Girson M, Twickler DM, Wendel GD et al. Acute obstructive hydrocephalus due to cysticercosis during pregnancy. *Infect Dis Obstet Gynecol.* 1994;1(4):198–201.

CHAPTER 16

Neurosurgery

Judith M. Wong[1], Anil Can[2], & Rose Du[2]

[1] Department of Neurosurgery, University of California Los Angeles, Los Angeles, CA, USA

[2] Department of Neurosurgery, Brigham and Women's Hospital, Harvard Medical School, Boston, MA, USA

Introduction

Neurosurgical disease during pregnancy is rare but poses particular diagnostic and therapeutic challenges with two lives at stake. Little is known of the epidemiology, natural history, and appropriate therapy for these disease states. The most common neurosurgical presentations in pregnant patients are neoplastic and vascular followed by trauma [1]. We review the literature and present cases from our own experience regarding intracranial hemorrhage (ICH), hypertensive disorders, trauma, and tumors during pregnancy.

Intracranial hemorrhage during pregnancy

ICH is a rare but serious complication of pregnancy. Mortality rates as high as 83% have been described, though most studies report maternal mortality at 40–50%. ICH accounts for 5–12% of maternal deaths [2]. Physiological hemodynamic changes during pregnancy, independent of hypertensive and/or coagulation disorders, may account for the increased risk of hemorrhage. Cardiac output increases by 60% during the first 30 weeks of gestation and plateaus thereafter. Maternal blood volume and arterial and venous pressure increase steadily throughout. More dramatic but transient changes occur during labor and delivery but with uncertain effects on ICH risk [3].

Skidmore et al. evaluated the presentation, etiology, and outcome of stroke in pregnancy and puerperium. Of more than 60,000 consecutive deliveries, there were 36 patients with stroke. Eleven of these were ICHs. The most common presentations were decreased levels of consciousness (8 of 11) and headaches followed by focal deficits and seizures. Thirty-one of the 36 events occurred after the onset of the third trimester, with 16 of these occurring in the first postpartum week. Events did occur during other periods, however. One eclamptic basal ganglionic hemorrhage occurred at 30 weeks, and the earliest ruptured arteriovenous malformation (AVM) occurred during a twin gestation at 25 weeks. The most common etiologies were ruptured AVMs and pre-eclampsia/eclampsia (four each). One was due to a ruptured aneurysm, and two were of unknown etiology. Six of the 11 ICH patients underwent a neurosurgical procedure during their hospitalization. Sixty four percent of the patients had a neurological deficit at the time of discharge, and the majority of patients required rehabilitation or nursing home [2].

Dias and colleagues reviewed the literature and found 154 patients with ICH associated with a vascular lesion during pregnancy. Of these, 77% were due to aneurysm rupture, and 23% were due to AVM rupture. Locations of the

Neurological Illness in Pregnancy: Principles and Practice, First Edition.
Edited by Autumn Klein, M. Angela O'Neal, Christina Scifres, Janet F. R. Waters and Jonathan H. Waters.
© 2016 John Wiley & Sons, Ltd. Published 2016 by John Wiley & Sons, Ltd.

causative lesions, as well as patient age at presentation, were similar to those reported in the general population. It should be noted that the mean parity of this group was approximately two, implying that many of the patients had previous uneventful pregnancies. Mean gestational age at hemorrhage was approximately 30 weeks for both types of vascular lesions. Both maternal and fetal mortality were higher in the nonsurgically managed group even after adjusting for other covariates including clinical severity. Overall maternal mortality from aneurysmal hemorrhage was no different from the general population (35%) and was directly related to Hunt and Hess grade. Overall maternal mortality from AVM rupture was higher than the nongravid population but possibly attributable to worse neurological status at presentation. No differences were observed in maternal or fetal outcome between cesarean and vaginal delivery. Generally, operative intervention should be based upon neurosurgical considerations, while mode of delivery should be based on obstetrical considerations [3].

Analysis of data from the Nationwide Inpatient Sample 1998–2002 revealed 423 patients with pregnancy-related ICH, an incidence of 6.1 pregnancy-related ICH per 100,000 deliveries, or 7.1 pregnancy-related ICH per 100,000 at-risk person-years. Control data revealed a baseline risk of 5.0 non-pregnancy related ICH per 100,000 person-years. Of these pregnancy-related ICHs, 58% occurred in the postpartum period. Risk factors associated with ICH in this population were coagulopathy, preeclampsia/eclampsia, preexisting or gestational hypertension, age ≥ 35, smoking, and African American race [4].

Arteriovenous malformations

Fifteen to 23% of peripartum ICH with associated mass lesion, is due to AVMs [1,3]. AVMs are significantly more likely to rupture during pregnancy, likely because of physiological hemodynamic changes. Radiosurgical series report 3–9% hemorrhage rate during pregnancy

compared with 3–4% when not pregnant [5,6]. Our own data corroborate these findings. In 54 women with angiographic diagnosis of an AVM, we found an overall annual hemorrhage and rebleed rate of 1.5 and 7%, respectively. Annual hemorrhage rate when not pregnant was 1%, while annual hemorrhage rate during pregnancy was 11% (8% during pregnancy itself), resulting in a hazard ratio for pregnancy as a time-dependent variable of 8 (18 when the analysis was restricted up to age 40) [7].

When rupture does occur, it tends to occur during the third trimester at a mean gestational age of 30 weeks [3] and has a similar clinical presentation as rupture in the nongravid patient [2]. One retrospective study of all cases presented in the literature suggested no benefit of operative intervention over nonsurgical management for either maternal or fetal mortality but did not have adequate numbers to detect such a difference. Similarly, there was no statistically significant difference between cesarean section (c-section) and vaginal delivery on fetal outcome [3].

Decisions regarding surgical management of ruptured AVM during pregnancy should be based on neurosurgical considerations, whereas mode and timing of delivery should depend on obstetrical considerations. Thus, initial operative intervention depends on rupture acuity. Acute hydrocephalus requires emergent ventriculostomy. Symptomatic mass effect and/or herniation requires emergent decompression with resection of the vascular lesion if surgically feasible. Non-operative AVMs without mass effect should be observed in the acute period.

Case 1: ruptured arteriovenous malformation

At 38 weeks gestation, 39-year-old G1P0 presented with acute headache, lethargy, and confusion. Examination was notable for lethargy and confusion. Head CT showed a large cerebellar hemorrhage with associated hydrocephalus and AVM with feeders from the posterior

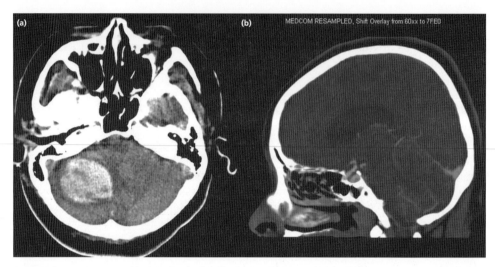

Figure 16.1 (a) Noncontrast head CT showing large right cerebellar hematoma from a ruptured arteriovenous malformation (AVM). (b) CT angiogram (CTA) demonstrating an AVM with feeders from the posterior inferior cerebellar artery.

inferior cerebellar artery (Figure 16.1). She underwent an emergent C-section with concurrent placement of an external ventricular drain, followed by a suboccipital craniotomy for clot evacuation and resection of the AVM. At follow-up 1.5 years later, she had mild residual left facial weakness and ataxic speech but was ambulatory and independent with activities of daily living. The baby was also thriving well.

Case 2: ruptured arteriovenous malformation

At 28 weeks gestation, 29-year-old G1P0 presented with acute headache and homonymous hemianopsia. Head CT showed a parietal ICH. Cerebral angiogram showed a right parietal AVM fed by the angular artery, with drainage into the superior sagittal sinus (Figures 16.2a–16.2c). She underwent surgical resection of the AVM and evacuation of the hematoma. Postoperative angiogram showed complete resection of the AVM (Figure 16.2d). Her visual field defect resolved over time. She went on to deliver at 36 weeks gestation. At two-year follow-up, the patient was neurologically intact and the child was healthy.

Intracranial aneurysms

Previous studies suggested an increase in aneurysm rupture risk during pregnancy and delivery, but more recent studies show no difference [8, 9]. Analysis of data from the NIS estimated a rupture risk of 1.4% during pregnancy and 0.05% during delivery. The rate of C-sections in these patients with unruptured aneurysms was almost twice the rate of vaginal deliveries [9].

If a pregnant patient presents with a ruptured aneurysm, however, the lesion should be treated promptly given that the risk of rerupture is highest within the first 24–48 hours. In Kassell and Torner's 1983 study, the risk of rebleed was 4.1% within the first 24 hours, then dropped sharply until the end of 48 hours at which time it was about 1.5% per day. The cumulative rebleed rate at 14 days was 19% [10]. Dias et al. evaluated maternal and fetal mortality associated with the treatment of ruptured intracranial aneurysms. They found a 63% and 27% maternal and fetal mortality, respectively, associated with untreated ruptured intracranial aneurysms, and an 11% and 5% maternal and fetal mortality in the case of treated aneurysms

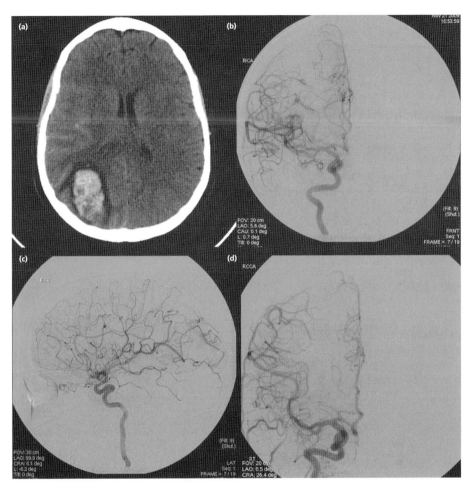

Figure 16.2 (a) Noncontrast head CT showing parietal ICH from a ruptured arteriovenous malformation (AVM). Cerebral angiography ((b) anteroposterior and (c) lateral views) shows an AVM with a feeding artery from the angular branch and drainage into the superior sagittal sinus. (d) Postoperative angiogram showing complete resection.

[3]. Similarly, Kim et al. found that the maternal mortality related to untreated aneurysmal rupture was significantly higher than in treated ruptured aneurysms [9]. The decision to operate in the emergent setting should be based on neurosurgical rather than obstetrical considerations.

Angiography

Catheter-based angiography during pregnancy poses particular risk to the developing fetus due to radiation. This risk depends on the stage of fetal development at the time of radiation exposure. Radiation damage during embryogenesis, the first 2 weeks of pregnancy, usually results in death of the embryo. Organogenesis occurs from weeks 2–7 of gestation. Exposure to radiation during this period results in congenital abnormalities. Fetal growth and development occurs from week 8 until birth, during which the radiation risk includes growth restriction, central nervous system effects such as microcephaly or eye malformations, developmental delay due to neuron depletion, and development of childhood cancer [11, 12]. All these effects appear to be dose dependent. Neuronal depletion is greatest during weeks 8–15, when neuroblast proliferation and migration to the cerebral cortex occurs [13]. On the other hand, there is no evidence to support mutagenic or teratogenic effects from iodinated contrast.

If angiography must be performed, numerous precautions may minimize radiation exposure to the fetus, including maternal abdominal lead shielding (both anteriorly and posteriorly), appropriate collimation, limiting fluoroscopy to cephalad of the aortic arch, use of low x-ray photon flux and low pulse frequency settings, and proper positioning of the equipment to maximize diagnostic data from each study [12]. Other non-ionizing radiation-based imaging modalities, including time-of-flight MRA, may also be considered.

Cavernous malformations

ICH from rupture of cavernous malformations (CMs) carries less risk than rupture of intracranial aneurysms or AVMs overall. Similar to that in non-pregnant patients, cavernoma rupture typically presents with seizure and less commonly with focal neurological deficit. Unlike AVM rupture, pregnancy does not appear to increase the risk of hemorrhage from CMs. In a recent study of 168 pregnancies in patients with one or more CMs, the overall risk of symptomatic hemorrhage was 3% per pregnancy or 3.4% per person-year. One prior study reported a hemorrhage rate of 1% per person-year. In comparison, hemorrhage risk has been reported to be as high as 4.2% per person-year in natural history studies. Of note, vaginal delivery was performed without complication in the majority of the patients with known CM [14–16].

Indications for surgery are similar to non-pregnant patients. As in the case of intracranial aneurysms and AVMs, the decision to operate should be based upon neurosurgical rather than obstetrical considerations. A history of CM is a contraindication to neither pregnancy nor vaginal delivery.

Moyamoya

Pregnancy outcomes in the setting of moyamoya disease are good, if the disease is known, and if the patient is well-managed throughout her pregnancy. In 70 reported cases of pregnancies in patients with known moyamoya disease, only 1 patient suffered poor outcome. She was diagnosed with moyamoya disease at age 10 and did not undergo extracranial to intracranial (EC–IC) bypass. She became pregnant at age 23. At 30 weeks gestation, she developed bilateral ventricular hemorrhage. Bilateral ventricular drainage was performed after C-section. She developed akinetic mutism, but the infant was normal. Two other patients with known moyamoya disease developed ischemic symptoms postpartum but recovered. Notably, both these patients had undergone previous bypasses [17]. There were only two poor fetal outcomes, both of which were attributable to congenital anomalies from medical therapy [18].

Pregnant patients with undiagnosed moyamoya disease fare much worse, underscoring the importance of close monitoring peripartum when the disease is known. In 25 patients with previously undiagnosed moyamoya, 16 presented with ICH and 5 with seizures or TIAs. Of the mothers, 3 died, 8 had poor outcome, and 12 had good outcome. Of the newborns, 2 died, 1 suffered hemiparesis, and 15 made a good recovery. For both newborns and mothers, poor outcome was related to maternal cerebral hemorrhage [18].

Management of moyamoya during pregnancy and postpartum focuses on the prevention of ischemic and/or hemorrhagic events. Appropriately timed C-section is the preferred method of delivery to avoid hypertension and hyperventilation, though there is no evidence to support this claim. It is important to maintain normocapnia and normotension during delivery.

Surgical management of hemorrhagic events is similar to non-pregnant patients, including decompression of mass effect from hematoma and ventriculostomy for treatment of resultant hydrocephalus. Similar to non-pregnant patients, bypass surgery is not indicated in the immediate post-ICH period.

Cerebral venous thrombosis

Similar to non-pregnant patients, cerebral venous thrombosis (CVT) carries a worse prognosis if associated with hemorrhagic venous infarction. In Skidmore's study of 36 patients with stroke during pregnancy, 4 had CVT. None of the cases had clear etiology other than hypercoagulability of the pregnant/puerperal state. One case was associated with systemic lupus erythematosus and another with dehydration. All four presented with headache, with the only one who had hemorrhagic venous infarction presenting with altered consciousness. Although there were limited data regarding neurological outcome, three of the four patients were discharged home. The patient with hemorrhagic venous infarction was discharged to a nursing home [2].

Lanska and Kryscio used National Hospital Discharge Survey data to evaluate pregnancy-associated CVT and found a risk of 11.4 for CVT per 100,000 deliveries with zero risk of mortality within their data set. Among demographic factors, including age, presence of hypertension, and stage of pregnancy, they were unable to find any risk predictors [19].

Anticoagulation remains both treatment and early secondary prophylaxis for CVT. During pregnancy, a heparin derivative typically comprises this anticoagulation. In cases refractory to medical management and or clinical deterioration, invasive endovascular techniques such as direct chemical thrombolysis and/or direct mechanical thrombectomy have been used. These procedures, however, are only supported by small case series and anecdotal reports [20].

Hypertensive disorders in pregnancy

HELLP syndrome is characterized by hemolysis, elevated liver enzymes, and low platelet count, and is associated with systemic derangements including disseminated intravascular coagulation, respiratory distress, acute renal failure, and

stroke. ICH secondary to coagulopathy and/or thrombocytopenia is a rare but feared complication of this syndrome and tends to occur antepartum, though it may also occur postpartum. Hemorrhages have been reported in various locations within the brain including brainstem, basal ganglia, and subcortical parenchyma with or without intraventricular extension.

Patients with HELLP syndrome should be managed as high risk. Early recognition and prompt treatment are critical to prevent intracranial and systemic complications. In addition to aggressive blood pressure management and seizure prevention, immediate correction of coagulopathy and thrombocytopenia with appropriate blood products may prevent or minimize neurological damage, though patients with ICH often have poor outcome [21].

Trauma

It is general consensus to treat neurotrauma in the setting of pregnancy similar to the non-pregnant patient. Intracranial pressure (ICP) may be managed medically or surgically with decompressive craniectomy. Mannitol is classified as Class B, meaning that animal reproduction studies have failed to demonstrate fetal risk though there are no adequate and well-controlled studies in pregnant women, while hypertonic saline is Class C, meaning that animal studies have shown an adverse effect on the fetus but that there are no adequate and well-controlled studies in humans. For Class C drugs, potential benefits may warrant use of the drug in pregnant women despite potential risks [22].

Tumors

The incidence of brain tumors does not appear to increase during pregnancy, though there is some evidence supporting symptomatic worsening from meningiomas secondary to hormonal changes [23]. In a study of eight women diagnosed with malignant brain tumors during pregnancy, all eight antenatal patients suffered neurologic crisis. Six were emergently delivered after maternal deterioration, and two were delivered electively in the early third trimester after fetal pulmonary maturity. Four mothers died, two had poor long-term outcome, and one infant died [24].

Similar to other neurosurgical issues during pregnancy, the decision to operate should be made on neurosurgical rather than obstetrical considerations. Benign and/or asymptomatic tumors should be observed. Malignant and/or symptomatic lesions (particularly from mass effect) should be treated in a manner independent of the pregnancy. The timing and mode of delivery should then be made based on obstetrical considerations.

Chiari malformations

Chiari malformations are a group of four congenital anomalies with type 1 CM (CM1) as the most common variant, typically presenting in adulthood and characterized by displacement of the cerebellar tonsils through the foramen magnum and, predisposing the patient to hydrocephalus, syringomyelia, and brainstem compression.

Most of the anesthetic risks to parturients with CM1 are related to an increase in cerebrospinal fluid (CSF) pressure associated with pregnancy and prolonged straining during the second stage of labor, or the potential complications of spinal or epidural anesthesia. The negative spinal pressure that could occur during spinal neuraxis anesthesia could cause cerebellar tonsillar herniation resulting in neurologic deterioration. In two case reports, spinal neuraxial anesthesia was performed in patients with uncorrected CM1, and only diagnosed subsequently because of neurological worsening [25, 26]. In cases of uncorrected CM without signs of increased ICP or syringomyelia, epidural anesthetic would be the technique of choice, avoiding the risk of

cerebellar herniation as a result of spinal anesthesia and potential airway compromise due to general anesthesia [27]. Nevertheless, a major risk of epidural anesthesia is inadvertent dural puncture. In addition, uneventful spinal anesthesia has been reported in women with surgically corrected CM1 [28–30]. In these cases, without syringomyelia or signs of increased ICP, spinal rather than epidural anesthesia may be preferable due to reduced risk of local toxicity and CSF leakage during an inadvertent wet tap. However, residual disease may result after incomplete surgical decompression, and the use of standard regional anesthetic techniques without careful preoperative neurological evaluation could have fatal consequences.

General anesthesia would be preferable over any type of regional anesthetic for patients with syringomyelia or signs of increased ICP, avoiding CSF pressure fluctuations [31, 32]. Coughing, neck movement, and hyperextension during intubation and extubation may lead to further compression at the foramen magnum and cervical spinal cord, with traction on the lower cranial nerves and elevation of CSF pressure. With the need to perform rapid-sequence induction and the usual precautions for patients with elevated ICP (e.g., hyperventilation, blood pressure control), general anesthesia can be challenging. As the literature is extremely limited, the safety of different anesthetic techniques in CM1 patients remains unclear, and each patient with CM1 requires an individual anesthetic plan using a multidisciplinary approach [33].

Conclusion

The management of neurosurgical disease during pregnancy is particularly challenging with an additional life at stake. The risk of ICH from an AVM is increased because of augmented maternal hemodynamics, particularly during the third trimester. This increased risk has not been demonstrated in other vascular lesions such as aneurysms and cavernous malformations. While some tumors may be hormone-related, the incidence of brain tumors does not appear to increase during pregnancy. Decisions regarding surgical and obstetrical management should be determined on an individual basis and based upon an understanding of the neurosurgical disease.

References

1 Cohen-Gadol AA, Friedman JA, Friedman JD, Tubbs RS, Munis JR, Meyer FB. Neurosurgical management of intracranial lesions in the pregnant patient: a 36-year institutional experience and review of the literature. *J Neurosurg.* 2009;111:1150–1157.

2 Skidmore FM, Williams LS, Fradkin KD, Alonso RJ, Biller J. Presentation, etiology, and outcome of stroke in pregnancy and puerperium. *J Stroke Cerebrovasc Dis.* 2001;10:1–10.

3 Dias MS, Sekhar LN. Intracranial hemorrhage from aneurysms and arteriovenous malformations during pregnancy and the puerperium. *Neurosurgery.* 1990;27:855–866.

4 Bateman BT, Schumacher HC, Bushnell CD, et al. Intracerebral hemorrhage in pregnancy: frequency, risk factors, and outcome. *Neurology.* 2006;67:424–429.

5 Horton JC, Chambers WA, Lyons SL, Adams RD, Kjellberg RN. Pregnancy and the risk of hemorrhage from cerebral arteriovenous malformations. *Neurosurgery.* 1990;27:867–871.

6 Forster DM, Kunkler IH, Hartland P. Risk of cerebral bleeding from arteriovenous malformations in pregnancy: the Sheffield experience. *Stereotact Funct Neurosurg.* 1993;61(Suppl 1):20–22.

7 Gross BA, Du R. Hemorrhage from arteriovenous malformations during pregnancy. *Neurosurgery.* 2012;71:349–356.

8 Jaigobin C, Silver FL. Stroke and pregnancy. *Stroke.* 2000;31:2948–2951.

9 Kim YW, Deal D, Hoh BL. Cerebral aneurysms in pregnancy and delivery: pregnancy and delivery do not increase the risk of aneurysm rupture. *Neurosurgery.* 2013;72:143–150.

10 Kassell NF, Torner JC. Aneurysmal rebleeding: a preliminary report from the cooperative aneurysm study. *Neurosurgery.* 1983;13:479–481.

11 Brent RL. Radiation teratogenesis. *Teratology.* 1980;21:281–298.

12 Meyers PM, Halbach VV, Malek AM, et al. Endovascular treatment of cerebral artery aneurysms during pregnancy: report of three cases. *Am J Neuroradiol.* 2000;21:1306–1311.

13 Little JB. Low-dose radiation effects: interactions and synergism. *Health Phys.* 1990;59:49–55.

14 Kalani YMS, Zabramski JM. Risk for symptomatic hemorrhage of cerebral cavernous malformations during pregnancy. *J Neurosurg.* 2013;118:50–55.

15 Witiw CD, Abou-Hamden A, Kulkarni AV, Silvaggio JA, Schneider C, Wallace MC. Cerebral cavernous malformations and pregnancy: hemorrhage risk and influence on obstetrical management. *Neurosurgery.* 2012;71:626–631.

16 Gross B, Lin N, Du R, Day AL. The natural history of intracranial cavernous malformations. *Neurosurg Focus.* 2011;30:E24.

17 Fukushima K, Yumoto Y, Kondo Y, et al. A retrospective chart review of the perinatal period in 22 pregnancies of 16 women with moyamoya disease. *J Clin Neurosci.* 2012;19:1358–1362.

18 Komiyama M, Toshihiro Y, Shouhei K, Sakamoto H, Fujitani K, Shigeki M. Moyamoya disease and pregnancy: case report and review of the literature. *Neurosurgery.* 1998;43:360–368.

19 Lanksa DJ, Kryscio RJ. Stroke and intracranial venous thrombosis during pregnancy and puerperium. *Neurology.* 1998;51:1622–1628.

20 Kernan WN, Ovbiagele B, Black HR, et al. Guidelines for the prevention of stroke in patients with stroke and transient ischemic attack: a guideline for healthcare professionals from the American Heart Association/American Stroke Association. *Stroke.* 2014; 45:2160–2236.

21 Yokota H, Miyamoto K, Yokoyama K, Noguchi H, Uyama K, Oku M. Spontaneous acute subdural haematoma and intracerebral haemorrhage in patient with HELLP syndrome: case report. *Acta Neurochir.* 2009;151:1689–1692.

22 Burkey BW, Holmes AP. Evaluating medical use in pregnancy and lactation: what every pharmacist should know. *J Pediatr Pharmacol Ther.* 2013;18:247–258.

23 Roelvink NCA, Kamphorst W, van Alphen HAM, Rao BR. Pregnancy-related primary brain and spinal tumors. *Arch Neurol.* 1987;44:209–215.

24 Tewari KS, Cappuccini F, Asrat T, et al. Obstetric emergencies precipitated by malignant brain tumors. *Am J Obstet Gynecol.* 2000;182:1215–1221.

25 Barton JJ, Sharpe JA. Oscillopsia and horizontal nystagmus with accelerating slow phases following lumbar puncture in the Arnold-Chiari malformation. *Ann Neurol.* 1993;33:418–421.

26 Hullander RM, Bogard TD, Leivers D, Moran D, Dewan DM. Chiari I malformation presenting as recurrent spinal headache. *Anesth Analg.* 1992;75:1025–1026.

27 Semple DA, McClure JH. Arnold-chiari malformation in pregnancy. *Anaesthesia.* 1996;51:580–582.

28 Landau R, Giraud R, Delrue V, Kern C. Spinal anesthesia for cesarean delivery in a woman with a surgically corrected type I Arnold Chiari malformation. *Anesth Analg.* 2003;97:253–255.

29 Mueller DM, Oro' J. Chiari I malformation with or without syringomyelia and pregnancy: case studies and review of the literature. *Am J Perinatol.* 2005;22:67–70.

30 Parker JD, Broberg JC, Napolitano PG. Maternal Arnold-Chiari type I malformation and syringomyelia: a labor management dilemma. *Am J Perinatol.* 2002;19:445–450.

31 Ghaly RF, Candido KD, Sauer R, Knezevic NN. Anesthetic management during Cesarean section in a woman with residual Arnold-Chiari malformation Type I, cervical kyphosis, and syringomyelia. *Surg Neurol Int.* 2012;3:26.

32 Agustí M, Adàlia R, Fernández C, Gomar C. Anaesthesia for caesarean section in a patient with syringomyelia and Arnold-Chiari type I malformation. *Int J Obstet Anesth.* 2004;13:114–116.

33 Chantigian RC, Koehn MA, Ramin KD, Warner MA. Chiari I malformation in parturients. *J Clin Anesth.* 2002;14:201–205.

CHAPTER 17

Sleep disorders

Sally Ibrahim & Nancy Foldvary-Schaefer

Cleveland Clinic Lerner College of Medicine, Cleveland, OH, USA

Introduction

The physiological alterations across the female reproductive lifespan and pregnancy impact wake and sleep, in some cases meeting diagnostic criteria for sleep disorders. The menopausal transition incurs dramatic and permanent hormonal changes affecting sleep, increasing the risk for sleep disorders. Sleep complaints are reported by at least one-third of pregnant women [1]. Emerging evidence suggests an adverse impact of sleep disorders on maternal-fetal health. Therefore, early diagnosis and treatment of sleep disorders in pregnancy may improve pregnancy outcomes. Herein, we discuss sleep disorders and sleep complaints in women with special attention to pregnancy and menopause. The classification and diagnostic criteria of sleep disorders are based on the *International Classification of Sleep Disorders*, 3rd edition (ICSD-3) [2].

Sleep duration quality, and architecture in reproductive women

Sleep duration and quality change dynamically across pregnancy. Prospective studies indicate that sleep duration increases in the first trimester in association with a subjective increase in daytime sleepiness. Sleep duration returns closer to pre-partum levels in the second trimester, then subsequently decreases reaching its nadir post-partum [3]. Subjective sleep quality also declines across pregnancy, starting in the first trimester [1, 4]. Similarly, objective measures using polysomnography (PSG) demonstrate alterations in sleep architecture in pregnant women. Pregnancy mainly impacts slow wave sleep, sleep efficiency, and wake after sleep onset (WASO). Slow wave (deep) sleep percentage decreases by late pregnancy [5]. Sleep efficiency, defined as the percentage of time asleep/time in bed, decreases especially near the end of pregnancy. Reduced sleep efficiency is likely related to nocturnal awakenings, increased WASO and cortical arousals [3, 5].

In the non-pregnant population, short sleep duration is a risk factor for a variety of adverse outcomes including hypertension (HTN), coronary artery disease (CAD), obesity, weight gain, and glucose intolerance [1, 6]. Similar adverse effects are recognized in pregnancy. Short sleep duration, variably defined as less than 5–7 hours of sleep, is associated with an increased incidence of gestational diabetes mellitus (GDM) (odds ratio [OR] 11.7), elevated third trimester blood pressure (BP) and risk of preeclampsia [6, 7]. Environmental (e.g., smoking), physical (e.g., higher body mass index [BMI]), and medical (e.g., sleep disorders) factors affect sleep duration and quality in pregnancy [1, 6]. Aging and menopause give rise to poorer sleep quality

Neurological Illness in Pregnancy: Principles and Practice, First Edition.
Edited by Autumn Klein, M. Angela O'Neal, Christina Scifres, Janet F. R. Waters and Jonathan H. Waters.
© 2016 John Wiley & Sons, Ltd. Published 2016 by John Wiley & Sons, Ltd.

and shorter sleep duration, especially in those with comorbid medical conditions [8].

Primary sleep disorders in reproductive and menopausal women

Sleep disorders are categorically outlined according to the diagnostic criteria of the ICSD-3. Over 80 disorders are recognized, each assigned to one of six general categories including insomnias, hypersomnias of central origin, parasomnias, sleep-related breathing disorders, circadian rhythm disorders, and sleep-related movement disorders. Isolated symptoms/normal variants and other sleep disorders largely associated with medical and psychiatric conditions are classified separately. The most common sleep disorders affecting pregnant and menopausal women are detailed below.

Insomnia

Insomnia is defined as a persistent sleep difficulty despite adequate sleep opportunity associated with daytime impairment [2]. Insomnia symptoms of sleep initiation/maintenance difficulties or poor quality sleep are reported in up 33–50% of the population, though 10–15% has impairment from their symptoms and therefore meets criteria for having an insomnia disorder [9].

The diagnostic criteria for insomnia include [2]:

- Difficulty with sleep initiation or maintenance, waking up too early, or sleep that is chronically non-restorative or perceived as poor in quality.
- The complaint/difficulty occurs despite adequate opportunity and circumstances for sleep.
- The complaint/difficulty is associated with some form of daytime impairment (fatigue, decreased energy, excessive concern/worry about sleep, mood disturbance,

poor school/work or social performance or other symptom of sleep loss).

Insomnia is classified as primary or comorbid with other medical or psychiatric conditions. Insomnia comorbid with a psychiatric disorder is the most common type of insomnia [2]. Insomnia symptoms can precede the onset of a mood disorder and are postulated to precipitate mood disorders in some people [8]. Risk factors for insomnia include female gender, advancing age, and comorbidities such as mood or medical disorders, shift work, substance abuse, and other sleep disorders. The female: male ratio is 1.4:1, increasing after the age of 45–1.7:1 [8]. The gender difference may be related to the higher prevalence of anxiety and depression in women [5, 8].

Insomnia is the most common sleep disorder in pregnancy. Self-reported insomnia increases across pregnancy from 38% in early pregnancy to 54% in late pregnancy and is likely due to adjustments to the physical, hormonal, and metabolic changes associated with the condition [1]. Sleep maintenance disturbances from nocturnal awakenings is reported in up to 72% of pregnant women [10]. Nocturia is the most common cause, while others include dreams, leg cramps, gastrointestinal problems (e.g., reflux), discomfort (e.g., back discomfort), and less commonly, fetal movements [3, 10]. Rising nocturnal oxytocin levels that peak at night may not only explain why labor and delivery typically occurs at night, but also why many women have insomnia in the latter part of the night [8]. Cortisol levels double in pregnancy and may also contribute to comorbid insomnia and depression [8]. Difficulty returning to sleep after awakenings is especially problematic in the third trimester [3]. As in the general population, sleep initiation difficulties are a significant predictor of mood disorders in pregnant women [11].

The prevalence of insomnia increases with age and menopausal status. In the study of Women's Health Across the Nation, nearly half of surgical menopausal women reported insomnia [8]. Causes of sleep disruption in this population include hot flushes, mood disorders, and sleep-related breathing disorders [5]. Hot flushes generally have a circadian rhythm, peaking in the evening and disrupting sleep continuity in some patients [5]. Hot flushes are responsive to estrogen treatment which has also been found to improve subjective sleep and mood in some women [5].

Insomnia management includes pharmacological (Table 17.1) and non-pharmacological therapies (Table 17.2) [9, 13]. Non-pharmacological therapies for insomnia include sleep-promoting behaviors such as relaxation and improvement in sleep hygiene, cognitive behavioral therapy for insomnia (CBT-I), and other complimentary therapies [9]. Since severe insomnia can lead to psychological distress and a variety of medical conditions, the risks and benefits of available treatments must be assessed on a case-by-case basis [9, 13]. Medications have the advantage of promptness of action in some patients, but disadvantages of potential side effects, dependence, and perceived stigma in their use. Sleep medications for insomnia are seldom prescribed during pregnancy due to concerns for adverse effects on fetal health. It is often medically preferable for patients with chronic insomnia to be treated with CBT-I by a clinically-trained sleep psychologist. While as effective as medications during short-term treatment, CBT-I is proven to be more effective in sustaining sleep improvements over time, and is usually rated by patients, significant others, and providers as more effective than pharmacotherapy alone [9]. Non-pharmacological treatments can be delivered by behavioral sleep therapists in individual or group formats or web-based programs [14]. Exclusion of other sleep disorders during pregnancy that affect sleep initiation and maintenance is required.

Sleep-related breathing disorders

Obstructive sleep apnea (OSA), the most common of the sleep-related breathing disorders, is characterized by repetitive episodes of upper airway obstruction resulting in partial or complete airflow cessation, oxygen desaturations and arousals from sleep. Patients report daytime fatigue or sleepiness, nocturnal awakenings, snoring, gasping or choking in sleep, witnessed apneas, nocturia, and unrefreshing sleep. Women are more likely than men to present with non-classical symptoms including depressed mood and anxiety, leading to a delay in diagnosis [8].

PSG is required to diagnose OSA and measure treatment efficacy (Table 17.3) [13]. In-laboratory PSG is the gold standard test for the diagnosis and involves recording of physiologic parameters important for staging sleep and scoring respiratory events and limb movements. These include electroencephalography (EEG), electrooculography (EOG), chin and limb electromyography (EMG), electrocardiography (ECG), airflow, respiratory effort, oxygen saturation, and carbon dioxide. Video monitoring is used to grade sleep positioning and is especially helpful in clarifying complex nocturnal behaviors of clinical concern. Portable devices that record heart rate, airflow, respiratory effort, and oxygen saturation are gaining utility for the confirmation of OSA in patients with a high suspicion of moderate-to-severe disease without comorbid medical and sleep disorders. Apneas (complete airway closure) and hypopneas (partial airway closure) are summed to produce the apnea–hypopnea index (AHI), the primary measure of disease severity (mild: 5–<15; moderate: 15–<30; severe: ≥30) (Table 17.3) [2, 13].

In general population, the prevalence of OSA is approximately 5% with a male to female ratio of about 2–3:1 [5, 8]. Gender differences are partially related to differences in upper airway tone and body fat distribution. The risk of OSA is 2.5 times greater in menopausal than premenopausal women. Rates of OSA in menopausal women reach values closer to men, while those taking hormone replacement therapy (HRT) are less likely to be affected [5, 8, 13]. However, HRT does not reduce obstructive respiratory events sufficiently to treat the disorder in women with OSA [8, 13]. The change

Table 17.1 Pharmacotherapy for insomnia

Drug class	Drug name (brand)	Dose (mg)	Pregnancy class[b]	Onset of action (min)	Elimination half-life (h)	Comments
Benzodiazepine receptor agonists	Eszopiclone (Lunesta)[a]	1–3	C	30	5–7	Approved for long-term use
	Zaleplon (Sonata)[a]	5–20	C	30	1	Short acting allows for midnight administration
	Zolpidem tartrate/extended release (Ambien/Ambien CR)[a]	5–10; 6.25–12.5	C	30	1.5–2.5 CR: 2.5–4	CR formulation approved for long-term use
Benzodiazepines	Estazolam (ProSom)[a]	0.5–2	X	8–24	8–24	Teratogenic effects, neonatal withdrawal, floppy infant syndrome; potential dependence
	Flurazepam (Dalmane)[a]	15–30	D	15–30	48–120	
	Temazepam (Restoril)[a]	7.5–30	X	60–90	8–20	
	Triazolam (Halcion)[a]	0.125–0.25	X	2–30	2–6	
	Clonazepam (Klonopin)	0.5–2	D	60–90	30–40	
	Lorazepam (Ativan)	0.5–2	X	30	10–20	
Melatonin receptor agonist	Ramelteon (Rozerem)[a]	8	C	30–69	1–2	Low potential for dependency
Sedating antidepressants	Doxepin (Silenor)[a]	3–6	C	30–60	8–24	Only antidepressant approved for insomnia
	Amitriptyline (Elavil)	25–75	C	30–60	10–25	Anticholinergic side effects
	Mirtazapine (Remeron)	15	C	30–120	13–40	Low doses effective
	Trazodone (Desyrel)	25–150	C	60–120	3–14	Low doses effective
Sedating antihistamines	Diphenhydramine (Benadryl)	25–50	B	30–60	4–8	Ingredient in OTC sleep aids; morning grogginess; may aggravate RLS
Other	Melatonin	1–3	—	3–60	1	More effective for phase shifting than sedation

[a]FDA labeled for insomnia.

[b]Food and Drug Administration safety classification: Pregnancy Categories A–D, X [12]:

A: Adequate/controlled studies in pregnancy fail to demonstrate a risk to fetus. Possible fetal harm appears remote.

B: Animal studies have not demonstrated a fetal risk or there are no controlled studies in pregnant women. Or, animal studies show possible risk, but controlled studies in women do not demonstrate risk.

C: Animal studies have revealed adverse effects on the fetus (teratogenic, embryocidal). There are no adequate/controlled studies in women. Despite potential risk, use only if the potential benefit justifies possible risk.

D: Evidence of human fetal risk. Use in pregnant women may be acceptable despite risk (e.g., drug needed in a life-threatening situation or for a serious disease when safer drugs cannot be used).

X: Evidence in animals/humans of fetal abnormalities or risk. Risk clearly outweighs any possible benefit; drug is contraindicated.

RLS, restless legs syndrome; OTC, over the counter.

Table 17.2 Non-pharmacological behavioral therapies and sleep hygiene for insomnia

Non-pharmacological therapies	Underlying principles
Bed time routine and at bed time	
Relax and perform soothing behaviors prior to sleep (e.g., progressive muscle relaxation, create calm environment).	Relaxation promotes sleep, reduces tension, and quiets the mind to prepare for sleep.
Avoid watching TV, electronic pads/computers, texting, and use of other electronics in the bed.	Light exposure and alerting activities diminish sleep initiation processes.
Avoid stimulants such as caffeine, smoking, and alcohol within 6 hours of bed time.	Stimulants interfere with sleepiness and sleep onset. Alcohol interferes with sleep quality.
While in bed and during the sleep period	
Use a comfortable bed and pillow support.	To support the back as the abdomen enlarges in pregnancy.
Use the bed only for sleep and sex.	This helps promote positive sleep associations.
Avoid any rumination or worry in bed. Avoid clock watching or being too alert about time.	Mental activities, especially negative, can alter the body's ability to sleep.
If one cannot sleep within 15–20 minutes, get out of bed. Do something calm and relaxing in dim lighting until feeling sleepy again.	This helps the body to avoid alertness while in bed, helps the body to positively associate the bed with sleep, and reinstate the sleep state.
Daytime practices	
Set consistent regular bed and wake times.	Helps to maintain a sleep rhythm that promotes sleep.
Avoid long and late evening daytime naps. Otherwise, take only short naps (~20 minutes).	Naps steal sleep pressure away from the night, making sleep initiation difficult.
Address mood concerns (i.e., anxiety, depression), and physical complaints, such as low back pain/discomfort.	These conditions promote insomnia. Pain and discomfort may alter usual sleeping position and limit comfortable sleep.
Consider implementation of complimentary therapies, such as relaxation and mindful yoga.	These may be helpful for anxiety, stress reduction, and promote sleep initiation.

Table 17.3 Diagnostic criteria of obstructive sleep apnea

Criteria: (A and B) or C satisfy the criteria

A   The presence of one or more of the following:

    1 The patient complains of sleepiness, nonrestorative sleep, fatigue, or insomnia symptoms.

    2 The patient wakes with breath holding, gasping, or choking.

    3 The bed partner or other observer reports habitual snoring, breathing interruptions, or both during the patient's sleep.

    4 The patient has been diagnosed with hypertension, a mood disorder, cognitive dysfunction, coronary artery disease, stroke, congestive heart failure, atrial fibrillation, or type 2 diabetes mellitus.

B   Polysomnography (PSG) or out of center sleep testing (OCST) demonstrates:

    1 Five or more predominantly obstructive respiratory events (obstructive and mixed apneas, hypopneas, or respiratory effort related arousals (RERAs)) per hour of sleep during PSG or per hour of monitoring (OCST)/portable monitoring.

    OR

C   PSG or OCST demonstrates:

    1 Fifteen or more predominantly obstructive respiratory events (apneas, hyopneas, or RERAs) per hour of sleep during a PSG or per hour of monitoring (OCST).

Adapted from American Academy of Sleep Medicine 2014. Reproduced with permission of American Academy of Sleep Medicine.

in body fat distribution in menopausal women resulting in an increased waist:hip ratio as well as larger neck girth likely contributes to the increasing risk for OSA in older women [5, 8]. Premenopausal women have higher BMIs compared with men of similar OSA severity which is likely the result of greater upper body mass distribution in men [8].

The prevalence of OSA in pregnancy is unknown, mainly due to the lack of epidemiological studies using objective measurements. Most studies rely on self-reported measures. Using the Berlin screening questionnaire, 10–25% of pregnant women are classified as high risk for OSA [7, 15]. OSA may emerge de novo or worsen in pregnancy. The percentage of women who report snoring nearly doubles from pre-pregnancy to the final month of pregnancy, and some women have emerging symptoms such as witnessed apneic episodes [16]. Weight gain, the enlarging gravid uterus and upper airway edema, and congestion likely contribute to the increased risk of OSA in pregnancy [8]. Pregnant women may be more susceptible to apnea due to the decrease in functional residual capacity and increase in oxygen consumption [17]. Higher BMI and neck girth are associated with the progression of OSA symptoms over pregnancy [15, 16].

A growing body of evidence supports the negative impact of OSA on maternal–fetal health and pregnancy outcomes. Snoring and OSA increase the risk of GDM, preeclampsia and pregnancy-induced HTN [1, 15, 18]. Even non-obese pregnant women with OSA symptoms have greater risk for preeclampsia [15]. Potential mechanisms include cyclical hypoxemia and re-oxygenation, promoting pro-inflammatory markers that underlie these conditions. Habitual snoring is associated with increased cord blood levels of nucleated red blood cells, interleukin-6, and other inflammatory markers [1, 19]. The severity of sleep-related breathing disturbances required to confer adverse pregnancy outcomes is unknown. Consequently, early diagnosis and treatment of OSA is recommended,

even in mild cases particularly in the presence of symptoms.

The severity of OSA guides therapeutic options. Conservative therapies including protective sleep positioning in the lateral decubitus position, treatment of nasal congestion, and avoidance of sedatives, alcohol, excessive weight gain and sleep deprivation should be recommended in all cases. For patients with moderate-to-severe OSA (AHI ≥15) or patients with mild OSA (AHI ≥5–<15) with respiratory events associated with severe oxygen desaturation, cardiac arrhythmia, or severe daytime sleepiness, positive airway pressure (PAP) therapy is the treatment of choice. PAP can be delivered continuously (CPAP), by auto-titrating devices (AutoPAP) or with bi-level delivery (Bi-level-PAP). An overnight titration study performed in the sleep laboratory establishes the therapeutic pressure setting for PAP devices. In patients with rapidly changing body habitus as in pregnancy, AutoPAP may be particularly suitable. Other therapies, such as oral appliances and upper airway surgery are alternatives to PAP in appropriately selected cases [13].

At present, there is a paucity of data guiding the evaluation and treatment of OSA in pregnancy. Given the prevalence of OSA in the general population, clinical screening of all pregnant women is recommended. Habitual snoring in the setting of daytime sleepiness or fatigue, witnessed apnea, or comorbidities (e.g., GDM, preecamplsia, HTN, obesity) should prompt formal evaluation. Women suspected of having OSA should be referred for PSG [7, 15]. Therapies for OSA have not been systematically studied in pregnancy. CPAP appears to be safe and effective in pregnant women [8, 13, 17]. In limited studies, women with OSA and preeclampsia treated with CPAP therapy showed improvements in BP and increase in cardiac output [8, 17]. Symptoms of OSA often improve or resolve post-partum [16]. In one study, post-partum AHI measured by PSG decreased by one-third compared with the final trimester of pregnancy [18]. Women with OSA during pregnancy should be re-evaluated post-partum as some may no longer require treatment and others may benefit from a change in therapy.

Restless legs syndrome

Restless legs syndrome (RLS), also known as Willis Ekbom Syndrome, is the most common sleep-related movement disorder. PSG is not required unless other comorbid sleep disorders are suspected. However, 80% of patients with RLS have frequent periodic limb movements during sleep on PSG [2, 13, 20]. RLS is defined by the following four criteria [2]:

- An urge to move the legs usually accompanied or caused by an uncomfortable and unpleasant sensations in the legs.
- The urge to move or the unpleasant sensations begin or worsen during periods of rest or inactivity (e.g., lying or sitting).
- The urge to move or the unpleasant sensations are partially or totally relieved by movement (e.g., walking or stretching) at least as long as the activity continues.
- The urge to move or the unpleasant sensations are worse, or only occur, in the evening or night.

RLS is classified as primary/idiopathic or secondary to a medical condition/medication. In the non-pregnant population, primary RLS is usual familial and occurs sporadically or by autosomal dominant inheritance. Secondary causes of RLS include pregnancy, iron deficiency, uremia, peripheral neuropathy, and medications (e.g., antihistamines, antidepressants, and dopamine antagonists). Risk of RLS increases with age. The prevalence of RLS in the general population is approximately 10% and is twice as common is women as in men. Gender differences are partially explained by parity. Women with more pregnancies tend to have more RLS, while nulliparous women have nearly similar prevalence to men [21]. Restless legs syndrome should be differentiated from other conditions associated with abnormal movements or sensations in sleep including nocturnal leg cramps, arthritic pain, positional discomfort/paresthesias, and unconscious foot movements (e.g., foot tapping).

The severity of RLS is graded clinically using the International RLS Study group rating scale (IRLS) from mild to severe [20]. The prevalence of RLS was recently found to be nearly three fold greater in people with cardiovascular disease with severe RLS more likely to be associated with HTN, cerebrovascular disease, and CAD [22]. In turn, treatment of RLS incurs a host of health benefits, such as improvement in quality of life, sleep quality, and mood [20].

Restless legs syndrome is the most extensively studied sleep disorder in pregnancy. The condition is highly prevalent, affecting 26–32% of pregnant women [21, 23]. Symptoms of RLS emerge or worsen with advancing pregnancy. Severe RLS increases from 15% in the first trimester to over 30% in the third trimester [1]. Interestingly, RLS severity tends to decline in the 2 weeks prior to delivery [24]. Two forms of RLS in pregnancy have been distinguished. One is the transient form of RLS which resolves rapidly within 1 month postpartum but can recur with subsequent pregnancies [21]. The other form which is present prior to pregnancy is most often the idiopathic form and worsens during pregnancy but returns to baseline severity after delivery. Despite its prevalence, RLS is frequently unrecognized by patients and providers alike [23]. As in non-pregnant women, moderate-to-severe RLS adversely affects sleep duration and quality as well as daytime functioning due to difficulty falling or staying asleep, in some cases increasing the likelihood of using sleep aids during pregnancy [21, 23]. Newer evidence suggests that even transient RLS in pregnancy can be a risk for subsequent development of idiopathic RLS [21].

During menses and menopause, RLS is also more pronounced in women. Hot flushes may coexist with RLS in menopausal women. Premenopausal RLS is strongly associated with migraine disorders [5]. At menopause, there is a decline in migraines but not RLS. HRT does not ameliorate RLS symptoms in menopausal women [21].

The pathophysiology of RLS in the general population involves iron and dopaminergic activity affecting nociceptive pathways in the nervous system [2]. Iron plays a role in the development of RLS during pregnancy. The hemodilution of pregnancy may reduce effective iron transport. Additionally, there is increased fetal demand for iron, and by the second trimester, levels of ferritin and hemoglobin fall regardless of adequate dietary intake [13]. Development or worsening of RLS during menopause, menses, and pregnancy, and the precipitous decline in RLS after delivery suggests that hormonal factors influence the expression of RLS [21]. The antidopaminergic effect of estrogen may underlie the increasing prevalence of RLS toward the end of pregnancy when estrogen levels peak. In a prospective study examining hormonal and metabolic changes in pregnancy, pregnancy-related RLS was associated with a more prominent physiological estradiol elevation compared with pregnant controls [24].

Goals of RLS therapy are to provide symptomatic relief, restore sleep quality and duration, and eliminate daytime consequences. Most mild cases of RLS require no more than conservative measures. These include behavioral modifications, such as avoidance of smoking, caffeine, excessive daytime motor activity, and prolonged erect posture [21]. Exercise, compression devices, and limiting use of medications that cause or exacerbate RLS are recommended [20]. Low serum ferritin prior to or during pregnancy is the best predictor of RLS during pregnancy even in women with normal iron levels and appropriate iron intake [21, 24]. In patients with ferritin levels <50 μg/L, iron replacement with oral ferrous sulfate dosed twice daily is beneficial [20]. Vitamin C (200–500 mg) should be taken with oral iron to increase absorption [13, 25]. Gastrointestinal distress, particularly constipation, is the usual limitation of adequate iron therapy [20].

Pharmacological therapy is typically required in moderate-to-severe cases of RLS (Table 17.4) [20]. FDA-approved agents for RLS include the non-ergot derived dopamine agonists, pramipexole, ropinirole, and rotigotine, as well as gabapentin enacarbil. Dopaminergic agents are considered first-line therapy for RLS. These agents should be administered at least 30 minutes prior to symptom onset and titrated up gradually to symptom resolution. Adverse effects of dopamine agonists include impulse control disorders such as gambling and compulsive eating, nausea at initiation and somnolence at higher doses [13, 20]. Dopamine agonists can produce augmentation, defined as the progression of symptoms earlier in the day or involving more parts of the body requiring discontinuation or change in the timing of treatment [13, 20]. Abrupt discontinuation of dopamine agonists can lead to rebound RLS symptoms. Levodopa is also effective for RLS, but is associated with a higher rate of augmentation and morning rebound [13, 20]. Other agents effective in the treatment of RLS prescribed off-label include opioids, benzodiazepines, and anticonvulsants such as pregabalin, carbamazepine, and gabapentin. Opioids are typically reserved for severe, refractory RLS when other agents are not effective or during withdrawal from dopaminergic agents in patients who develop augmentation. Their use is limited by constipation and concerns of dependency and tolerance [13]. Benzodiazepines improve RLS symptoms and sleep continuity in some patients, particularly in RLS patients with insomnia [13]. Gabapentin and gabapentin enacarbil are effective for symptom control without risk of rebound, withdrawal, or impulse control, although daytime somnolence has been reported [20].

Therapeutic interventions for RLS during pregnancy have not been formally studied. When severe, RLS can impact sleep duration and quality and may impact pregnancy outcomes [25]. Therefore, treatment in severe cases in the third trimester using low doses of

Table 17.4 Pharmacotherapy for restless legs syndrome

Drug class	Drug name (brands)	Dosage (mg)	Pregnancy class	FDA use	Comments
Dopaminergic agents (*agonists)					
	Ropinirole (Requip, Requip XR)*	0.25–4	C	Yes	Nausea, orthostatic hypotension
	Pramipexole (Mirapex, Mirapex ER)*	0.125–1.5	C	Yes	
	Rotigotine (Neupro)*	1–3/patch	C	Yes	
	Levodopa (L-dopa) or Carbidopa/levodopa (Sinemet)	10/100–50/200	C	No	Risk for augmentation
	Cabergoline (Dostinex)*	0.5–2	B	No	Ergot derivative; used for hyperprolactinemia
Anticonvulsants					
	Gabapentin enacarbil (Horizant)	600–1200	C	Yes	Once daily in evening taken with food
	Gabapentin (Neurontin)	200–2000	C	No	Useful for painful RLS; associated neuropathy
	Pregabalin (Lyrica)	50–450	C	No	
	Carbamazepine	200–400	D	No	Based on small series/case reports
Opioids					
	Oxycodone (Oxycontin, Roxicodone)	10–20	B	No	Scheduled controlled substances; lowest
	Codeine	≥15	C	No	dose should be used; abuse potential;
	Tramadol	50–150	C	No	shorter acting can aid with breakthrough
	Methadone	5–15	C	No	symptoms
Benzodiazepines					
	Clonazepam (Klonopin)	0.5–2	D	No	Sedation; dependency
Alpha-adrenergic agonists					
	Clonidine (Catapres, Kapvay)	≥0.1	C	No	Rebound hypertension, sedation
Vitamins and minerals					
	Ferrous sulfate (+ vitamin C)	325 mg BID/TID	—	—	Used for iron deficiency (ferritin <50 µg/L)
	Magnesium oxide	~300 mg/12.4 mmol	—	No	Dietary supplement

medication may be warranted [25]. The dopaminergic agents have theoretical risks on lactogenesis due to inhibitory properties of prolactin secretion by the dopamine receptor, and should not be used while breast feeding [13, 25]. Cabergoline is the only Pregnancy Class B dopaminergic agent, but has not been studied in pregnant women with RLS [12]. Benzodiazepines are generally avoided in pregnancy due to concerns of teratogenicity [13]. Similarly the use of anticonvulsants in pregnancy should be determined on a case-by-case basis and may be indicated if the benefits of therapy outweigh the risk of neonatal exposure [26]. Some opioids have a long history of safety in pregnancy, but carry risk of neonatal withdrawal syndrome with chronic use [13, 26]. Oxycodone is rated as a Pregnancy Class B drug and may be considered in small doses in severe cases. Intravenous magnesium sulfate used in pre-term labor completely resolved RLS symptoms in a single case report [27]. Magnesium has a depressant effect on neuronal excitability. In an open-label, unblinded study in non-pregnant patients with RLS taking oral magnesium nightly for 4–6 weeks, subjective improvement in sleep quality, reduced periodic limb movements, and increased sleep efficiency were observed [28].

Narcolepsy and the central hypersomnias

Hypersomnia is defined as the inability to sustain an alert and wakeful state during the usual waking part of the day. Fatigue, on the other hand, is the perception of lack of energy without an increased ability to fall asleep. The Epworth Sleepiness Scale (ESS) is a widely used subjective scale that ascertains one's self-reported propensity to doze during usual daytime activities. Abnormal sleepiness (ESS ≥10) and napping is commonly reported in pregnant women [10]. One-third of pregnant women have elevated ESS scores in the first trimester, and nearly half in the final trimester [16]. Daytime impairment due to hypersomnia is commonly reported

in the first trimester, remitting somewhat in the second trimester, and then increasing again by the third trimester of pregnancy [10, 16]. Postpartum, daytime sleepiness is magnified by the nocturnal demands of neonatal care. Women with more nocturnal sleep disturbance and less sleep in the post-partum period are more likely to have depressive symptoms [13].

The etiology of hypersomnia during pregnancy is likely multifactorial. In the general population, insufficient sleep is the most common cause of daytime sleepiness. In pregnancy, other sleep disorders such as OSA and RLS should be considered. Circadian rhythm disturbances can also cause daytime impairment due to the malalignment of sleep times with the normal circadian rhythm. Central disorders of hypersomnia should be considered in patients with severe daytime sleepiness not due to other more common disorders. Central disorders of hypersomnia include idiopathic hypersomnia, narcolepsy with and without cataplexy, narcolepsy or hypersomnia secondary to medical conditions, and hypersomnia secondary to drugs or substance abuse [2].

Severe daytime sleepiness is the hallmark of narcolepsy and the central hypersomnias. Narcolepsy is estimated to affect 0.02% of the population [2]. Narcolepsy is characterized by a pentad of symptoms including daytime sleepiness often accompanied by disturbed nocturnal sleep, sleep-related hallucinations, sleep paralysis, and cataplexy. Cataplexy is episodic, sudden, transient weakness resulting from loss of muscle tone that is triggered by strong emotions which are usually positive (e.g., laughing). It is generally bilateral, brief, and associated with a transient loss of deep tendon reflexes. Episodes can vary in frequency and intensity. Cataplexy, like rapid eye movement (REM) sleep, is regulated by adrenergic and cholinergic pathways involved in sleep–wake physiology [13]. The intrusion of REM into the waking state produces sudden, reversible muscle atonia and areflexia during a cataplectic attack [13]. Loss of hypothalamic hypocretin-secreting neurons is the primary pathophysiological defect of narcolepsy. Most narcolepsy patients, and especially those with cataplexy, have low cerebrospinal fluid hypocretin [13]. The loss of hypocretin contributes to instability of sleep- and wake-promoting pathways in the central nervous system, the so-called "flip flop" switch, causing REM intrusion into wakefulness (sleep-related hallucinations, sleep paralysis, and cataplexy), excessive sleepiness, and disturbed nocturnal sleep at night [13]. Though the cause of hypocretin deficiency is unknown, autoimmune destruction of these cells by unknown environmental triggers in susceptible patients with HLA DQB1*0602 predisposition has been hypothesized [13].

The diagnostic criteria for narcolepsy are shown in Table 17.5 [2]. Confirmation with objective sleep testing is recommended, though not required in patients with definite cataplexy [13, 29]. Overnight PSG followed by a multiple sleep latency test (MSLT) is used to exclude other sleep disorders and confirm the presence of daytime sleepiness. The MSLT consists of 5 nap trials performed at 2-hour intervals beginning no sooner than 1.5–3 hours after the morning awakening. During a nap trial, the propensity to sleep is recorded and sleep latency is measured. Mean sleep latency (MSL) across the nap trials and REM sleep periods (SOREMPs) are calculated. Results of the MSLT can be affected by REM suppressant medications and alcohol, environmental factors, and sleep timing/duration prior to testing. Thus, the use of sleep logs or actigraphy, a portal device worn on the wrist that estimates sleep and wake patterns, is recommended for 1–2 weeks prior to testing [2].

Table 17.5 Diagnostic criteria for narcolepsy I (with cataplexy) and narcolepsy II (without cataplexy)

Classification	Diagnostic criteria
Narcolepsy (without cataplexy)	
A	The patient has daily periods of irrepressible need to sleep or daytime sleepiness lapses into sleep occurring for at least 3 months.
B	A mean sleep latency of ≤8 minutes and two or more sleep onset REM periods (SOREMPs) on an MSLT performed according to standard techniques. SOREMP (within 15 minutes of sleep onset) on the preceding nocturnal polysomnogram may replace one of the SOREMPs on the MSLT.
C	Cataplexy is absent.
D	*Either* CSF hypocretin-1 concentration has not been measured *or* CSF hypocretin-1 concentration measured by immunoreactivity is either >110 pg/mL or >1/3 of mean values obtained in normal subjects with the same standardized assay.
E	The hypersomnolence and/or MSLT findings are not better explained by other causes such as insufficient sleep, obstructive sleep apnea, delayed sleep phase disorder, or the effect of medication or substances or their withdrawal.
Narcolepsy (with cataplexy)	
A	The patient has daily periods of irrepressible need to sleep or daytime sleepiness lapses into sleep occurring for at least 3 months.
B	The presence of one or both of the following: 1 Cataplexy *and* a mean sleep latency of ≤8 minutes and two or more sleep onset REM periods (SOREMPs) on an MSLT performed according to standard techniques. SOREMP (within 15 minutes of sleep onset) on the preceding nocturnal polysomnogram may replace one of the SOREMPs on the MSLT. 2 CSF hypocretin-1 concentration measured by immunoreactivity is either ≤110 pg/mL or <1/3 of mean values obtained in normal subjects with the same standardized assay.

Adapted from American Academy of Sleep Medicine 2014. Reproduced with permission of American Academy of Sleep Medicine [2].

The treatment of narcolepsy and other central nervous system hypersomnias is limited to optimization of wakefulness using conservative approaches combined with strategic use of caffeine, naps, and pharmacological agents, as no therapies yet exist that are targeted to correct the hypocretin deficiency. Regular timing of adequate sleep, avoidance of shift work, and regular naps are recommended. Unintentional sleep episodes impacting work or school performance or driving or interfering with personal and social commitments require pharmacological strategies. Drug therapy for narcolepsy best targets daytime sleepiness and cataplexy (Table 17.6) [13]. Agents effective for cataplexy are generally also effective for the other REM manifestations of narcolepsy but not for daytime sleepiness. According to the American Academy of Sleep Medicine practice parameter, modafinil/armodafinil and sodium oxybate, both FDA-approved for treatment of daytime sleepiness in narcolepsy, are standards of therapy for wake promotion [29]. Sodium oxybate is the only agent FDA approved for both daytime sleepiness and cataplexy. Traditional stimulants (e.g., dextroamphetamines and methylphenidate) have a long history of clinical utility for wake promotion. The goal of wake promotion is to use the lowest dose possible to achieve maximal daytime functioning while minimizing side effects [29]. Dosing and timing need to be individualized, as medication effects vary widely [13]. Typical first-line agents are modafinil/armodafinil and methylphenidate [29]. Initial dosing is daily in the morning, though repeated administration may be required to optimize wakefulness throughout the day. Close clinical monitoring is required for adverse effects, dependence, and tolerance. When taken late in the day, wake-promoting agents can cause insomnia [13, 29].

Management of narcolepsy during pregnancy is based on anecdotal observations as no prospective studies or large series are available. Sodium oxybate is the only Pregnancy Class B agent and warrants consideration. The use of pharmacotherapy for the treatment of daytime sleepiness in pregnant women with narcolepsy and other hypersomnias should be considered carefully, weighing the risks and benefits on a case-by-case basis. Some women may elect to withhold medical therapy that can result in the need to curtail employment obligations and limit driving [30]. In others, the risks and consequences of severe daytime sleepiness necessitate ongoing therapy, despite the uncertainties of its effect on the fetus [31]. Frequent episodes of significant or uncontrollable cataplexy may incur risk to the mother and interfere with labor and delivery, rarely leading to C-section [31]. In women with significant cataplexy, elective C-section delivery may be warranted. Cataleptic episodes are typically improved with medication, but symptoms return or rebound off medications. Sodium oxybate is the only FDA-approved treatment for cataplexy. Other agents used for cataplexy, such as the tricyclic antidepressants and selective serotonin reuptake inhibitors are generally less effective and prescribed off-label. Nearly all stimulants are excreted in breast milk, while excretion of non-traditional stimulants (e.g., modafinil, sodium oxybate) is unknown.

Conclusions

Sleep and its associated disorders are profoundly affected by pregnancy and menopausal status. The high prevalence of sleep disorders including insomnia, RLS, and OSA in pregnant and menopausal women warrant attention in clinical practice. Women are particularly vulnerable to insomnia and RLS, and prevalence rates of these disorders increase in menopause and pregnancy. Though some changes in sleep during pregnancy may be physiological, awareness of the emergence of sleep disorders in this population is growing. Worsening sleep quality, nocturnal awakenings, and daytime sleepiness should prompt further evaluation of sleep disorders. Finally, preliminary findings implicating

Table 17.6 Pharmacotherapy for narcolepsy

Drug class	Drug name (Brand)	Dosage (mg)	Pregnancy class	Indication[a]	Comments
Non-stimulant wake promoting agents	Modafinil (Provigil)	100–400	C	Narcolepsy[a], EDS in OSA[a], shift workers[a]	Headaches, nausea; nervousness; reduces efficacy of OCs
	Armodafinil (Nuvigil)	150–250			
CNS depressant	Sodium oxybate (Xyrem): *administered in 2 divided nightly doses*	4.5–9	B	EDS and cataplexy in narcolepsy[a]	Nausea edema due to high salt content, sleep walking, respiratory depression; may not combine with CNS depressants
Stimulants	Methylphenidate: Short acting: (Metadate, Methylin, Ritalin); Intermediate acting: (Metadate/Methylin ER, Ritalin SR); Long acting: (Metadate CD, Concerta, Ritalin LA)	10–60	C	Narcolepsy[b]	Schedule II controlled substances; potential for abuse; risk of neonatal toxicity/withdrawal; stimulant effects (e.g., headaches, palpitations)
	Dexmethylphenidate: (Focalin, Focalin XR)	10–60			
	Dextroamphetamines: (Dexedrine, Dextrostat, Dexedrine SR)	5–60			
	Mixed Dextro and Amphetamine Salts: (Adderall, Adderall XR)	5–60			
	Methamphetamines: (Desoxyn)	5–40			
Tricyclic antidepressant	Protriptyline (Vivactil)	25–200	C	Cataplexy	Dry mouth, urinary retention, constipation
	Clomipramine (Anafranil)	10–150			
	Desipramine (Norpramin)	25–100			
	Imipramine (Tofranil)	5–30			
Selective serotonin reuptake inhibitors	Fluoxetine (Prozac, Sarafem)	20–80	C	Cataplexy	Sexual dysfunction, dry mouth, nausea
	Venlafaxine (Effexor)	75–225			
Xanthine adenosine antagonist	Caffeine	<200	C	—	Small doses not associated with neonatal risk

[a]FDA approved.

[b]Methylphenidate and amphetamines are chemicals indicated for the treatment of narcolepsy symptoms. Newer drug formulations comprising these compounds are not specifically FDA approved for narcolepsy.

EDS, excessive daytime sleepiness; OCs, oral contraceptives; CNS, central nervous system; OSA, obstructive sleep apnea.

some sleep disorders as operative in poor pregnancy outcomes underscores the importance of basic research and prospective clinical studies in this important area of women's health research.

References

1 Facco FL, Kramer J, Ho KH, Zee PC, Grobman WA. Sleep disturbances in pregnancy. *Obstet Gynecol.* 2010;115(1):77–83.

2 Sateia M, ed. International *classification of sleep disorders*, 3rd ed. Westchester, IL: American Academy of Sleep Medicine, 2014.

3 Wilson DL, Barnes M, Ellett L, Permezel M, Jackson M, Crowe SF. Decreased sleep efficiency, increased wake after sleep onset and increased cortical arousals in late pregnancy. *Aust N Z J Obstet Gynaecol.* 2011;51(1):38–46.

4 Hedman C, Pohjasvaara T, Tolonen U, Suhonen-Malm AS, Myllylä VV. Effects of pregnancy on mothers' sleep. *Sleep Med.* 2002;3(1):37–42.

5 Moline ML, Broch L, Zak R, Gross V. Sleep in women across the life cycle from adulthood through menopause. *Sleep Med Rev.* 2003;7(2): 155–176.

6 Williams MA, Miller RS, Qiu C, Cripe SM, Gelaye B, Enquobahrie D. Associations of early pregnancy sleep duration with trimester-specific blood pressures and hypertensive disorders in pregnancy. *Sleep.* 2010;33(10):1363–1371.

7 Facco FL, Grobman WA, Kramer J, Ho KH, Zee PC. Self-reported short sleep duration and frequent snoring in pregnancy: impact on glucose metabolism. *Am J Obstet Gynecol.* 2010;203(2): 142.e1–142.e5.

8 Collop NA, Adkins D, Phillips BA. Gender differences in sleep and sleep-disordered breathing. *Clin Chest Med.* 2004;25(2):257–268.

9 Schutte-Rodin S, Broch L, Buysse D, Dorsey C, Sateia M. Clinical guideline for the evaluation and management of chronic insomnia in adults. *J Clin Sleep Med.* 2008;4(5):487–504.

10 Neau JP, Texier B, Ingrand P. Sleep and vigilance disorders in pregnancy. *Eur Neurol.* 2009;62(1): 23–29.

11 Swanson LM, Pickett SM, Flynn H, Armitage R. Relationships among depression, anxiety, and insomnia symptoms in perinatal women seeking mental health treatment. *J Womens Health (Larchmt).* 2011;20(4):553–558.

12 Drugs in: UpToDate, Post T (Ed), UpToDate, Waltham, MA; 2015.

13 Kryger M, Roth T, Dement W, eds. *Principles and Practice of Sleep Medicine.* 4th ed. Philadelphia: Elsevier, 2005.

14 Cheng SK, Dizon J. Computerised cognitive behavioural therapy for insomnia: a systematic review and meta-analysis. *Psychother Psychosom.* 2012;81(4):206–216.

15 Olivarez SA, Ferres M, Antony K, et al. Obstructive sleep apnea screening in pregnancy, perinatal outcomes, and impact of maternal obesity. *Am J Perinatol.* 2011;28(8):651–658.

16 Pien GW, Fife D, Pack AI, Nkwuo JE, Schwab RJ. Changes in symptoms of sleep-disordered breathing during pregnancy. *Sleep.* 2005;28(10):1299–1305.

17 Bourjeily G, Ankner G, Mohsenin V. Sleep-disordered breathing in pregnancy. *Clin Chest Med.* 2011;32(1):175–189.

18 Champagne K, Schwartzman K, Opatrny L, et al. Obstructive sleep apnoea and its association with gestational hypertension. *Eur Respir J.* 2009;33(3):559–565.

19 Tauman R, Many A, Deutsch V, et al. Maternal snoring during pregnancy is associated with enhanced fetal erythropoiesis–a preliminary study. *Sleep Med.* 2011;12(5):518–522.

20 Aurora RN, Kristo DA, Bista SR, et al. The treatment of restless legs syndrome and periodic limb movement disorder in adults–an update for 2012: practice parameters with an evidence-based systematic review and meta-analyses: an American Academy of Sleep Medicine Clinical Practice Guideline. *Sleep.* 2012;35(8):1039–1062.

21 Manconi M, Ulfberg J, Berger K, et al. When gender matters: restless legs syndrome. Report of the "RLS and woman" workshop endorsed by the European RLS Study Group. *Sleep Med Rev.* 2012;16(4):297–307.

22 Winkelman JW, Shahar E, Sharief I, Gottlieb DJ. Association of restless legs syndrome and cardiovascular disease in the Sleep Heart Health Study. *Neurology.* 2008;70(1):35–42.

23 Neau JP, Porcheron A, Mathis S, et al. Restless legs syndrome and pregnancy: a questionnaire study in the Poitiers District, France. *Eur Neurol.* 2010;64(5):268–274.

24 Dzaja A, Wehrle R, Lancel M, Pollmächer T. Elevated estradiol plasma levels in women with restless legs during pregnancy. *Sleep.* 2009;32(2): 169–174.

25 Manconi   M, Ferini-Strambi L, Hening WA. Response to Clinical Corners case (Sleep Medicine 6/2: 83–4): Pregnancy associated with daytime sleepiness and nighttime restlessness. *Sleep Med.* 2005;6(5):477–478.

26 Djokanovic N, Garcia-Bournissen F, Koren G. Medications for restless legs syndrome in pregnancy. *J Obstet Gynaecol Can.* 2008;30(6):505–507.

27 Bartell S, Zallek S. Intravenous magnesium sulfate may relieve restless legs syndrome in pregnancy. *J Clin Sleep Med.* 2006;2(2):187–188.

28 Hornyak M, Voderholzer U, Hohagen F, Berger M, Riemann D. Magnesium therapy for periodic leg movements-related insomnia and restless legs syndrome: an open pilot study. *Sleep.* 1998;21(5):501–505.

29 Morgenthaler TI, Kapur VK, Brown T, et al. Practice parameters for the treatment of narcolepsy and other hypersomnias of central origin. *Sleep.* 2007;30(12):1705–1711.

30 Hoque R, Chesson AL. Conception, pregnancy, delivery, and breastfeeding in a narcoleptic patient with cataplexy. *J Clin Sleep Med.* 2008;4(6):601–603.

31 Soltanifar S, Russell R. Neuraxial anaesthesia for caesarean section in a patient with narcolepsy and cataplexy. *Int J Obstet Anesth.* 2010;19(4):440–443.

CHAPTER 18

Neurourology of pregnancy

Kimberly L. Ferrante, Victor W. Nitti, & Benjamin M. Brucker

New York University School of Medicine, New York, NY, USA

Introduction

There are many pathophysiologic changes that occur in pregnancy. These include changes in the neurologic pathways to the lower urinary tract. In order to understand the changes that occur, we must first understand the normal neurophysiologic control of micturition.

A review of the neurophysiologic control of micturition

Innervation of the lower urinary tract is supplied by the autonomic nervous system, both the sympathetic system and parasympathetic system, as well as the somatic sensory and motor systems. This complex interaction of neurologic control, along with anatomic relationships and biomechanical properties, should allow for low-pressure storage of urine and voluntary complete expulsion of urine at an acceptable time interval (Figure 18.1).

Sympathetic innervation

The sympathetic nervous system acts on the detrusor muscle, the primary muscle of the bladder, as well as the bladder neck and intramural bladder ganglia. Preganglionic fibers of the sympathetic nervous system originate in the thoracolumbar spinal segments and synapse with both the prevertebral and paravertebral pathways. The postganglionic neurons then run through the lumbar splanchnic nerves to the inferior mesenteric ganglia and continue on through the hypogastric plexus to the upper posterior lateral pelvic wall in the presacral fascia. Here the neurons join the pelvic nerves forming the pelvic plexus. The pelvic plexus runs with the internal iliac vessels, which overlie the lower rectum anteriorly and laterally close to the anorectal junction. The pelvic plexus also innervates the lateral wall of the upper third of the vagina, bladder, and both the proximal urethra and lower ureter [1].

The preganglionic nerves release acetylcholine chiefly as a neurotransmitter while the postganglionic nerves release norepinepherine. The amount of norepinepherine released determines which receptors respond. Lower doses of norepinepherine stimulate the β-adrenergics located in the bladder body and promote detrusor muscle relaxation. Higher doses of norepinepherine stimulate α-receptors causing contraction in the bladder base as well as the smooth muscle of the urethra. Norepinepherine also works at the α-receptors of the parasympathetic ganglia and inhibits release of presynaptic acetylcholine thus minimizing parasympathetic pelvic ganglion firing. This acts to promote urine storage along with the noradrenergic effects of relaxation of the detrusor with contraction of the urethra and bladder base [2]. Thus the

Neurological Illness in Pregnancy: Principles and Practice, First Edition.
Edited by Autumn Klein, M. Angela O'Neal, Christina Scifres, Janet F. R. Waters and Jonathan H. Waters.
© 2016 John Wiley & Sons, Ltd. Published 2016 by John Wiley & Sons, Ltd.

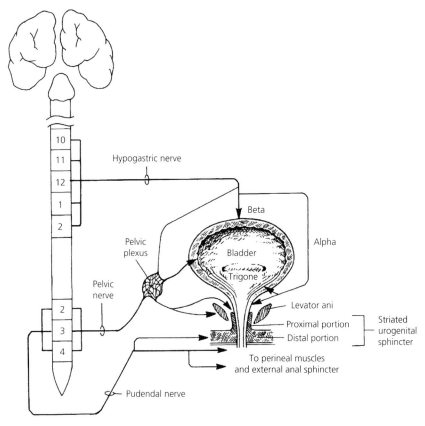

Figure 18.1 Peripheral innervation of the female lower urinary tract. Reproduced from Reference 1 with permission of Elsevier.

sympathetic effect is mostly facilatory on the sphincter mechanism and inhibitory on the detrusor promoting urine storage.

Parasympathetic innervation

Preganglionic fibers of the parasympathetic system arise in the nerve roots of S2–S4 in the conus medullaris. These fibers reach the presacral fascia running along the piriformis muscle overlying the sacral foramina. They merge with the pelvic plexus at the level of the ischial spine posteriorly in the hypogastric sheath. Like the sympathetics of the pelvic plexus, these parasympathetics innervate the rectum, genitalia, and the lower urinary tract. Those innervating the bladder terminate in pelvic ganglia within the wall of the bladder [1].

The nicotinic acetylcholine receptors are primarily responsible for excitatory transmission at the ganglia, however, some ganglia also have secondary muscarinic receptors. The predominant muscarinic receptors within the detrusor muscle are the M2 and M3 subtypes. Smooth muscle contraction of the bladder is thought to be mediated in large part by M3 receptors. Therapies for overactive bladder and urgency incontinence target these receptors. Stimulation of M2 receptors inhibits bladder relaxation by inhibiting adenyl cyclase release. Transmission of all of the neurotransmitters within the bladder wall is not yet fully understood, but is also thought to involve the neuropeptides vasoactive intestinal polypeptide (VIP) and substance P [3]. Thus the parasympathetic effect primarily facilitates detrusor contraction and is inhibitory to the sphincter mechanism promoting bladder emptying.

Innervation of the trigone and urethra

At birth, the trigone of the bladder is predominated by cholinergic receptors. This however changes and eventually the α-1 receptors (sympathetic) predominate. The urethra is also laden with α receptors. Along with norepinepherine, acetylcholine, VIP, and histamine are all neurotransmitters which act in the urethra [4]. Parasympathetic postganglionic neurotransmission is mediated mainly by nitric oxide, which acts to relax the smooth muscle of the urethra. Studies in cat bladders have also suggested that urethral relaxation is mediated in part by β adrenergics [5].

Somatic innervation

The neurons supplying somatic innervation to the lower urinary tract originate in Onuf's somatic nucleus, located laterally in the anterior horn gray matter from S2–S4. This nucleus is the origin of the pudendal nerve, which supplies efferent innervation to the striated sphincter (also known as the external sphincter, voluntary sphincter, or rhabdosphincter) of the urethra. The pudendal nerve releases acetylcholine resulting in contraction of the urethral sphincter by activating nicotinic cholinergic receptors. Controversy surrounds the exact pathways that innervate the skeletal muscle of the urethral sphincter. Somatic efferent branches of the pelvic nerves, which come from the pelvic plexus, innervate the proximal intramural portion of the rhabdosphincter. This innervation is thought to have both somatic and autonomic components [6]. The pudendal nerve then innervates the more distal periurethral striated muscles of the compressor urethra and urethrovaginal sphincter, other muscles that contribute to urethral support and urinary continence.

Regulation of somatic motor activity of the urethral skeletal muscle is different than the norm in that the muscle does not contain spindles. Typically the afferent arm of the spinal reflex would originate in the muscle spindles, synapse in the spinal cord and then an efferent arm would send the signal back to the muscle. The pudendal nerve innervates the periurethral striated muscle via one of its branches, the deep branch of the perineal nerve. Several spinal cord segments are involved in the spinal reflex response leading to pudendal nerve function. The afferent fibers of the reflex are transmitted both segmentally and via supraspinal routing. The receptors at this neuromuscular junction are nicotinic.

Sensory

When a normal bladder fills, there is little or no increase in intravesical pressure due to the compliance of the bladder wall. The filling process causes a stretch in the muscle cells up to 4 times their length. Thus the somatic sensors in the bladder wall respond primarily to stretch or contraction. The urothelium, once thought to be a passive barrier to urine, has been found to have a role in sensing bladder distention and chemical stimulation. Noxious stimuli (i.e., chemical stimuli) activate receptors or ion channels in the urothelial cells, which result in the release of mediators such as adenosine triphosphate, nitric oxide, acetylcholine, and nerve growth factor. These target adjacent nerves and myofibroblast and may have a paracrine effect on adjacent urothelial cells.

Urgency is transmitted via the parasympathetic system, but the sensory innervation can also follow the sympathetic pathway. The pudendal nerve is responsible for primarily carrying the signals of urethral sensation with help from the pelvic nerve. This innervation is both contralateral and ipsilateral in its supply.

Central nervous system

Central nervous system (CNS) control over the lower urinary tract is complex and not completely understood, however it involves primarily both the spinal cord and the brainstem [7]. The suprapontine brain is also involved in inhibition of the detrusor muscle and facilitates urine storage. The brainstem also exerts control on the detrusor muscle while the periurethral muscles are connected to the sacral spinal cord. Both cortical and subcortical pathways are involved with bladder activity as a whole with glutamate and gama-aminobutyric acid (GABA) being the chief neurotransmitters in these pathways. Cortical pathways include the precentral gyrus, lateral prefrontal cortex, anterior cingulated gyrus, while subcortical pathways involve the basal ganglia, brainstem raphe nuclei, locus ceruleus, hypothalamus, and midbrain periaqueductal gray. These specifically affect the medial and lateral pons in the brainstem. The pontine micturition center (or the M region), located in this area, is responsible for motor tone of the bladder, while the L region (the pontine storage center) plays a large role in continence [8].

Bladder filling and storage

Storage is controlled by the sympathetic system (Figure 18.2). McGuire (1986) demonstrated three responses to afferent adrenergic stimulation associated with increasing bladder volume [9]. These include a β receptor mediated relaxation of the detrusor muscle, an α-mediated contraction of urethral smooth muscle, as well as an inhibition of the pelvic ganglia to prevent parasympathetic signaling back to the bladder. Somatic innervation via a spinal reflex also contributes to storage by increasing the urethral pressure so that it maintains a pressure greater than that of the detrusor. As stated previously, the L region of the pons also contributes to the voluntary component of storage.

Voiding

Voiding is largely controlled by the parasympathetic system, however the precise pathways remain controversial. Most of our understanding comes from animal models [10]. In normal voiding, there is voluntary relaxation of the urethra with a coordinated contraction of the bladder. The M center of the pons is likely involved with this effort. Connections between the frontal cortex and the pons are what supply voluntary control of the micturition reflex. The external urethral sphincter on the other hand is controlled by the voluntary pathway from the frontal cortex to the pudendal nucleus located in the ventral horn of the spinal cord. There are thought to be complex connections mediating the connection between the sensorimotor cortex and the pudendal nucleus via the frontal cortex, thalamus, hypothalamus, basal ganglia, as well as the mesencephalic-pontine-medullary reticular formation in order to control

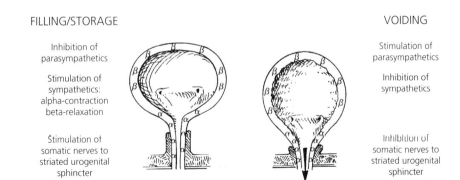

FILLING/STORAGE

Inhibition of parasympathetics

Stimulation of sympathetics: alpha-contraction beta-relaxation

Stimulation of somatic nerves to striated urogenital sphincter

VOIDING

Stimulation of parasympathetics

Inhibition of sympathetics

Inhibition of somatic nerves to striated urogenital sphincter

Figure 18.2 The role of the autonomic and somatic nervous systems in bladder filling and storage, as well as voiding. Reproduced from Reference 1 with permission of Elsevier.

voluntary sphincter activity [11]. Somatic stimulation from the bladder as it fills sends an afferent signal to the pelvic nerves which synapse with the spinal cord, connecting to the pontine mesencephalic reticular formation. This sends the sensation of bladder fullness to the brain. The external urethral sphincter then relaxes voluntarily to initiate voiding via inhibition of somatic motor neurons in the ventral horn of the spinal cord. This is controlled by efferent firing from the M center in the pons inhibiting pudendal firing and thus relaxing the sphincter while stimulating detrusor contraction by activating parasympathetic neurons in the intermediolateral cell column at the level of S2 through S4. Sympathetic efferents are inhibited during voiding, opening the bladder neck via postganglionic parasympathetic stimulation.

Changes to the urinary system during pregnancy

The urinary system is not spared by the multitude of physiologic changes seen during pregnancy. The specific neurologic changes and potential nerve injuries are described below within this section, but first we provide a summary of other physiologic changes to the urinary system.

The kidney length is increased by approximately a centimeter, the renal pelvis, calyces and ureters all dilate. There is an increased glomerular filtration rate and renal plasma flow increases by approximately 50%. There are also changes in acid–base metabolism and renal water handling [12]. Focusing, however, on the lower urinary tract, the bladder is greatly affected by the growing uterus. Before 12 weeks of gestational age, there are few changes seen. However, after the first trimester, the size of the uterus causes bladder pressure to increase from 8 cm H_2O to 20 cm H_2O at term [13]. To compensate for this, the urethral length increases by approximately half a centimeter and the maximal urethral pressure increases from 70 to 93 cm

H_2O in an effort to maintain continence. However, this is not always successful. Over 90% of women will have one or more urinary symptoms in pregnancy, with frequency of urination and stress urinary incontinence being the most common [14]. Approximately 20% of women will report new onset stress incontinence during pregnancy and leakage can be elicited on physical examination [15].

Other lower urinary tract symptoms include increased urine output and urinary frequency. Frequency is present at some stage of pregnancy in 81% if women [16]. This is in part due to the increased glomerular filtration rate and also increased fluid intake. While the trend amongst the lay public is to drink more water in recent years, these observations go back to the 1960's [16]. Pregnant women take in on average approximately half a liter more fluid than non-pregnant women. This is likely a response to increased fluid output [17]. The enlarging uterus would also presumably make bladder capacity smaller, however this has proven not to be the case. Bladder capacity as tested by cystometry, does not decrease during pregnancy for the majority of women [16]. Symptoms of frequency usually begin in the first trimester and worsen throughout the pregnancy [18].

Pregnancy also increases the mobility and descent of the bladder. Pregnant women have more descent of the bladder neck with valsalva than non-pregnant controls [19] and there is evidence that stage II anterior wall prolapse (to within 1 cm of the hymen) is present in almost half of women in their first pregnancy [20, 21]. This prolapse usually resolves with delivery and does not require treatment.

The bladder and urethral mobility can also be tested by a retroverted uterus. Although urinary retention is an uncommon occurrence (approximately 1 in 3000–8000 pregnancies) [22, 23], it is important to understand the etiology. The most common gestational age for this to occur is 12–14 weeks and the cause is usually a retroverted uterus which has become incarcerated in the pelvis. This can happen secondary to the presence of uterine fibroids, uterine anomalies, as well as a contracted pelvis. When attempting to place a catheter in this situation, the practitioner should know that the catheter usually passes quite easily. One hypothesis is that the fixed retroverted positioning places the bladder base on so much stretch that the urethra cannot relax in order to allow voiding [16]. This theory has been supported by urodynamic data in these patients who show an inability to void and lack of urethral contraction along with absence of detrusor activity. Another hypothesis involves the elevated progesterone levels found in pregnancy. In other high progesterone states such as assisted reproductive technology, patients have experienced urinary retention in the absence of pregnancy and urodynamic testing has again shown that the urethra is unable to relax and the detrusor unable to contract when attempting to void. A study in rabbits also shows that progesterone affects the adrenergic response of the bladder [24]. Urinary retention, although more common in the first trimester, can happen at any gestational age in pregnancy because of the high levels of progesterone throughout.

Treatment of urinary retention secondary to a retroverted uterus involves bimanual manipulation into an anteverted position. Placing the patient in a knee–chest position can help with this. In the case of patient intolerance, anesthesia should be used. Rarely, intra-abdominal surgery is necessary to relieve the position. In the majority of cases, the uterus remains in the anteverted position. In the rare case that the uterus resumes its retroverted position and continued stretch of the bladder neck, the patient will require intermittent self catheterization usually for a period of 1–2 weeks until the uterus no longer fits within the pelvis and can no longer become incarcerated. An alternative therapy involves the placement of a Smith–Hodge lever pessary to maintain an anteverted uterine positioning.

Physiologic changes to the lower urinary tract in pregnancy also include changes in the neurotransmitter receptors. Many of these documented changes are going to be extrapolated from animal studies. The lack of human studies may come from the difficulties and ethical consideration of studying pregnant women. One of the changes of neurotransmitter receptors was described by Baselli and colleagues [25]. This study looked at pregnant rabbit bladders and showed that muscarinic receptors decrease in density by 24%, further contractile response was lessened in pregnancy. In addition, Wilfehrt and colleagues in 1999 found smaller bladder contractions of parous rats when compared to age-matched virgins. Parous rats also showed diminished relaxation response to norepinepherine when compared to controls [26].

Although limited, some human data have been published. In 2012, Frederice and colleagues found that decreased basal tone in the urinary bladder was associated with irritative bladder symptoms amongst women in the third trimester [27]. They looked at 91 nulliparous women between 30–34 weeks of gestational age evaluating both pelvic floor muscle function via surface electromyography (EMG) as well as irritative bladder symptoms. Symptoms were elicited with questioning using the International Continence Society's terminology [28]. Nocturia was reported by 80% of women, with increased daytime frequency reported by 59%. And both stress and urge incontinence were present in 51% and 25% of women, respectively.

Disorders resulting from parturition

There are few neurourologic disorders described in the antenatal period. However, during parturition and the postpartum period there is a greater potential for neurologic disruption affecting the lower urinary tract. The pudendal nerve is the most likely nerve to be injured in this period resulting in a pudendal neuropathy. This can occur via direct injury to the pelvic nerves from compression by the fetal head or secondary to assisted delivery with forceps, a traction injury during the second stage of labor with descent of the fetal head. In addition, prolapse occurring for a prolonged period after vaginal delivery can also result in injury secondary to excessive stretch placed on the nerve. This prolapse also causes disruption of the pelvic floor muscles which play an intimate role in voiding function. Some degree of pudendal neuropathy can occur in up to 80% of women having their first baby [29].

Pudendal nerve damage is usually a result of demyelination, although rarely it can involve axonal disruption in severe cases [30]. In a study of nerve conduction by Snooks et al. in 1984, women who delivered vaginally had significantly prolonged mean pudendal nerve terminal motor latency, implying nerve damage, when compared to those women who delivered via cesarean section or non-parous controls [31]. Interestingly, the latency tended to be even longer in multiparous women compared to primiparous women. However, primiparous women who delivered with the aid of forceps had the longest latencies. The abnormalities in nerve conduction were mostly resolved by the 2-month follow-up visit. The exception was multiparous women, who were delivered via forceps. In contrast to these finding Allen et al. (1990) found minimal improvement of pudendal nerve latency at 2 months [29]. In a study of direct pudendal nerve crush in a rat model, there was incomplete recovery at 2 weeks, while there was evidence of neuroregeneration at the 6-week mark [32]. Clinical practice suggests that most pudendal injuries resolve with time however, studies with longer follow up are needed. Risk factors for pudendal nerve injury include increasing parity, the use of forceps, and increasing birth weight [33].

As described above in the section Somatic innervation, the external urethral sphincter is innervated by the perineal branch of the pudendal nerve. The normal function of the external sphincter can be affected by nerve injury. In a rat model of pudendal nerve injury, they found that it resulted in decreased urethral outlet resistance as well as striated muscle atrophy in the external urethral sphincter [34]. Snooks et al. in 1985 showed that women with stress urinary incontinence had increased motor nerve latency of the perineal branch of the pudendal nerve to the urethral striated sphincter muscles [35]. While risk of persistent stress urinary incontinence after delivery is <1% [36], in the immediate postpartum period up to 25.5% of women experience stress incontinence [37]. This study also showed that 31.4% of women in the immediate postpartum period experienced *de novo* urgency incontinence. There is a rat model of pudendal nerve injury that showed an association with detrusor overactivity, which is the usual underlying cause of urgency incontinence [38]. Human data also support the notion of pudendal nerve injury's association with overactive bladder. This comes from a study showing that women who undergo a forceps delivery (and thus increase risk of pudendal nerve injury) have an almost 3 times higher risk of having overactive bladder [39]. We know that a connection exists between the pelvic floor and anal sphincter muscles. This is demonstrated by the use of the 'knack' or 'quick-flick' maneuvers for overactive bladder. This is when women perform quick contractions of their pelvic floor muscles, including the anal sphincter, and it can help to temporarily abort involuntary detrusor contractions that may lead to urgency incontinence [40]. Therefore disruption of the anal sphincter or the nerves innervating the sphincter or pelvic floor may release some inhibitory effect on the bladder ultimately affecting continence. Forceps delivery is a large risk factor for anal sphincter injury.

Urinary retention, defined here as the inability to urinate 6 hours after delivery, can also occur as a result of nerve injury during delivery, although it is more uncommon than incontinence occurring in only 0.7–4% of vaginal deliveries [41, 42]. In these cases the injured nerve is the pelvic nerve. The mechanism of injury to the pelvic nerves is the same as described above, via both compression and stretch. Aside from the potential pelvic nerve injury there are other factors that may contribute to urinary retention after labor. This includes physiologic changes resulting in hypotonia and increased post-void residuals as well as pain, constipation, and iatrogenic medication (i.e., narcotics, epidurals). Risk factors for urinary retention in the postpartum period include primarily, prolonged labor, instrumental delivery, epidural anesthesia (which can incidentally lead to bladder overdistention), and perineal lacerations. These women should be treated with intermittent self-catheterization, as the great majority resolve within 72 hours after delivery. Long-term urinary retention is poorly reported in the literature, although Ching-Chung reports a case that lasted 15 days [42].

Although there are no case reports in the literature, anecdotally, postpartum women will also complain of the lack of the sensation of the urge to void. This is presumably a result of damage to pelvic nerves by the mechanisms described above. These women can be treated with timed voids every 2–3 hours and reassured that the sensation should return with time. In researching the natural history of urinary retention in young women, Swinn et al. (2002) polled 91 women with urinary retention in the absence of neurologic disorders. Of those, 15% identified childbirth as the precipitating event [43].

Evaluation and treatment

Most stress and urgency incontinence found during pregnancy is transient. However, should it be persistent after delivery, first-line conservative therapy includes behavioral modification and pelvic floor exercises. The diagnosis can be made clinically or in some cases urodynamic studies can be helpful. Clinically, patients with stress incontinence will complain of leakage with cough, laugh, sneeze, or exercise, while patients with urgency incontinence will complain of an overwhelming urge to urinate and not making it to the bathroom in time.

Physical examination is useful as well in that stress urinary incontinence can also be elicited by examining the urethra for leakage while a patient with a full bladder increases intra-abdominal pressure by valsalva or cough. A patient's ability to tighten pelvic floor muscles, rectal tone, and perineal sensation should also be assessed. A post void residual (by catheterization or ultrasound) can be useful to ensure that persistent urinary symptoms are not caused by retention of urine (a failure to empty the bladder.) In some cases the physician may elect to perform pressure/flow urodynamics in order to understand the underlying cause of the bladder/urethral dysfunction. Pressure flow urodynamics involves the filling of the bladder with a small catheter at a steady rate while measuring the pressure within the bladder. The sensation of the bladder is noted and the urodynamicist can observe for any impairment in compliance of the bladder, involuntary detrusor contraction, stress incontinence, etc. The patient is then asked to void and the flow rate and detrusor pressure are recorded. Surface EMG can be helpful to ascertain the relaxation of the sphincter and pelvic floor during micturition. In some case simultaneous fluoroscopy is used (Videourodynamics) to capture additional information about bladder filling and bladder emptying. The bladder is filled with a radio-opaque dye which allows for visualization of the bladder and urethra during the examination. Videourodynamics are particularly helpful when looking for neurologic causes of bladder dysfunction.

For both stress urinary incontinence and overactivity of the bladder (with or without incontinence) behavioral modification includes limiting excessive fluid intake as well as voiding on a schedule to try to avoid a full bladder. For urgency and urgency incontinence, avoidance of bladder irritants can also help. Pelvic floor exercises (with or without a pelvic floor physical therapist) can also strengthen the pelvic floor muscles. This can help prevent stress urinary incontinence and help reduce urgency and urgency incontinence. As describes above in the Disorders resulting from parturition section, the "knack maneuver" of quickly squeezing the anus can calm urge long enough to let the patients void in a socially accepted location (i.e., the bathroom). If patients do not gain satisfactory improvement with conservative therapy, stress urinary incontinence is most commonly treated with synthetic midurethral slings. Patients that have persistent bother from urgency or urgency incontinence will often find benefit from anticholinergic medication (i.e., oxybutynin).

Urinary retention after pregnancy can be managed with indwelling catheter or clean intermittent catheterization, however the latter is preferred. When retention is refractory, urodynamics may help determine an underlying reversible etiology. Some cases of urinary retention, which do not improve over time, may be successfully treated with sacral neuromodulation. However, this should not be initiated until the patient has completed childbearing and she should be managed with clean intermittent catheterization until that time. If the most recent pregnancy was the patient's last, we know that it can take up to a year for women to recover from pelvic nerve injury after childbirth, so the procedure should not be considered until this time. The exception to this is if a patient develops Fowler's syndrome postpartum. This disorder involves urinary retention secondary to failure of the urethra to relax and can occur postoperatively or postpartum [44]. The cause of Fowler's syndrome is not well-understood, but is classically diagnosed with urethral needle EMG. Sacral neuromodulation works very well for Fowler's syndrome [45]. Sacral neuromodulation involves stimulation of the S3 nerve (pelvic plexus), which innervates the bladder, pelvic floor muscles and rectum. In addition to urinary retention, sacral neuromodulation can be used to treat refractory frequency urgency, urge incontinence, and fecal incontinence. The exact mechanism of this therapy is unknown, but is thought to be due to afferent inhibition [46]. The procedure is usually performed in two stages. Stage I involves a temporary wire with external stimulation to ensure improvement before Stage II placement of a subcutaneous implantable pulse generator. The procedure is performed by placement of a percutaneous lead in the S3 foramen. The lead is then connected to an external pulse generator and trialed by the patient for at least a period of several days. If the patient notes an improvement, they may proceed to Stage II, otherwise the lead is removed. In a study by Jonas et al. (2001), 38% of patients treated for urinary retention qualified to move on to Stage II of the procedure. Of those, 69% were able to completely stop self-catheterization. Seventy one percent of patients had sustained improvement at 18 months of follow-up [47].

Conclusions

The neurologic pathways in the control of bladder filling, storage, and voiding are complex and not completely understood. Changes to the bladder seen in pregnancy include decreased tone and increased pressure with symptoms of urgency, frequency, and sometimes incontinence. Urinary retention may also occur at any time during pregnancy due to high progesterone states, although most commonly in the first trimester. The birth process will frequently disrupt pelvic nerves, most commonly the pudendal resulting in incontinence, retention, and impaired sensation. An understanding or the innervation of the lower urinary tract may allow for the potential location of injury to be deduced based on the deficit. This pathology should be treated with supportive treatment with the knowledge that the nerves usually regenerate with time.

References

1 Benson JT, Walters MD. Neurophysiology and pharmacology of the lower urinary tract. In:

Walters MD, Karram MM, eds., *Urogynecology and Reconstructive Pelvic Surgery*, 3rd ed. Philadelphia: Mosby Elsevier, 2007; pp. 31–43.

2 Blaivas JG. The neurophysiology of micturition: a clinical study of 550 patients. *J Urol*. 1982; 127(5):958–963.

3 de Groat WC, Yoshimura N. Pharmacology of the lower urinary tract. *Ann Rev Pharmacol Toxicol*. 2001;41:691.

4 Andersson KE, Mattiasson A, Sjögren C. Electrically induced relaxation of the noradrenaline contracted isolated urethra from rabbit and man. *J Urol*. 1983;129(1):210–214.

5 McGuire EJ, Herlihy E. Bladder and urethral responses to isolated sacral motor root stimulation. *Invest Urol*. 1978;16(3):219–223.

6 Elbadawi A. Autonomic muscular innervation of the vesical outlet and its role in micturition. In: Hinman F Jr, ed., *Benign Prostatic Hypertrophy*. New York: Springer-Verlag, 1983; pp. 330–348.

7 Barrington FJ. The relation of the hind-brain to micturition. *Brain*. 1921;44:23.

8 Holstege G, Kuypers HG, Boer RC. Anatomical evidence for direct brain stem projections to the somatic motoneuronal cell groups and autonomic preganglionic cell groups in cat spinal cord. *Brain Res*. 1979;171:329.

9 McGuire EJ. The innervation and function of the lower urinary tract. *J Neurosurg*. 1986;65:278.

10 Kruse MN, Belton AL, de Groat WC. Changes in bladder and external urethral sphincter function after spinal cord injury in the rat. *Am J Physiol*. 1993;264(6 Pt 2):R1157–1163.

11 Bradley WE, Timm GW, Scott FB. Innervation of the detrusor muscle and urethra. *Urol Clin North Am*. 1974;1:3.

12 Cunningham FG, Leveno KJ, Bloom SL, Hauth JC, Gilstrap L III, Wenstrom KD. Maternal physiology. In: Rouse D, Rainey B, Spong C, Wendel GD Jr, eds., *Williams Obstetrics*, 22nd ed. USA: McGraw Hill, 2005; pp. 137–140.

13 Iosif S, Ingemarsson I, Ulmsten U. Urodynamic studies in normal pregnancy and in puerperium. *Am J Obstet Gynecol*. 1980;137(6):696–700.

14 Stanton SL, Kerr-Wilson R, Harris VG. The incidence of urological symptoms in normal pregnancy. *Br J Obstet Gynaecol*. 1980;87(10): 897–900.

15 Nel JT, Diedericks A, Joubert G, Arndt K. A prospective clinical and urodynamic study of bladder function during and after pregnancy. *Int Urogynecol J Pelvic Floor Dysfunct*. 2001;12(1):21–26.

16 Francis WJ. The onset of stress incontinence. *J Obstet Gynaecol Br Emp*. 1960;67:899–903.

17 FitzGerald MP, Graziano S. Anatomic and functional changes of the lower urinary tract during pregnancy. *Urol Clin North Am*. 2007;34(1):7–12.

18 Aslan D, Aslan G, Yamazhan M, Ispahi C, Tinar S. Voiding symptoms in pregancy: an assessment with international prostate symptom score. *Gynecol Obstet Invest*. 2003;55(1):46–49.

19 Dietz HP, Benness CJ. Voiding function in pregnancy and puerperium. *Int Urogynecol J Pelvic Floor Dysfunct*. 2005;16(2):151–154.

20 O'Boyle AL, Woodman PJ, O'Boyle JD, Davis GD, Swift SE. Pelvic organ support in nulliparous pregnant and nonpregnant women: a case control study. *Am J Obstet Gynecol*. 2002;187(1):99–102.

21 O'Boyle AL, O'Boyle JD, Ricks RE, Patience TH, Calhoun B, Davis G. The natural history of pelvic organ support in pregnancy. *Int Urogynecol J Pelvic Floor Dysfunct*. 2003;14(1):46–49; discussion 49.

22 Keating PJ, Walton SM, Maouris P. Incarceration of a bicornuate retroverted gravid uterus presenting with bilateral ureteric obstruction. *Br J Obstet Gynaecol*. 1992;99(4):345–347.

23 Weekes AR, Atlay RD, Brown VA, Jordan EC, Murray SM. The retroverted gravid uterus and its effect on the outcome of pregnancy. *Br Med J*. 1976;1(6010):622–624.

24 Tong YC, Broderick G, Hypolite J, Levin RM. Correlations of purinergic, cholinergic and adrenergic functions in rabbit corporal cavernosal tissue. *Pharmacology*. 1992;45(5):241–249.

25 Baselli EC, Brandes SB, Luthin GR, Ruggieri MR. The effect of pregnancy and contractile activity on bladder muscarinic receptor subtypes. *Neurourol Urodyn*. 1999;18(5):511–520.

26 Wilfehrt HM, Carson CC 3rd, Marson L. Bladder function in female rats: effects of aging and pregnancy. *Physiol Behav*. 1999;68(1–2):195–203.

27 Frederice CP, Amaral E, Ferreira ND. Urinary symptoms and pelvic floor muscle function during the third trimester of pregnancy in nulliparous women. *J Obstet Gynaecol Res*. 2013;39(1): 188–194.

28 Abrams P, Artibani W, Cardozo L, Dmochowski R, van Kerrebroeck P, Sand P. Reviewing the ICS 2002 terminology report: the ongoing debate. *Neurourol Urodyn*. 2009;28(4):287.

29 Allen RE, Hosker GL, Smith ARB, Warrell DW. Pelvic floor damage and childbirth: a neurophysiological study. *Br J Obstet Gynaecol*. 1990;97:770–779.

30 Fitzpatrick M, O'Herlihy C. The effects of labour and delivery on the pelvic floor. *Best Pract Res Clin Obstet Gynaecol*. 2001;15(1):63–79.

31 Snooks SJ, Swash M, Setchell M, Henry MM. Injury to innervation of pelvic floor sphincter musculature in childbirth. *The Lancet*. 1984;8: 546–550.

32 Damaser MS, Samplaski MK, Parikh M, Li Lin D, Rao S, Kerns JM. Time course of neuroanatomical and functional recovery after bilateral pudendal nerve injury in female rats. *Am J Physiol Renal Physiol*. 2007;293:F1614–F1621.

33 Snooks SJ, Swash M, Henry MM, Setschell M. Risk factors in childbirth causing damage to the pelvic floor innervation. *In J Colorectal Dis*. 1986;1: 20–24.

34 Peng CW, Chen JJ, Chang HY, de Groat WC, Cheng CL. External urethral sphincter activity in a rat model of pudendal nerve injury. *Neurourol Urodynam*. 2006;25:388–396.

35 Snooks SJ, Badenoch DF, Tiptaft RC, Swash M. Perineal nerve damage in genuine stress urinary incontinence: an electrophysiological study. *Brit J Urol*. 1985;57:422–426.

36 Viktrup L, Lose G, Rolff M, Barfoed K. The symptom of stress incontinence caused by pregnancy or delivery in primiparas. *Obstet Gynecol*. 1992;79(6):945–949.

37 Dolan LM, Hosker GL, Mallett VT, Allen RE, Smith ARB. Stress incontinence and pelvic floor neurophysiology 15 years after the first delivery. *BJOG*. 2003;110:1107–1114.

38 Furuta A, Kita M, Suzuki Y, et al. Association of overactive bladder and stress urinary incontinence in rats with pudendal nerve ligation injury. *Am J Physiol Regul Integr Comp Physiol*. 2008;294:R1510–R1516.

39 Handa VL, Blomquist JL, McDermott KC, Friedman S, Munoz A. Pelvic floor disorders after vaginal birth. *Obstet Gynecol*. 2012;119(2):233–239.

40 Miller JM, Perucchini D, Carchidi LT, DeLancey JO, Ashton-Miller J. Pelvic floor muscle contraction during a cough and decreased vesical neck mobility. *Obstet Gynecol*. 2001;97(2):255–260.

41 Bouhours AC, Bigot P, Orsat M, et al. Postpartum urinary retention. *Prog Urol*. 2011;21(1):11–17.

42 Ching-Chung L, Shuenn-Dhy C, Ling-Hong T, Ching-Chang H, Chao-Lun C, Po-Jen C. Postpartum urinary retention: assessment of contributing factors and long-term clinical impact. *Aust N Z J Obstet Gynaecol*. 2002;42(4):367–370.

43 Swinn MJ, Wiseman OJ, Lowe E, Fowler CJ. The cause and natural history of isolated urinary retention in young women. *J Urol*. 2002;167(1):151–156.

44 Fowler CJ, Kirby RS. Abnormal electromyographic activity (decelerating burst and complex repetitive discharges) in the striated muscle of the urethral sphincter in 5 women with persisting urinary retention. *Brit J Urol*. 1985;57:67–70.

45 Elneil S. Urinary retention in women and sacral neuromodulation. *Int Urogynecol J*. 2010;21(Suppl 2):S475–483.

46 Hassouna M, Elmayergi N, Abedelhady M. Update on sacral neuromodulation: indications and outcomes. *Curr Urol Rep*. 2003;5:391.

47 Jonas U, Fowler CJ, Chancellor MB, et al. Efficacy of sacral nerve stimulation for urinary retention: results 18 months after implantation. *J Urol*. 2001;165:15–19.

Index

Neurological Illness in Pregnancy: Principles and Practice, First Edition.
Edited by Autumn Klein, M. Angela O'Neal, Christina Scifres, Janet F. R. Waters and Jonathan H. Waters.
© 2016 John Wiley & Sons, Ltd. Published 2016 by John Wiley & Sons, Ltd.